DENTAL ETHICS

DENTAL ETHICS

Bruce D. Weinstein, Ph.D.

Center for Health Ethics and Law
West Virginia University

Lea & Febiger
Philadelphia • London 1993

Lea & Febiger
Box 3024
200 Chester Field Parkway
Malvern, Pennsylvania 19355-9725
U.S.A.
(215) 251-2230

Executive Editor—Darlene Barela Cooke
Development Editor—Sharon R. Zinner
Production Coordinator—Peter J. Carley
Manuscript Editor—Jessica Howie Martin

Library of Congress Cataloging-in-Publication Data

Dental ethics / [edited by] Bruce D. Weinstein.
        p.   cm.
    Includes bibliographical references and index.
    ISBN 0-8121-1444-2
    1. Dental ethics.   I. Weinstein, Bruce D.
    [DNLM: 1. Ethics, Dental.   WU 50 D414]
  RK52.7.D46 1993
  174'.2--dc20
  DNLM/DLC
  for Library of Congress   92-49537
                                                                 CIP

NOTE: Although the author(s) and the publisher have taken reasonable steps
to ensure the accuracy of the drug information included in this text before
publication, drug information may change without notice and readers are advised
to consult the manufacturer's packaging inserts before prescribing medications.

PRINTED IN THE UNITED STATES OF AMERICA

Print number: 5   4   3   2   1

Reprints of chapters may be purchased from Lea & Febiger in quantities of 100 or more.
Contact Sally Grande in the Sales Department.

To W. Robert Biddington,
with deep respect and gratitude

Preface

What does it mean to be a good dentist? Is a dentist ethically obligated to care for persons with AIDS? What are the limits of the duty to protect patient confidentiality? What kinds of advertisements are ethically acceptable, and why? How should dental hygienists and dentists resolve some of the ethical conflicts they face together? Is there a right to dental care? What are the moral implications regarding the low number of women and minorities in the profession? Dentists and hygienists are increasingly asking themselves these questions, but they have not had a book available to help them find answers. This volume was prepared to meet this need.

The topics chosen for inclusion were derived from the Curriculum Guidelines on Ethics and Professionalism in Dentistry developed by the American College of Dentists, the American Association of Dental Schools, and the American Dental Association's Council on Dental Education.* These guidelines recognized that the questions in the first paragraph raise fundamental issues about professional life and the relationship one has with patients. They are *ethical* questions because they concern the appropriate conduct of dentists and refer directly to the welfare and rights of patients and others.

Answering ethical questions in dentistry requires expertise in clinical dentistry as well as philosophical ethics. Much of the literature in bioethics, however, is written by persons with expertise in only one component. To avoid this problem, every chapter in this book represents a collaboration between both an expert in ethics and an expert in clinical dentistry or dental hygiene. The authors are leaders in their respective fields, and their work has already helped to establish dental ethics as a legitimate and valuable discipline. Because they recognize that dental ethics is above all a *practical* endeavor, they have integrated realistic cases into their discussions.

The book is divided into three sections. The first section introduces the reader to the field of dental ethics and provides a framework for approaching ethical problems in the clinical setting. The second section examines topical issues in depth. Included here are ethical analyses of the dentist-patient relationship; informed consent; AIDS; duties toward incompetent or chemically dependent colleagues; relationships with dental hygiene and auxiliary personnel; issues concerning race, gender, and class, advertising; and research. The third section presents two extensive case commentaries as examples of how one might think through a case from an ethical perspective. The American Dental Association's *Principles of Ethics and Code of Professional Conduct,* and a comprehensive bibliography, comprise the appendices.

This book is intended for students and practitioners alike. Students in dental school or hygiene or assistant programs will learn about issues that they will face as clinicians (if they have not already done so), and practitioners will have the opportunity to reflect with other dentists and ethicists on issues that are among the most important facing the profession today. Although reflection on ethical issues does not guarantee morally sensitive behavior, the conscientious reader who grapples with the material presented here will be taking important steps toward being a better provider of care.

Dental ethics is a maturing specialty, and continuing interaction between clinicians and ethicists will strengthen the field. Readers are cordially invited to send to the editor comments about this book, as well as reports of cases they have encountered that raise challenging ethical issues.

Bruce D. Weinstein
Center for Health Ethics and Law
P.O. Box 9022
West Virginia University Health
  Sciences Center
Morgantown, WV 26506-9022

* Curriculum Guidelines on Ethics and Professionalism in Dentistry. J. Dent. 53:144, 1989.

Acknowledgments

Editing a book is a lot like directing a film. There are a lot of people behind the scenes without whose diligent efforts the project could not be completed, and *Dental Ethics* is no exception. Alvin H. Moss granted me a generous amount of time to complete this book, and my secretary, Cynthia F. Jamison, provided superb clerical assistance. Sharon R. Zinner, Darlene Barela Cooke, and Jessica Howie Martin of Lea & Febiger were exceptionally supportive throughout, and Ray Kersey helped me to get started. The faculty, residents, and students of the West Virginia University School of Dentistry have allowed me to observe their work in the dental clinic, and I have learned much from students in our dental ethics classes. I am especially thankful to Abe Getty, Rashida Khakoo, Mary Logan, Bill McCutcheon, Michael Perich, Shelia Price, David Puderbaugh, Ted Stevens, and Mary Ellen Waithe for their support and good cheer. My friends and family, as always, helped me in innumerable ways.

A special word of thanks is in order to the contributors. I am grateful for the enthusiasm with which each of them greeted my invitation, for their patience in working through several drafts of their manuscripts with me, and most of all for producing essays that will make an important contribution to the field. This book would not have been possible without the pioneering work of two of the contributors, David T. Ozar and John G. Odom.

W. Robert Biddington, former Dean of the West Virginia University School of Dentistry, provided me with an entree into the world of academic dentistry and supported my proposal for developing an extensive curriculum in dental ethics. I dedicate this book to him.

B.D.W.

Contributors

Thomas H. Boerschinger, LL.B.
Associate General Counsel and Director,
  Council on Ethics, Bylaws and Judicial
  Affairs
American Dental Association
Chicago, Illinois

Donald F. Bowers, D.D.S., M.S.D.
Ohio State University College of Dentistry
Columbus, Ohio

Courtney S. Campbell, Ph.D.
Department of Philosophy
Oregon State University
Corvalis, Oregon

Teresa A. Dolan, D.M.D., M.P.H.
University of Florida at Gainesville
Dental School
Gainesville, Florida

Mary Alice Gaston, R.D.H., M.S.
Department of Dental Hygiene
University of Tennessee at Memphis
Memphis, Tennessee

John A. Gilbert, D.M.D.
Quality Assurance
UM-KC School of Dentistry
Kansas City, Missouri

Marcia A. Gladwin, R.D.H., Ed.D.
Department of Dental Hygiene
West Virginia University
Morgantown, West Virginia

Thomas K. Hasegawa, Jr., D.D.S., M.A.
Baylor College of Dentistry
Department of General Dentistry
Dallas, Texas

B. Bizup Hawkins, R.D.H., M.A.
Thomas Jefferson University
College of Allied Health Sciences
Philadelphia, Pennsylvania

Jeffrey Hollway, Ed.D.
Office of Educational Planning
School of Dental Medicine
State University of New York, Buffalo
Buffalo, New York

Jeffrey P. Kahn, Ph.D., M.P.H.
The Center for the Study of Bioethics
Medical College of Wisconsin
Milwaukee, Wisconsin

Gordon G. Keyes, D.D.S., M.S., J.D.
Department of Oral Pathology
West Virginia University
Morgantown, West Virginia

Mary B. Mahowald, Ph.D.
Center for Clinical Medical Ethics
University of Chicago
Chicago, Illinois

Patricia A. Main, D.D.S., D.D.P.H., M.Sc.
Director, Community Dental Service
City of North York Public Health Department
North York, Ontario, Canada

Eric M. Meslin, Ph.D.
University of Toronto
Centre for Bioethics
Tanz Neuroscience Building
Toronto, Ontario, Canada

Linda C. Niessen, D.M.D., M.P.H.
Department of Community Health and
  Preventive Dentistry
Baylor College of Dentistry
Dallas, Texas

John G. Odom, Ph.D.
Ohio State University College of Dentistry
Columbus, Ohio

David T. Ozar, Ph.D.
Department of Philosophy
Loyola University of Chicago
Chicago, Illinois

Lisa S. Parker, Ph.D.
Department of Human Genetics
University of Pittsburgh
Pittsburgh, Pennsylvania

Vincent C. Rogers, D.D.S., M.P.H.
Department of Community Dentistry
Temple University School of Dentistry
Philadelphia, Pennsylvania

Linda S. Scheirton, R.D.H., Ph.D.
Malden, The Netherlands

Mary Ellen Waithe, Ph.D.
Department of Philosophy
Cleveland State University
Cleveland, Ohio

Bruce D. Weinstein, Ph.D.
Center for Health Ethics and Law
West Virginia University
Morgantown, West Virginia

Margaret Welch, M.A., Ph.D. (Cand.)
Department of Philosophy
Loyola University of Chicago
Chicago, Illinois

Contents

SECTION I. The Foundations of Dental Ethics

SECTION II. Topical Issues

SECTION III. Case Studies and Commentaries

Foundations of Dental Ethics

Chapter 1

Virtues, Values, and Norms in Dentistry

David T. Ozar

SUMMARY

This chapter introduces the theme of this book, careful reflection on ethical and professional obligations of dentists, by examining a number of possible views that a person might take regarding such reflection, and by identifying three important resources that a dentist, or anyone else, has available to assist in making complex ethical judgments.

Such reflection might be viewed as something wholly limited to one's feelings and views at the present moment, whenever that is. But many people find it valuable to ask about actions they are considering, "Is this the way that the sort of person who I want to be would act in this situation?" This question cannot be answered solely in terms of what I feel at this moment or what seems good right now. It requires me to ask myself what sort of person I want to be over the longer run, by the end of my life, for example, or at least from some vantage point later on when I can look back over the present part of my life and judge how I have done. Asking questions of this sort is one important resource for ethical decision makers. It is examined in this essay under the title "Personal Virtues."

Some people view ethical reflection as an activity to which other people can make no meaningful contributions. They consider the bases of ethical reflection for each person to be completely unique to that person. They believe that there is no transfer value whatsoever between the experience of values, goals, ideals, etc., of one human being and another. But no dentist can seriously adopt this view if he or she believes that dentistry provides genuine benefits to its patients, for example, in the form of relief of pain and the preservation and restoration of oral functioning. Beginning with this starting point, it is worth asking whether there are any other important values, goals, principles, etc., that are experienced by human beings generally. Asking questions of this sort is another important resource for ethical decision makers. It is examined in this essay under the title "Intrinsic Values."

Most professionals begin their ethical reflections, especially when the issue at hand pertains to their professional practice, by considering the obligations they have undertaken in becoming professionals. Although there is an alternative view that being a professional entails nothing special about obligations, and although this view deserves to be examined, the role and practice of professionals in our society seem to hold instead that professions and professionals have obligations.

But more than this is needed by the practicing professional who faces a difficult ethical judgment. One needs to understand in more detail what a profession is, and especially to understand the most important categories of professionals' obligations. Thoughtful answers to these questions are a third important resource for decision makers facing complex professional ethical decisions. This resource is examined in this essay under the title "Professional Norms."

In the final section of this chapter, the

case described in the introduction is discussed in more detail, and connections among the three resources (personal virtues, intrinsic values, and professional norms) are considered in relation to it.

CASE HISTORY

"Who's next, Sarah?" asked Dr. Beth Evans. It was 9 am on Monday.

"Mr. McIlwain is in Operatory 2. He was the emergency on Friday; you gave him medication for pain and told him to come back. Janice just seated him; you told her not to do anything else till you talked to him. The file's on the door."

"Thank you, Sarah. I certainly remember Mr. McIlwain; I've been thinking about him a lot."

In fact, Beth Evans had thought about this conversation with John McIlwain many times over the weekend. She had even called Dr. Bruliak to ask his advice. She had worked as Bruliak's associate for 1 year before the opportunity to buy this practice arose 6 months ago. She considered Dr. Bruliak a bit old-fashioned in many ways, but she still called him to talk over patients, sometimes just to let him know that she still thought of him, for she had learned a great deal from him in their year together. Sometimes she called because she needed to talk to someone who had been around longer and had seen more; that was her reason for calling about John McIlwain. She hoped Dr. Bruliak would have some words of wisdom for her.

John McIlwain had walked in the door on Friday afternoon and explained that he was in pain. Sarah had given him a health history and other forms and had told him he'd be seen within 45 minutes. There had been time for only a quick examination because Dr. Evans had to be out of town for the weekend. Her plane departed at 7 pm. While Dr. Evans was finishing with her 4 o'clock patient, Janice had taken McIlwain to the other operatory. At 4:35 Dr. Evans went in to see him.

The state of McIlwain's dentition was not the worst she had ever seen, but it was in very bad condition. Obviously, he had not had any dental care for a long time, and his oral hygiene was extremely poor. In her clinical examination, she saw that there were obviously carious lesions in half a dozen teeth and periodontal involvement at many sites as well. McIlwain said he was experiencing severe pain in the lower right quadrant, and that he had had pain there three times in the last two weeks. Aspirin had relieved it, and it had gone away. This was the first time that taking aspirin did not relieve it, and his boss had persuaded him to seek a dentist's help. At first look, it seemed likely that most of the teeth were restorable, but every quadrant needed restorative and periodontal treatment of some kind.

Dr. Evans focused her examination on the lower right teeth. The first molar was mobile and sensitive to touch. Pus came from a bump on the gum next to the tooth. There was no facial swelling, and much of the tooth was so decayed that he could not bite with it. Root canal therapy or an extraction would be necessary.

Unfortunately, McIlwain appeared to be a man of very limited means. In fact, at first sight, Beth wondered if he might live on the streets. But Sarah's notes on the intake card indicated that McIlwain lived and worked at a shelter for the homeless that was about a mile from Dr. Evans' office, on the other side of an expressway that separated two very different parts of the city.

"I only came because it hurt so bad," McIlwain said. "My boss said I'd better get it looked at, and you were the first dentist I found who would take me."

"You have so many problems here," she told him. "I believe the first molar may be the immediate source of pain. We'll need an x ray." Dr. Evans directed Janice to expose a periapical x-ray film of the tooth. "You must have a high tolerance for pain overall, considering how many of your teeth have problems. I'm surprised that some part of your mouth doesn't hurt almost all the time."

"You're right, it hurts pretty often," said McIlwain, "but not terrible pain like this. I even took aspirins for it, but now they aren't working either."

"What you really need is a complete examination, and that molar will need a root canal or extraction soon," said Dr. Evans. "You'll probably need a lot of dental treatment after that if you want to avoid crises like this in the future. I can tell you for sure that it's only a matter of time before you have another crisis like this, and the pain might even be worse. You need to get your whole mouth examined carefully, and we'll develop a plan to get all the problems fixed."

"Well, I'm broke, you know," said McIlwain. "I'm working steady and have a place to live, and I'm off the bottle, and I'm going to stay there. But I don't have any money."

"We'll cross that bridge when we come to

it," she had said. Dr. Evans viewed the x-ray film that Janice had brought. It confirmed that the molar was salvageable, and showed bone loss that would explain the drainage. Antibiotics would suppress the infection and make later extraction or root canal therapy easier. She described the situation to McIlwain, then told him, "I have a patient in the other chair and other patients with appointments coming in, so I can't do a comprehensive examination and x rays for you right now."

"Well, I've got to get back, too, to set up dinner, anyway," said McIlwain. "But it hurts terribly bad; can't you help that?"

"Oh, yes, certainly," said Dr. Evans. "I wouldn't let you leave here in pain. I will give you an anesthetic injection to stop the pain. It will last 8 to 12 hours. I will also give you some antibiotics for the infection, along with some pain medication. Will you come back on Monday to have a full examination? I have to be out of town over the weekend, so I can't see you until then, unless you prefer that I send you to another general dentist in the area who could see you tomorrow."

"No, it can wait till Monday if your pills and the shot will help me with the pain."

"They will," said Dr. Evans, "but I want to be sure that you come back." She gave the long-acting anesthetic injection, assured McIlwain that she'd return, and left the patient with Janice.

"If you want me to, I'll come back," he told Janice. "My boss will let me come; he knows how bad it's been hurting me." McIlwain felt along the side of his right jaw, then exclaimed, "Say, that stuff is working already. It don't hurt now at all! You know, I went to a dentist once when I was a kid, and he told my Mom I had strong teeth. So I sort of took him at his word." Janice was writing notes in the chart for Dr. Evans to read later. "The only other time I went was when I was in the service; we all had to see the dentist before they sent us over. They didn't want guys over in Vietnam having toothaches, I guess. Those military dentists fixed all my teeth in four appointments, and I never thought I'd need any more dental work. We were sent to 'Nam right afterwards, and I never went to another dentist. I just didn't have the money, and the VA was too far away."

Dr. Evans returned. "Feeling better?" she asked.

"I'll say. Maybe I can sleep tonight!" he replied.

"Well, take one of these antibiotic tablets every 6 hours until they are all gone, and take one of these pain capsules every 4 hours. They will help once the numbness wears off. The instructions are written on the packets. Also, talk to the receptionist to set up an appointment for a full examination on Monday. If the pain worsens, or if you notice swelling in your face, call my emergency number, and you will be referred to another doctor who is covering for me while I'm away. I will see you on Monday."

Dr. Evans was sure that McIlwain would need a lot of expensive treatment, or at the very minimum, would require several extractions, leaving some gaps that would affect his chewing function. The infected molar would have to be dealt with once the antibiotics began to take effect. Dr. Evans thought it doubtful that he would consent to a root canal procedure because of the cost. With his apparent change to a more stable sort of life, she surmised, perhaps he could learn proper oral hygiene. He was only 48, so it would be a shame to extract good teeth just because he couldn't afford restorative and prosthetic treatment.

After her last patient, she called Dr. Bruliak to see what he thought she ought to do in the case.

Dr. Bruliak's advice was not crystal-clear. "You know what I'm going to say, Elizabeth," he said. "I say it all depends on your personal values. Either you make great sacrifices and do everything this fellow needs in the best way; or you find a way to help him somewhat, but not in the best way possible, so it costs you less; or you find a way to get him to pay for some of it and you take the rest as a loss; or you tell him what he needs and leave it up to him, if he can afford it or not."

"But I know he can't afford it," Dr. Evans said. "He can't afford anything; there's no question about that."

"I understand that," said Dr. Bruliak. "All I'm saying is that there is no right answer to your question. You ought to do whatever your values tell you to do. It is a matter of *your* personal values. I would not criticize you either way and neither should anyone else. It is all a matter of your personal values."

Most of us have received advice like this fairly often, but it is not immediately clear what the advice is intended to communicate. One way of introducing the theme of this book is to examine some of the possible meanings of this sort of advice and to ask which make sense and are supported by the data of our own experience, and which do not make sense and do not hold up. We can ask, for example, if Dr. Bruliak is correct in saying that there are no right answers, no standards besides purely personal ones, that a dentist can look to in determining the ethically correct action in a complex situation. Or are their sources of standards besides the purely personal, especially those of the moment when one is facing the situation at hand?

This chapter proposes that a dentist has three sets of resources to look to for assistance in determining morally and professionally correct actions. These three sets of resources are "virtues, values, and norms," or more fully, "personal virtues, intrinsic values, and professional norms." Each of these resources for ethical judgment is examined in the sections that follow, with special emphasis on professional norms, which have the most to say specifically about the professional practice of dentistry.

PERSONAL VIRTUES

When Dr. Bruliak says, "You ought to do whatever your values tell you to do," and, "It is a matter of *your* personal values," he might be saying: "Do what feels best at the time; do whatever seems best to you at the moment." On the other hand, Dr. Bruliak might be quite chagrined to be understood in this way. He might be urging Beth Evans precisely *not* to decide the matter solely on the basis of her feelings or concerns *at this moment,* but rather to look at the choice from the perspective of her life as a whole. That is, he might be advising her to examine each way of responding to the situation and ask this question: "Is this the way that the sort of person I want to be would act in this situation?"

This is a very different question from "What feels good or seems good to me at this moment?" It cannot be answered solely in terms of what you feel at this moment or what seems good just now, because it requires you to ask yourself what sort of person you want to be over the longer run, by the end of your life, for example, or at least from some vantage point later on

when you can look back over the present part of your life and judge how you have done.

The point of this question is to take account of the fact that human actions are not isolated in narrow "present moments." Every one of our actions leaves a permanent mark on us developmentally, no matter how old we are, and it is reasonable for thoughtful persons to examine the actions they might perform from the perspective of the developmental effects of these actions upon them as they move through their lives.

This does not say much, if anything, as yet about what a thoughtful person would want to be or become over the long run. So this question does not automatically identify any particular criterion of rightness or wrongness that a thoughtful person ought to employ in determining what to do in a given situation. But it asks a question that forces the person to think about such criteria. It forces him or her to compare the alternative courses of action presently available in the light of the alternative futures to which they would lead, and the alternative kinds of person that the individual might become from acting in one way or another just now.

If Dr. Bruliak intends his advice in this way, the term "personal" in the expression "personal values" does not refer to how one is, feels, etc., at a given moment. It refers instead to the person choosing as someone with a past that has been moving in a certain direction—to be affirmed and supported or criticized and changed in the present situation—and with a future, or rather many possible futures, to be shaped and selected by acting in one way or another. So the word "personal," when intended in this way, emphasizes the fact that choices made in the present become part of who one is as one moves into the future. It urges us to take this aspect of ourselves very seriously.

The term "values" in the expression "personal values" refers—if Dr. Bruliak intends his advice in the manner just explained—to the conception or conceptions of oneself that one must consider in taking this developmental aspect of human reality seriously. "Values" here represents all the various kinds of goals, satisfactions, ideals, principles of conduct, and other criteria for acting that a person might incorporate as relatively permanent parts of "who I am and want to be." In this interpretation of Dr. Bruliak's words, the term "values" is neutral as to the many different goals, satisfactions, ideals, etc. that Beth Evans might choose to make a part of her life. But, of course, *she* cannot remain neutral about this; she must reflect on *which* kind of person she chooses to be and to become.

Although many people still seem to consider the developmental aspect of human life important, it is not something that is commonly talked about in today's public culture. The older terms for it, "virtue" and "character," sound old-fashioned and strange to our ears. This makes it harder for us to communicate about, and even to think carefully about, this aspect of our lives. In fact, our lack of easy vocabulary on this point is one reason why we might not be sure if this is in fact what someone like Dr. Bruliak is referring to when he speaks of "personal values," or if he is really just saying the more common thing, "Do what feels best at the moment."

To highlight the difference between asking the sort of question being discussed here and asking, "What seems good at the time?," the older term "virtue" is used in this essay, and modified by the term "personal," understood in the sense just described. The point of interpreting Dr. Bruliak's words in this way, then, is that one of the most important resources a dentist has for judging how to act correctly in a complex situation is the perspective of *personal virtue*. This perspective approaches a choice of action in terms of one's life as a larger whole, and it bids us ask about each available way of responding to the situation at hand, "Is this the way in which the sort of person who I want to be and to become would act?"

INTRINSIC VALUES

When Dr. Bruliak says, "there is no right answer to your question," another interpretation of his words should be considered. He might be saying that no goals, values, or ideals have any kind of *general* meaning for human beings, but only each

one's *own* chosen goals, values, etc. If this is so, even when a person thinks in terms of his or her whole life, no one's choice of what sort of person to be and to become can benefit from other people's experiences. There is no transfer value among human experiences of value; that is, no learning from one another about value. Each of us must then make the choice of who to be and to become solely on the evidence available in his or her own set of personal experiences. It is very important to ask if we humans really are this isolated in our decisions about what sort of persons to be and, on the basis of that, how we ought to act in each given set of circumstances.

If we are this isolated, it also follows that none of us can ever justifiably criticize or commend any other human being for how he or she acts, or for the kind of person that he or she is or is becoming. Both criticism and commendation depend on a common basis of judgment, some criteria for judging actions or character that are common to the two (or more) parties to the conversation. If each one's only evidence about goals, values, etc., were limited to his or her own personal experiences, there would be no such common basis of judgment. So the question here is twofold: can human beings learn from each other's experiences of goals, values, etc., so that we have more to go on in our decisions than just our own personal experiences; and is there enough transfer value between human beings' experiences of goals, values, etc., that at least some of our criticisms and commendations of other people's actions and character, and theirs of us, are justifiable?

A great deal of our conversation about ourselves and others takes it for granted that there is some transfer value and that we can learn from one another's experiences of goals, satisfactions, ideals, principles of conduct, etc. It takes it for granted that we are not so isolated in these matters as answering the preceding questions negatively would require. Some moral philosophers call a negative answer to these questions "moral subjectivism," because it involves a fundamental relativism about the criteria to be used in determining what actions are right, wrong, good, bad, moral, immoral. The moral subjectivist believes that, in all the circumstances in which we take transfer value and the possibility of learning from one another for granted, we are making a fundamental mistake. The reality, such thinkers hold, is that we are profoundly isolated in regard to goals, values, etc., and have no data to rely on but our own personal experiences.

This is not the place to try to formulate a detailed response to the moral subjectivist. It seems clear, however, that dentists presuppose some commonality of values among human beings. They believe that relief of pain and adequacy of oral function are genuine benefits for their patients, and this is something they could not possibly affirm unless there were transfer value between their own and other human beings' experiences. It is doubtful, in other words, that any dentist would ever be a thoroughgoing subjectivist, even if he or she were not sure whether or how far our common human values extend beyond the absence of pain and the maintenance of ordinary oral functioning. For this reason, it is quite doubtful that Dr. Bruliak really intends to recommend a subjectivist point of view to Dr. Evans when he says, "There is no right answer."

This reflection on Dr. Bruliak's words suggests another resource for the thoughtful dentist to consider when a particular case seems morally complex. As soon as it is acknowledged that there are some common human values, for example, the relief of pain and the value of ordinary oral functioning, it is reasonable to continue the discussion of common human values and to examine other possible values as well. There is substantial evidence to support the claim that truth, self-determination, justice, friendship, and keeping one's promises are also common human values. The thoughtful decision maker inquires whether any of these candidates has bearing on the situation that he or she faces, and then asks whether the evidence supporting their status as common human values is stronger than the evidence to the contrary. If it is, there is a second resource, other than personal virtue, to apply in resolving a situation.

The phrase used in this essay to represent this resource is "intrinsic value." The word "intrinsic" refers to the idea that there are goals, satisfactions, ideals, principles of conduct, etc., which are worth pursuing *for their own sake,* and not only as a means of achieving some other goal, satisfaction, ideal, etc. (i.e., not only as "instrumental values"). Although they may also sometimes function as means to something else, the things classified as being of *intrinsic* value are specifically worthy of being chosen by human beings *for their own sake.* They are the characteristics of a human life, whatever they may be, that are worth a human being's choosing to make them a permanent part of his or her life, and so they are the measure of the sort of person a human being ought to choose to be and to become.

The term "value" in the phrase "intrinsic value" is simply used as a place-holder here for the whole range of candidates— goals, satisfactions, ideals, principles of conduct, etc.—that might be common features of human life in terms of which we can discuss the rightness or wrongness, goodness or badness, or morality and immorality of human actions, i.e., the general category of what a human ought and ought not to do and be. Other terms, e.g., "norm" or "standard" and a number of others, might perform this place-holding function just as well as "values."

The point of these comments is certainly not to try to resolve the question of what is valuable for human lives generally, much less to limit the list of candidates by selecting the particular word "value." The point is, rather, to propose, by speaking of intrinsic values as a resource for a dentist facing a complex decision, that the dentist make use of what human beings have discovered about what is worth pursuing, doing, and being in human life. It is to propose that human beings have already learned quite a bit about this, and continue to do so, and that what *other* human beings have learned about this is also valuable for the individual.

In any given situation, of course, it may not be exactly clear what lessons of common human experience and the intrinsic values are relevant to the case at hand. In fact, when Dr. Bruliak says, "there is no right answer," he may mean precisely that, when he looks at Dr. Evans' situation in terms of the common human values that he is familiar with, these values do not enable him to readily identify one course of action as the best. In this connection, it is important to note the vast difference between a person's saying, "The intrinsic values that I am considering do not point clearly toward one action rather than another," and making the subjectivist claim that "There are no intrinsic values, so there is no point in looking for guidance of that sort."

We all have experienced situations in which the intrinsic values that we regularly refer to have not yielded a single clear answer to the question, "What should I do?" But within the notion of intrinsic value is a further suggestion, in the form of a *procedural* suggestion, for us to follow in such situations. The notion of intrinsic value reminds us that we are talking about *transfer value* among human experiences of value; that is, about *learning from one another*. So when our own grasp of intrinsic values leaves us still without enough understanding of our situation, it makes sense for us to seek out other humans whose different experiences of life may be able to complement our own and assist us in the situation at hand.

So, if Dr. Bruliak's experience does not yield helpful guidance, perhaps Dr. Evans should talk to other fellow human beings, whether dentists or not; i.e., she might look for assistance from human lives of other sorts. In the matter of how we ought to act, the life experience amassed by every one of us—even when we include the vicarious experience along with the personal—is very limited. This is why one human goal that seems truly worth pursuing is to learn as much as we can about intrinsic value by a continuing effort to broaden the base of human experience on which our judgments about values and actions are formed, meaning both our own personal experience and experiences learned from others.

But apart from the general worth of broadening the bases of our judgments about value, when we need to determine what we should do in a given situation, there is often no better procedure to follow than to seek out those whose experiences of life we judge rich and whose judgments

about those experiences we consider wise. The point is not to ask them to judge our obligations for us, of course, but to enrich our understanding of the intrinsic, transferable human values that might be found in the situation we face. Moreover, it often turns out that we learn the most when those we consult do not spontaneously view the matter exactly as we do, because they are often the ones most likely to see values in the case that we ourselves have missed.

PROFESSIONAL NORMS

There is one way in which Dr. Bruliak's response to Dr. Evans is certainly incorrect, at least on any straightforward reading of his words. There is one way in which it is simply *not true* that "It all depends on your personal values." For there are certainly standards of *professional* conduct that are relevant to Dr. Evans's actions as a dentist, standards that exist independently of her personal values or choices of personal virtue. In fact, for most dentists, such *professional* norms of conduct are the most important determinants of what they ought and ought not to do in their practice. That is why professional norms are the central focus of most chapters of this book and of most other discussions of dental ethics. Therefore, these professional norms deserve careful examination here as well.

What is the basis of professional norms and how can we determine their content, so that a dentist can use them as a resource in a particular situation? The answer to these questions requires a brief reflection on the nature of a profession, which then returns us to the topic of the basis of professional obligations and professional norms. Then seven categories of professional obligations are identified. The final section of this chapter talks about how the three resources, personal virtue, intrinsic values, and professional norms, fit together.

What is a Profession?

A great many occupational groups describe themselves as "professions." Nevertheless, for most of them, the appropriateness of speaking of the group as a profession can be called into question. That is, an explanation can be legitimately demanded for applying the term "profession" to the group. But for a few occupational groups, most notably at present physicians, lawyers, and dentists, no such explanation is needed. In fact, doubts about their being professions would need to be explained. I shall say that these three occupational groups are *central instances* of profession in our society at present, and that the question, "What is a profession?" is to be understood as asking what are the key features of these central instances of *profession.*

What, then, are the chief features that these central instances of *profession* have in common and that distinguish them, sometimes more, sometimes less, from other occupational groups?

There are four key features of the central instances of *profession:* important and exclusive expertise, internal and external structure, autonomy in practice, and professional obligation.

IMPORTANT AND EXCLUSIVE EXPERTISE

For an occupational group to be a profession, it is prerequisite that its occupational activity be such that it provides its clients with something that the larger community widely judges to be *extremely valuable* because it is of high-ranking intrinsic value, because it is a necessary condition of any person's achievement of whatever he or she values, or both. This is one reason why investment counselling, for example, is not a central instance of a profession. It is fully possible for people to achieve their goals in life without the particular benefits that investment counsellors provide to their clients.

But health and the preservation of life, to take two commonly identified goals of the medical profession, are held by almost everyone to be values of the highest order, either as valuable in and of themselves ("intrinsically valuable") or else as necessary conditions of people's achievement of whatever else they value (necessary "instrumental values"). In a similar way, security—e.g., security of one's property and person against the errors of others and

against the adverse workings of government and of the legal system—as one defensible description of the goal of the legal profession, is also widely valued as a necessary means for achieving whatever other goals one has within the context of constraining social structures, and some people would hold that the experience of security is valuable in itself. If we focus on the most obvious value that dentistry secures for its patients, namely, oral health in the sense of pain-free oral functioning, this too is a very important human value. Adequate oral functioning is a necessary condition of nutrition and therefore of other valued aspects of human life, and being free of pain is valuable both intrinsically and instrumentally (i.e., as a means to something else), more so when pain is of greater intensity.

Moreover, it is a key feature of a profession that its members are *expert* in securing this value for its clients. Of course, occupations of all sorts are performed better by persons who understand them and have performed them for some time. But it is a characteristic of the expertise of a profession that it is subtle and complex enough that only persons fully educated in both the knowledge and the practice of it can be depended upon to correctly judge the need for expert intervention in a given situation, or to judge the quality of such an intervention as it is being carried out. Judgments of need and judgments of the quality of the expert's performance by those not so trained are not dependable. Nor, because of the importance of what is at stake, is it sufficient to judge the performance solely on the basis of its long-term outcomes, even when the non-expert can accomplish such a judgment unaided. For long-term judgments will not be known for some time, and the risk of severe negative consequences in the meantime, in a matter of great importance, means that delayed judgments are simply not enough.

The concept of *need* that is relevant here is a very subtle and complex concept. On the one hand, it clearly refers to the objective facts about a client that the professional takes into account in judging whether to do something for a client and what to do. But *need* also always implies a value judgment, a reference to what is a *normal* condition for this patient, or what is a *better* situation for this client. That is why the question, "What are the central values of this profession?" is so important. In addition, because patients and clients may hold other values to be important to them, besides those central to a profession, it is crucial to examine carefully the various relationships that are possible between practitioner and patient, professional and client, in regard to decisions about the actual goals and the professional's actual interventions for each client. Both of these issues are discussed subsequently.

Thus, only those who have been properly educated can be depended on to provide a correct judgment of need or of the quality of an intervention for a client as it occurs, and similarly, only those so educated can be depended on to teach others in the knowledge and especially in the practice of the profession's expertise. Because of this, within the society's division of labors, a profession's expertise is also unavoidably exclusive.

INTERNAL AND EXTERNAL STRUCTURE

The second key feature concerns the internal and external structure of a profession. As an occupational group made exclusive by reason of its particular body of expertise, a profession is also therefore characterized by a set of internal relationships of which the most important is a *mutual recognition of expertise* on the part of those who are expert in its practice. These internal relationships may be quite informal or may become quite formal.

In addition, when we speak of a profession, we most often have in mind not only a community of experts mutually recognizing each other's expertise, but also an institutionalization of this relationship in a formal organization. The expression "the profession of dentistry" thus refers most properly to all those who are expert in the practice of dentistry and mutually recognized as such by one another, within relevant geographic limits.

Another aspect of this feature of a profession is the recognition by the larger community that only those expert in the relevant knowledge and practice are ca-pable of rendering dependable judgments regarding the need for it and regarding the quality of an expert intervention. Thus, they alone are recognized as capable of dependably providing clients with the benefits derived from this expertise. That is, the expertise of a profession is not only mutually recognized by those who possess it, but by the members of the larger community as well.

Because of the exclusive nature of professional expertise and the importance for the community of its being properly applied, the external recognition of a profession is often expressed in formal actions of the larger community, such as certification, licensure, etc. Moreover, because students of the profession must undertake lengthy and specialized training to master its expertise, external recognition of the profession by the larger community tends naturally to include a grant of exclusive authority to train and certify new members of the profession. But, as with internal recognition, it is not the formal actions of the community as such, but the more fundamental reality of the community's recognition of this as an expert group that is essential to the character of a profession.

AUTONOMY IN PRACTICE

The third key feature concerns the profession's and its members' measure of control over various aspects of their expert practice. Because the activity of a profession is so valued by its clients, and because proper performance and dependable judgments about performance depend upon expertise that is unavoidably exclusive, and therefore is not available to the ordinary person, a profession's clients routinely grant its members extensive *autonomy* in the actual performance of the profession's practice. In particular, the judgments of the professional are ordinarily held by clients to be controlling on any matter that is within the range of the professional's expertise.

This grant of autonomy of judgment to the professional in his or her professional practice goes beyond the general recognition by the larger community ("external recognition") that the professional group possesses the relevant expertise. It depends on the further assumption that each member of the expert community possesses this expertise and is therefore a dependable provider of its benefits. This grant of autonomy to the individual professional includes three elements: first, determination of the specific *needs* of the client in matters within the range of the professional's expertise; second, determination of the likely *outcomes* of various courses of action that the client, the professional, or some other party might undertake in response to these needs; and third, judgment of which of the *possible courses of action* is most likely to best meet the client's needs.

A fourth judgment, the judgment about which intermediate, *instrumental steps* are appropriate in carrying out the chosen course of action, is often carried out by the professional as well. But this fourth judgment is also frequently relegated to a technician, who is capable of performing instrumental actions but lacks the expertise to judge when they are needed.

Many professional-client encounters do not involve explicit evidence of all three (or four) of these elements. The point here is not that all three are always explicitly present. The point is rather that whenever any of them are present, they are seen by clients to be matters in which the professional's judgment is controlling, precisely by reason of the professional's expertise. These are the elements of professional practice over which the professional most clearly and most characteristically exercises autonomy.

Consider, for example, the encounter between a dentist and a patient. The patient ordinarily accepts as controlling the dentist's judgments regarding the nature of the patient's present condition and need for care, if any; the range of courses of action that might be taken in response; the likelihood the one of these courses of action will best meet the patient's needs; and the determination of the various instrumental actions to be taken in carrying out that course of action.

Although this grant of autonomy to the professional is from each client individually, clients do not ordinarily make this grant of autonomy simply on the basis of their individual judgment of the expertise of the individual professional. They make it, rather, on the basis of a more complex set of factors involving the community's (external) recognition of the professional group's expertise and the professional group's (internal) recognition of the expertise of the particular professional. Thus, even though this grant of professional autonomy takes place above all between the individual client and the professional, its full meaning can be understood only against the background of the whole, complex institution of the profession.

In addition, at the level of the whole profession's dealings with the whole community, there is a further grant of autonomy to the profession in the areas of its expertise. It is also characteristic of professions that the larger community not only recognizes their collective and individual expertise, in the senses already discussed, but permits the professional group to be self-regulating in the determination of who shall be considered a member of the expert group, what counts as appropriate expert practice, and the like.

PROFESSIONAL OBLIGATIONS

The fourth key feature of a profession is, for the purposes of this essay, the most important. It is a central characteristic of the institution of profession that membership in a profession implies the acceptance by the member of a set of norms of professional practice.

To make this point clearer, contrast this Normative Picture of a profession with a Commercial Picture. According to the Commercial Picture, being a member of a profession is no different in principle from the activity of any producer selling his or her wares in the marketplace. On this view, the professional has a product to sell and makes whatever agreements with interested purchasers that the two parties are willing to make. Consequently, beyond some fundamental obligation not to coerce, cheat, or defraud others in the marketplace, the professional would have no other obligations to anyone except such obligations as he or she voluntary undertakes with specific individuals or groups. In other words, according to the Commercial Picture, there are no specifically professional values or obligations in any profession. There is nothing to which a person is obligated *because* he or she is a professional.

The Commercial Picture of professions is supported by more than a few writers about dentistry, some considering it an accurate description of what professions are like, others maintaining that professionals or the community at large would be better off if professions conformed to it more thoroughly. But recall the point made earlier, that all professional groups have an exclusive corner on some valuable form of knowledge within a society. Wherever there is exclusive and valuable knowledge, there is power, power to control the knowledge itself, and especially power over the aspects of human life that depend upon the knowledge. Now compare how various powerful groups are dealt with in our society. Contrast the members of professions with politicians, for example.

We accept without too much complaint the terribly inefficient system of periodic re-election, to take one example, because we want to keep close watch over those with political power. Experience has taught us that those with power are tempted to misuse it, and we want to keep a close eye on them. We tolerate the excesses of a free press that, for example, leaves public figures with very little privacy for the same reason, because such a free press makes it harder for politicians to misuse their power.

But the professions, although they do face some slight measure of regulation through licensing boards and the like, are subjected to remarkably little oversight in our society. In fact, even when there is regulation, who regulates them? For the most part, it is their own members, as has already been noted. Of course, this is reasonable in one way because the members of a profession know the profession's expertise far better than anyone else. But the point is that the larger community does not regulate professions in the same ways as it does other powerful groups. It assures itself that the power of the profession will not be misused by another means, by means of the institution of profession.

But this means that the way in which a profession functions within the larger community is inherently normative. It means that, when a person enters a profession, he or she assumes obligations, obligations whose content has been worked out—and is continually being affirmed or adjusted—through an ongoing dialogue between the expert group and the larger community. Professions, to put it briefly, are normative. Professions and professionals have obligations.

The Basis of Professional Obligations

This view of the nature of profession is not news to most dentists, who take this view of profession for granted as they practice their professions, even though they rarely stop to articulate it. But this view has an important implication regarding the basis of professional obligations and the way in which we are to identify their content.

Some people take the position that the content of a profession's obligations is determined by the members of that profession and no one else. The view of profession just offered, however, implies that the content of a particular profession's obligations at a given time is the product of a dialogue between the profession and the larger community. Not only does the community at large have an immense stake in what a profession does, but it is by reason of the larger community's grant of professional autonomy and self-regulation to the professions that the professions have the characteristics that they have. Thus it is important to stress that the content of the obligations of a profession is not determined by the profession alone.

The dialogue between the profession and the larger community that determines this content is subtle and complex, only occasionally explicit or made formal, and it is ongoing in time, never completed, as the profession and the larger community gradually address the profession's obligations in the face of new opportunities and new challenges. But such a dialogue is nevertheless the source of the current contents of dentists' professional obligations.

As a consequence of this fact, no one can adequately determine a dentist's obligations in some matter simply by asking what dentists say about the situation or what organized dentistry says about it. We must also ask what the larger community understands dentists to be committed to. To many, this may seem an awfully vague test of a person's professional obligations. Particularly when dentistry is faced with new opportunities or difficult new challenges, like HIV and AIDS, for example, this dialogue can be agonizingly slow, and members of the profession may wonder if they have any guidance, from either party to the dialogue, much less from both in some sort of consensus, about how they ought to act. Nevertheless, if a profession's obligations are in fact the work of the profession and the larger community together, as has been argued, this is a test that may not be set aside.

Seven Categories of Professional Obligation

Although there are probably other useful ways of dividing the general topic of professional obligation, one valuable and informative way to study professional obligations in dentistry is in terms of the following seven categories. A useful way to understand these categories is to think of each as posing a question to the profession.[1]

1. The Chief Client

    Every profession has a chief client or clients. This is the person or set of persons whose well-being the profession and its members are chiefly committed to serving. The patient in the chair is certainly one of a dentist's chief clients. But a dentist has professional obligations to the patients in the waiting room and beyond, and perhaps even to the whole larger community, the public. Just who is included among a dentist's chief clients, then, and how do a dentist's obligations to one of these compare with and weigh against the dentist's obligations to the others?

2. An Ideal Relationship between Professional and Patient

    What is the proper relationship between the professional and the client as they make judgments and choices about the patient's care? There are many different ways of conceiving this ideal relationship, including the model of informed consent, when it is a relationship between the dentist and a fully competent adult.[2] It is worth asking whether the model of informed consent expresses this ideal fully or not. In addition, what is the proper relationship between the dentist and a patient who is incapable of fully participating in treatment decisions? What is the dentist's role, the role of the patient, up to the limit of his or her capacity, and the role of other parties?

3. A Hierarchy of Central Values

    Every profession is focused only on certain aspects of the well-being of its clients. Therefore a dentist is not really committed to advance the client's well-being *entirely*, even if taking account of "the whole patient" is essential in the achievement of even this partial goal. Rather, there is a certain value or set of values that are the specific focus of this profession and its particular expertise. These can be called the *central values* of that profession. They are the basis of what is *normal* and *needed* in the profession's practice. What, then, are the central values of dentistry and dental practice? If there are more than one, as there almost certainly are, are they ranked, and if so, in what order?[3]

4. Competence

    Every professional is obligated both to acquire and to maintain the expertise needed to undertake his or her professional tasks, and every professional is obligated to undertake only those tasks that are within his or her competence. This is probably the most obvious category of professional obligations. But even here it is valuable to try to articulate the standards involved. For example, what counts as sufficient or minimally adequate competence on the part of a dentist to perform a particular, nonroutine procedure for a patient? Is dentistry right to recognize a variety of clinically acceptable but very different kinds of treatment for a number of dental care needs? And so on.

5. The Relative Priority of the Client's Well-being

Most sociologists who study professions, and most of the literature of professions about themselves, speak of "commitment to service" or "commitment to the public" as one of the characteristic features of a profession. But these expressions admit to many different interpretations with very different implications for actual practice. What sorts of sacrifices are dentists professionally committed to make for the sake of their clients? What sorts of risks to life, health, financial well-being, reputation, etc., is a dentist obligated to face when meeting a patient's dental care needs?

6. Relations With Co-Professionals

Each profession has norms, usually largely implicit and unstated, concerning the proper relationship between members of the profession. For example, should dentists relate to other dentists in the same area of practice as competitors in the marketplace? Should they work to support one another's practices even if patients have to pay more as a result? How should a dentist deal with another dentist's inferior work? And so on. In addition, there are situations in which members of different professions are caring for the same patients. What are the proper relationships between them?

7. Relations Between the Profession and the Larger Community

In addition to relationships between professionals and their clients, the activities of every profession involve relationships between both the profession as a group and its members and the larger community as a whole or various significant subgroups of it. What obligations does dentistry have, and what obligations to individual dentists have to the larger community regarding inferior work or unethical practice, or regarding dentists who are substance-dependent or substance abusers? What is the proper standard for professional advertising? Do dentists have special public health obligations when the larger community faces a serious epidemic? How should health care resources be distributed, and what role should dentistry and dentists play in working toward or supporting that proper mode of distribution? These and many other difficult questions need to be asked about dentists' and dentistry's place within the larger community.

PUTTING PERSONAL VIRTUE, INTRINSIC VALUES, AND PROFESSIONAL NORMS TOGETHER

There are two ways in which these three resources for moral reflection interact, one general and substantive, the other more concrete and procedural.

First of all, it is worth asking why societies have professions and why individuals become professionals. The answer is in terms of intrinsic values. That is, societies develop and support professions in order to secure certain values, such as the absence of pain and appropriate oral functioning and the benefits that these, in turn, lead to (e.g., nutrition and the support of life and health, aesthetic values, communication, and human relationship). These values have widespread standing in human experience, and hence are what have here been called intrinsic values. They are also values that cannot be secured for a society's people without specialized expertise. Therefore societies establish and support professions.

Individuals become members of professions in part for the same reasons, in order to secure the same intrinsic values for others. They also become professionals to secure other intrinsic values for themselves, e.g., the satisfaction of meaningful work, and to secure other values for their families and other persons, e.g., the instrumental (and possibly intrinsic) value of security in the resources needed for life, for health, and the other intrinsic values that these resources serve.

At the most fundamental level, then, professional norms exist for the sake of certain intrinsic values, and must be tested against them. This is not only true when a professional norm must be adapted to meet changing circumstances or at the outset of a new profession when its norms are the object of dialogue between expert group and large community for the first time. It is also true when other obligations that a professional has in a particular situation come in conflict with his or her professional obligations in that situation. For it is not the case that the professional obligations *always* "win." It is not part of what we mean by a profession that one's professional obligations are always the determining factors of what the person ought to do.

But how does one judge that some other obligation outweighs one's professional obligations in a given situation? If we find ourselves in a situation in which it is perfectly clear that our professional obligation is to do X, but we have other obligations to do Y instead, what resources do we have for determining which of these obligations is more important? The answer is the intrinsic values that are at stake in the situation: the intrinsic values that are the reasons why this professional obligation exists at all; the intrinsic values that are the reasons why X is a professional obligation for the professional in the first place; and the intrinsic values that are at stake, and the commitments and aspects of personal virtue that are related to them, concerning other persons affected by our actions in the situation. No simple algorithm can be given for weighing all these matters properly. But the point remains that professional norms exist for the sake of intrinsic values; and it is to these that we must turn when the question at hand is whether we are morally justified, or even

morally required, to conscientiously disobey our professional obligations.

Secondly, the three resources of personal virtue, intrinsic values, and professional norms interact in important procedural ways in many concrete situations. That is, by turning to each of these three resources in turn, the practicing dental professional can find guidance in moral reflection, regarding both particular actions that he or she is considering, and the habits and patterns of action that the professional supports in his or her life, or else criticizes and tries to change.

It is not true, of course, that a person can run through the list once—looking at professional norms, then intrinsic values, then personal virtues—and consider the task of moral reflection done. The "procedure" requires that each category of resources for reflection be used repeatedly and that the resources be allowed to correct and amend each other in one's reflections. Each of these three categories offers the thoughtful professional a set of questions that enables him or her to reflect more and more clearly and carefully about what ought and ought not to be done.

The case proposed at the beginning of this essay is far too complex to be fully resolved here. But a sample of the kind of moral reflection that Dr. Evans might engage in could be useful. It can show how the three resources for moral reflection can enrich a dental professional's understanding.

Markers are inserted into the text here to suggest which of the three resources is most operative at that point: PN for professional norms, IV for intrinsic values, and PV for personal virtues.

Suppose, then, that Beth Evans reflected on her obligations towards Mr. McIlwain in this way:

"First of all, Mr. McIlwain is my patient. He is so because he needs my professional services and because he has sought me out; and also, given the opportunity to seek professional services elsewhere, if he does return on Monday, he will have specifically chosen to be cared for by me (PN).

"Now, I have a special obligation to my patients, not just those actually in the chair—although that is where he will be when I speak to him—but to all my patients of record (PN). I have an obligation to meet their dental needs, at least up to the standards of minimally competent practice in my profession. So, from this point of view, I have an obligation to provide Mr. McIlwain with minimally adequate oral care (PN). This would surely include a lot of cleaning and prophylaxis that Janice would do; but because McIlwain could not pay for it, I would have to absorb the cost myself. It would also require either quite a bit of expensive restorative work, or maybe pulling some healthy teeth and providing him with dentures, if that could be justified in so young a man and if I believed he has developed sufficient self-discipline to care for his new dentition properly. I'd have to pay for all of that out of my pocket, too, either way (PN).

"Of course, the question of money aside, I might ask whether he *can* take care of his teeth properly if I provide him with the care he needs (PN). Would I be pouring my money down a hole to help him? If so, perhaps I could justifiably claim that it would be a waste and I am not obligated to try to do the impossible (IV).

"Unfortunately for that line of thinking, I really do think he is trying to get his life in order, and I think that pain-free oral functioning will probably help him in that. I could actually imagine his successfully developing good hygiene habits, and his successfully getting his teeth properly restored by coming faithfully for a series of appointments here, could really contribute to the formation of a positive self-image for him (IV). So I can't honestly take that easy way out of my dilemma (PV).

"But what about the financial side? Do I really have an obligation to treat him if he cannot pay anything for my services? (PN) Maybe in some ideal world, society would care enough about people's health that some sort of system would be set up to ensure appropriate health care for everyone (IV). I would personally support a tax-based system of national health insurance if it included dental coverage (PV). But it is not my responsibility to personally attend to every unmet need when the fault lies in the larger social system; I am sure of that (PN and PV).

"One possibility is to provide only emergency treatment. That is all I am most seriously obligated to provide to patients who are not yet patients of record (PN). But in this case, determining the proper emergency treatment will practically make him a patient of record; I can't claim that I fulfilled that obligation when I gave him the pain pills and sent him away because I had to catch a plane (PN).

"Besides, when someone who has not trusted many people and who needs to establish some solid social relationships makes the move of returning—as I really think he will—don't I have some deeper obligation besides my professional one to help him change his life? (IV and PV)

"But does my professional obligation therefore include everything Mr. McIlwain needs? I am surely not obligated to bankrupt myself for patients whom our society doesn't provide for properly. What would happen to my other patients if I did that? As a dentist, I have committed myself to placing my patients' well-being ahead of my own to a considerable degree. But that commitment is not unlimited, even if the profession talks as if it is in its P.R. literature. But, then, where are the limits? (PN) I already have a number of patients who fall into the category of receiving charity care. Most try to pay something or I find out afterwards that they are charity care because they don't pay all their bills. Mr. McIlwain's situation is more dramatic because he seems so completely unable to pay, and because I know about his circumstances up front. But he is not the only patient I have who needs charity care, and he needs a great deal more care than most patients of this sort. Would I be fulfilling my professional obligation better, the obligation to accept some sacrifices for my patients' sake, if I declined to provide extensive treatment for Mr. McIlwain in order to provide less expensive charity care for a larger number of other patients? Or is it unprofessional to count people and dollars in this way? (PN)

"Actually, I never thought about it in this way before, that I should think about tradeoffs among my charity patients. Suppose I figured out a set amount of charity care that I would provide per year or, preferably, per quarter (PN). I could calculate it from my costs and what I need to save for better equipment and what would be a just payment to myself for my services. Anything else is profit, and it would be appropriate that my obligation to provide some charity care should come out of that (PN and IV). On the other hand, if I allow a certain amount for charity care each quarter, that will have a regular effect on my income, and that means it will affect my family. So I had better talk this over with my husband, before I set the amount of charity care that I will provide each quarter, or rather the upper limit, because it may not always be that much (IV and PV).

"The nice thing about doing it this way is that, when a patient needs charity care, I would know if the needed care was within the range of the sacrifices that I professionally owe my patients, or if doing this case for partial payment or no payment or doubtful payment would be taking me beyond that amount (PN and PV). Also, I could honestly say to a patient that I can't afford to help just now. I could be more forthright about it, too, and more confident in what I said to patients about it, instead of hemming and hawing (PV). I would also be able to tell them they could return in the next quarter, at least for treatment that could wait, because if I didn't borrow too much from future quarters, there would always be something there that a patient could come back for (PN and PV).

"All of that sounds great, but I don't have time to figure all of that out before I see Mr. McIlwain. What shall I do about him?

"One possibility is that he needs so much care, to fully restore his mouth to its proper state, that I am almost sure it would put me over any reasonable limit for this quarter and soak up a lot of what would be budgeted for next quarter (PN). On the other hand, I really admire his efforts to get his life in order; and I would like to help him do that, even if it does require more charity than I professionally owe right now (IV and PV).

"But I also wonder if simply giving him dental care, without asking for something in return, is the right thing. I wonder if he has any skills that he could donate in return for care, either something I could personally use, or maybe something he could do for some church or other group in return for my dental care. I want to help him; but I want to do it in the right way, the way that will help him the most (IV and PV)."

Few of the views about professional obligation and intrinsic values that have been attributed to Dr. Evans here have been carefully argued for in this chapter, although all of them can be carefully defended. But many readers have alternative views about professional obligation and intrinsic values that deserve careful reflection as well. The statements of Dr. Evans should be taken instead as a starting point for the reader's own reflection on the case posed. How should a dentist in Dr. Evans' situation act, and do the reflections attributed to Dr. Evans here make sense? Whether the reader agrees with them, in whole or in part, or not, these statements can in any case serve as an example of how the resources of personal virtues, intrinsic values, and professional norms can guide a person's reflections on what ought and ought not to be done.

Human powers of moral reflection grow most when they are exercised, and above all when thoughtful people exercise them together. The cases and essays in this book are aimed at your exercising your moral reflective powers, both individually and with others. In each instance, ask what the case or essay suggests to you in terms of the sort of person you choose to be and to become (personal virtues), in terms of the values that human life supports across a broad range of human experience (intrinsic values), and in terms of the obligations that each dental professional undertakes, whose content is the product of ongoing dialogue between the larger community and dental practitioners committed to the well-being of their patients (professional norms).

DISCUSSION QUESTIONS

1. Why should a thoughtful decision maker ask, "Is this the way that the

sort of person who I want to be would act in this situation?"

2. What are some candidates for intrinsic values that have the support of many humans' experience? What reasons could be given for and/or against adopting each of these as a stable criterion of decision making in one's life?

3. What are the seven categories of professional obligation identified in this chapter?

4. Each category of professional obligation provides a set of questions to be answered by a profession like dentistry. What is dentistry's current answer to each of these seven sets of questions?

5. Every profession changes—ideally, improves—over time. Are there any answers to these seven sets of questions about professional obligation in dentistry that ought to be changed, improved? Why or why not?

6. How could dentistry bring about a more articulate and effective dialogue with the larger community about the contents of dentistry's professional obligations? Should dentistry try to do this? Why or why not?

REFERENCES

1. Ozar, D.: Ethics and the practicing dentist: A framework studying professional ethics. J. Am. Coll. Dent., 58(1):4, 1991.
2. Ozar, D.: Three models of professionalism and professional obligation in dentistry. J. Am. Dent. Assoc., 110:173, 1985.
3. Ozar, D., Schiedermayer, D., and Siegler, M.: Value categories in clinical dental ethics. J. Am. Dent. Assoc., 116:365, 1988.

Chapter 2

The Normative Principles of Dental Ethics

Courtney S. Campbell
Vincent C. Rogers*

SUMMARY

The moral integrity and identity of dentistry are grounded in an individual and collective profession of commitment to the welfare and needs of patients. Because dentistry is inherently a moral profession, moral questions and issues are at the core of clinical practice. This chapter addresses the role of normative principles in dental practice in clarifying and justifying moral choices in dentistry. The normative principles of dental ethics, including nonmaleficence, beneficence, justice, and respect for autonomy, set out guides and standards of required, prohibited, or permitted conduct.

The first section differentiates three kinds of moral problems that can emerge in dental practice, including moral weakness, moral uncertainty, and moral dilemmas, which can be distinguished by the differing role of principles. In instances of moral weakness, a normative principle requires or prohibits certain action that conflicts with personal self-interest. In situations of moral uncertainty, a dentist may inquire whether a moral responsibility exists or how far it extends. Finally, situations of moral dilemmas arise when two normative principles come into conflict. Although all three problems are present in dental practice, much of the dental ethics literature has focused on moral dilemmas.

Several debates in dental ethics concern which principles are recognized or affirmed, which principle or principles have priority in dilemmatic situations, and the content or meaning of these principles. The recognition of certain principles as normative for dentistry is related to how dentistry as a moral profession and practice is conceived. Different principles are implicit in a commercial, guild, or partnership model of dentistry. Major views addressing whether certain values or principles have priority in dentistry are considered, and the meaning of principles of nonmaleficence, beneficence, justice, and respect for autonomy, as well as derivative rules, such as veracity or truthfulness, informed consent, and confidentiality, are explored through illustrative cases drawn from clinical practice.

The concluding section proposes several elements required for responsible ethical decision making in dental practice, including an assessment of the medical and social context, clarification of the ethical problem, determination of the stakeholders, identification of options and alternatives, examination of the process of decision making, and justification of decisions through balancing conflicting principles and obligations. Throughout the chapter, the authors contend that the normative principles of dental ethics can help dentists shape their care and practice in ways that are genuinely responsive to the needs and welfare of the persons who present themselves as patients.

* The clinical cases in this chapter were drawn from the experiences of this author.

THE NORMATIVE PRINCIPLES OF DENTAL ETHICS

Fundamental moral commitments underlie the professional practice of dentistry, as exemplified in the preamble to the ADA's *Principles of Ethics and Code of Professional Conduct,* which calls upon the profession to provide quality care in accordance with patient benefits and patient needs.[1] Dentists offer a wide array of services to achieve these objectives, ranging from furnishing advice and consultation, to education about effective methods of preventive oral health care, to applying professional knowledge in the use of specialized techniques to correct dental problems and restore full dental functioning insofar as possible. The social esteem of the dental profession in large measure reflects broad recognition of both the importance of these commitments and the success of the profession in devising methods, nontechnical and technical, that manifest these commitments in clinical interactions with patients.

It is not, however, always possible for dentists to benefit patients and to meet patient needs simultaneously. The following example illustrates how moral conflicts may emerge for dentists in the clinical setting.

CASE 1

D.C. is a 35-year-old salesperson who is married and has two children, ages 7 and 5. A "patient of record" who has made regular visits to his dentist, Dr. M., D.C. could be termed an exemplary patient, were it not for his smoking habit. D.C. smokes roughly a pack a day, despite Dr. M.'s consistent warnings.

On this occasion, D.C. presented to his dentist with a chief complaint of a painful irritation on the posterior lateral border of his tongue. Upon examination, Dr. M. located an ulcerative lesion, about 12 mm in diameter, with "rolled" borders; upon palpation, there was evidence of cervical lymphadenopathy, which could be described as a firm, nontender, but movable mass. The patient had "noticed" the soreness for about 6 weeks, but thought he had merely sustained some sort of injury to the tongue that would heal over time.

Dr. M. was reasonably confident that the lesion was malignant, and suggested an incisional biopsy. This recommendation aroused fears in D.C., who questioned the dentist at length about the possibility that the area was "cancerous." Dr. M. hesitated to reveal his suspicions completely and replied that the area was probably not carcinoma but that a biopsy was necessary for a correct diagnosis.

The conflict between patient benefit and patient need confronted by Dr. M. is revealed by his less-than-candid disclosure of the rationale for his professional recommendation. Regardless of the outcome of the biopsy, Dr. M. appears convinced that his patient would benefit from the procedure. That benefit may take several forms, such as obtaining knowledge that can resolve the diagnostic and prognostic uncertainties that currently exist, as well as providing a basis for the design of a treatment plan. However, the commitment to patient need likewise exerts itself in the form of the patient's request for information. D.C. has a need "to know" about the possibility that a portion of his tongue may be cancerous; moreover, because obtaining the biopsy will require an invasive procedure, Dr. M. has a responsibility to provide that level of knowledge necessary for D.C. to give an informed consent to the procedure.

Dr. M.'s hesitant reply might also be seen as consistent with the commitment to patient benefit because his answer seeks to reassure and protect D.C. from the fear and anxiety he has already expressed, and which could likely be exacerbated by a full disclosure of the dentist's rationale for the biopsy. Indeed, Dr. M.'s answer could suggest an underlying concern that his patient would not consent to the biopsy if he completely unveiled his suspicions. He may seek to compromise on the disclosure of information to obtain the patient's consent. This compromise, however, appears to reduce D.C.'s need to *Dr. M.'s* view of what would benefit D.C., generating a conflict of "paternalism" in which a professional claims to know the best interests of his or her patient.

In considering these competing considerations and the moral strategy of Dr. M.'s reply, we are engaged in a process of ethical *deliberation,* or what the American philosopher John Dewey referred to as an "imaginative rehearsal in the mind" of alternative courses of action when confronted with a difficult moral choice. When we choose one course of action, and give reasons—patient benefit, truthfulness, informed consent, etc.—for our choice, we are involved in moral *justification,* defending our actions by citing moral and professional principles. The focus of this chapter is on the role of moral justification in dental ethics and the ways in which normative principles can illuminate and, sometimes, resolve moral conflicts in the practice of dentistry. We focus particularly on the significance of four principles—nonmaleficence, beneficence, justice, and respect for autonomy—in illustrative clinical cases. We conclude by highlighting several essential elements of ethical decision making in clinical dental practice.

MORAL PROBLEMS AND JUSTIFICATION

It is important at the outset to distinguish different kinds of problems we encounter in the moral life generally and in dentistry more specifically. A first category we might refer to as a problem of *moral weakness,* in which moral responsibilities point in one direction and personal inclinations in another. If, for example, on a day when a professor is supposed to be inside a classroom teaching students, he or she decides that, because of the warm sunshine and bright, blue sky, his or her time is better spent on the beach, we can rightfully say that the person has failed to meet moral and professional responsibilities. Similarly, if in Case 1, Dr. M.'s reply had been motivated by a concern to end his conversation with D.C. as expeditiously as possible to make his weekly tee time at the local country club, we would not think that this was a compelling moral reason for his actions. Because the demands of morality and personal self-interest appear so diametrically opposed in such instances, many moral philosophers would not consider such cases to involve a genuine moral conflict.

Although we may be confronted with such choices somewhat routinely in our personal lives, an important part of dental ethics focuses on a quite distinct kind of issue, what we may call problems of *moral uncertainty.* In such instances, a dentist may be uncertain whether there is a moral obligation or, if there is, how far it extends. Do individual dentists have responsibilities to provide uncompensated care for medically indigent patients? If a dentist has previously accepted a patient under his or her care, are there any grounds for limiting or terminating care? These are uncertainties about the *existence* of an obligation or its *scope.* The following case illustrates choices about the scope of an obligation with respect to noncompliant patients.

CASE 2

Ms. C., a 35-year-old business executive, is under the care of a periodontist, Dr. G., for severe periodontal disease. Dr. G.'s "policy" is to initiate patient contracts in which he would "spell out" the patient's responsibilities in adhering to his recommendations for personal oral hygiene maintenance while under his care. If a patient does not meet his "standards," he terminates treatment. Dr. G. insists that the patient, in addition to routine flossing and brushing, use adjunctive perio aids such as the "proxy brush, Butler loops, and gingival stimulators." Plaque scores and a gingival bleeding index are used to monitor patient progress and compliance.

Although Ms. C. feels that she was trying to conform to this policy, her condition does not show improvement. In addition, her busy schedule, commitments to family, and social obligations often preclude adherence to a strict oral hygiene regimen. Dr. G. now questions whether it is a "waste" of his time to continue treatment and whether he should continue to treat Ms. C.

Dr. G.'s question is in part about the scope or extent of his obligation to provide treatment for a particular patient. His moral commitment to benefit patients by providing quality care may well require the demanding standards he insists upon in his treatment of periodontal disease. He perhaps feels that his time will be put to better use by devoting more attention to patients who do live up to the contractual agreement. We might well ask whether the standards imposed by his patient contracts are fair and whether, in entering into this agreement, Ms. C. understood that noncompliance risked terminating the relationship.

At another level, the alternatives before Dr. G. (terminate a relationship because of nonfulfillment of a contract, continue treating a not fully compliant patient, etc.) raise deeper questions about the underlying model of dentist-patient relationships. David Ozar has insightfully developed a typology of three models of professionalism and professional-patient relationships in dentistry—the commercial, the guild, and the interactive—and supported the emphasis of the interactive model on decisionmaking in a "partnership of equals."[2] Dr. G. could cite Ms. C.'s noncompliance as indicative of her unwillingness to assume the responsibilities of this partnership, but his policy of initiating patient contracts requiring specific performance reflects less a sense of equality than a commercial model, under which failure to comply with the terms of a contract constitutes grounds for terminating a relationship. At the least, his professional commitment to patient benefit should temper his insistence on fulfillment of contractual obligations to the extent that, if he determines that he is unable to provide further care for Ms. C., he should assist her in finding a dentist who will.

We sometimes can resolve conflicts of moral uncertainty about the existence or the scope of an obligation by appealing to normative ethical principles or professional norms articulated by the ADA. Yet, as the latter considerations mentioned in Case 2 illustrate, such questions can easily shade into a third kind of moral problem, which can be described as *moral dilemmas.* A moral dilemma is constituted by existing obligations or responsibilities that come into conflict. A dentist, confronted with making a choice about treatment, may find good moral reasons to support alternative but conflicting courses of action. To choose one course will necessarily mean precluding the other course, and hence means that the dentist is unable to act fully on his or her responsibilities.

Much of the dental ethics literature has in fact focused on moral dilemmas, a feature that gives a prominent role to moral justification. In instances of moral dilemmas, the question is less about violating moral responsibilities out of personal inclination (moral weakness), or determining the existence and/or scope of responsibilities (moral uncertainty), than about determining which of many values in conflict should take *priority.* In Case 1, for example, should more emphasis be given to patient benefit or to patient need? In Case 2, does an actual ongoing relationship with one patient outweigh the potential benefits to other patients?

Moral justification involves the articulation of defensible reasons for actions in this "grey area" of dental ethics; moral dilemmas arise where it is not unreasonable to expect that reasonable persons may initially differ. We may engage in a justificatory process before various audiences, including our conscience, patients, professional colleagues, or peer review committees. However, ethics requires us finally to move beyond these limited audiences and to be willing to defend our decisions and choices before a general public audience. As Laurence McCullough has maintained, ". . . ethics should appeal to the broadest possible intellectual base so that the analyses it offers will be accessible to all regardless of their particular beliefs and commitments."[3]

Justification is essential to all areas of ethics because, unlike the use of force, it provides a rational basis for others to alter their views or change their actions. Offering defensible reasons most typically assumes the form of appealing to normative rules and principles of ethical decisionmaking, which set out standards and obligations of right conduct.

A common conceptual model of the process of moral justification has suggested that judgments about particular choices of actions, moral rules, and moral principles are related in a hierarchical structure,[4] illustrated as follows:

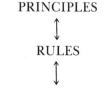

For example, in Case 2, assume that Dr. G. decided to terminate his relationship with his patient. If challenged by others to justify or defend his decision, he might have cited some form of rule along the lines of "Patients must keep their promises to dentists about treatment programs," and he might have justified such a rule by appealing to more general moral considerations about justice (fulfilling contracts), or beneficence (maximizing patient welfare), particularly in light of his concern about "wasting" time treating Mrs. C. In this instance, Dr. G.'s justification could be structured as follows:

PRINCIPLE: Justice or Beneficence

↑

RULE: Fidelity or Keeping Promises

↑

JUDGMENT: Termination of Relationship

The process of justification is also dialectal and corrective. We might start, for example, at the level of a particular choice and, in the course of defending that choice, discover other more compelling rules or principles that lead us to modify our original judgment. If we found that Ms. C. did not understand her agreement with Dr. G., or that contracts requiring specific performance are unfair in the context of dental practice, we might claim his decision to terminate the relationship unjustifiable because it violates principles of justice and respect for patient choices.

Alternatively, we might start our reasoning at the level of normative principles and work down to a specific choice or treatment recommendation. In Case 1, for example, one might contend that the principle of respect for patient autonomy (self-determination) generates rules of informed consent and veracity or truthfulness, which in turn support an obligation of full disclosure by Dr. M. to D.C. The reasoning behind this conclusion might be structured along the following lines:

PRINCIPLE: Respect for Patient Autonomy

↓

RULE: Informed Consent or Veracity

↓

JUDGMENT: Full Disclosure

This discussion illustrates that clarification and resolution of moral dilemmas in dental ethics may be conditioned by several considerations, including which values are recognized as ethical principles, their ethical priority, and their meaning. Let us examine these issues in turn.

MORAL PRINCIPLES AND PROFESSIONAL RELATIONSHIPS

Although the literature on dental ethics has frequently invoked both normative principles[3] (for example, beneficence, respect for autonomy, justice) and rules (veracity, fidelity, confidentiality) that are acknowledged in other realms of general social morality, the recognition of these as principles and rules *for dentistry* may be influenced by different conceptions of dentistry as a profession and of dentist-patient relationships. Let us build on themes in Ozar's typology to illustrate this point.

In the commercial model, for example, in which dental care is seen as a commodity sold by dentists and bought by patients as "consumers," the moral standards that would apply would be those appropriate to any conventional relationship of commercial exchange. That is, the morality of the relationship would be structured by principles that preserve and promote the decision making and autonomy of both parties and that prohibit the injury of one party by the other (nonmaleficence). These principles may generate rules about "consent" to contracts that are agreed upon, although this rule would more likely be modified by a stipulation of *caveat emptor* ("let the buyer beware") than by the concept of "informed consent."

Under such a model, moreover, it is not clear that a principle of patient benefit or beneficence would be recognized in any morally meaningful sense. Patients in dental practice would become the occasion by which professionals obtain self-referential benefits, such as financial gain or collegial esteem. Justice as a normative principle would be limited to the mutual fulfillment of responsibilities specified in a contractual agreement. All in all, the morality of the commercial model appears quite barren and minimalistic.

The guild model on Ozar's account is concerned above all with the preservation of the privileges and esteem of the profession of dentistry from intrusions by society, the law, and even patients. This view impacts not only on the recognition of normative principles, but also on their sources and grounding, as well as on the audience of justification. Thus, as historians of dentistry have observed, professional statements of dental ethics traditionally recognized the so-called "Golden Rule"—do unto others as you would have done to yourself—as the encompassing moral obligation for dentists.[5] The Golden Rule (which is often considered by moral philosophers to express a requirement of the principle of formal justice that we treat similar cases similarly) does not, unfortunately, provide much in the way of specific guidance for clinical decisions, and what is provided seems to suggest that the orientation for ethical actions is self-referential, that is, how the dentist would wish to be treated.

The implications of such a view are (1) that the *profession* by itself must articulate a more detailed and explicit account of ethical obligations; (2) that this account should be designed with the interests of the profession and how *it* wishes to be treated held in paramount importance; and (3) that the moral audience is limited to members of the profession. The guild model of dentistry thus culminates in an ethics by the profession, for the profession, and of the profession. The interests of others are ethically extraneous.

The interactive model articulated by Ozar provides the basis for a much fuller account of dentistry as a *moral* practice. The language of "partnership of equals" presupposes that principles of respect for (patient and professional) autonomy and patient benefit are at the core of what makes dentistry a profession. The idea of justice in the practitioner-patient relationship is likewise acknowledged in the appeal to equality.

Moreover, the interactive model also encompasses a dimension of social justice as a part of dentistry that is simply not present in the commercial or guild model. This is because it is ultimately "the community . . . which confers on the dentist the status

of professional."[2] The relationship between the community and the profession as a whole is therefore based on trust and assumes a fiduciary character. This trust allows the profession broad control over matters of self-regulation on the assumption that the principal purposes of dentistry are patient-oriented, rather than as in the guild model, professional self-interest. This sense of professional ethical responsibility toward the community entails that questions of justice with a social dimension are an appropriate domain for dental ethics.

MORAL PRINCIPLES AND THEIR PRIORITIES

One source of disagreement about the normative principles of dental ethics, then, may be attributed to differing images of the profession held by dentists, patients, or others in the professional and moral communities. However, if, as is implicit in the preceding discussion, more than one principle is recognized as normative, questions about priorities among conflicting principles are sure to arise when a moral dilemma is experienced in clinical decision making. The scholarly literature in dental ethics has not, however, always arrived at the same conclusions on this matter.

For example, David Ozar, David Schiedermayer, and Mark Siegler have identified seven distinct "value considerations" in the moral choices faced by dentists: life and health of the patient; appropriate and pain-free oral functioning; patient autonomy; preferred practice values; esthetic values; cost; and external considerations, including the patient's life-style, the patient's family, allocation of resources, and public safety and welfare. This account is in part *descriptive* ethics; it intends to portray the values that "dominate ethical reflection" in clinical decisionmaking.[6]

How, then, should dentists proceed when these considerations come into conflict? Ozar and colleagues formulate a serial ranking of the values in the order listed above. That is "as a general principle, . . . the value of life and health takes priority over and ranks above the six other categories of value,"[6] and a similar structuring is offered for the remaining considerations. Appropriate and pain-free dental functioning takes priority over patient self-determination, which itself limits the extent that professionals' practice values can control decisions about dental treatment.

Laurence McCullough, by contrast, contends that "three ethical principles emerge as fundamental to the practice of dentistry," which he identifies as beneficence, respect for autonomy, and justice.[3] McCullough does not offer any advance ranking of these normative principles out of a sense that the priorities may be conditioned by the particular circumstances at hand, and because of the current absence of a more general theory of value in dental ethics.

It is tempting to see in this terminological difference of "values" or "principles" a substantial methodological disagreement in dental ethics. Yet, if we push beyond the terminology to examine the *meaning* of both the value considerations described by Ozar and colleagues and the principles articulated by McCullough, we will find stronger indications of convergence than of divergence. Indeed, the considerations can be arranged in terms of the principles. For example, a dentist's commitment to the values of patient life and health, appropriate and pain-free oral functioning, and preferred practice values would be encompassed by the meaning of the beneficence principle. Similarly, the values of "patient autonomy" or "esthetics" are compatible with the principle of respect for autonomy, whereas the content of the justice principle would include issues of cost and "external considerations."

Moreover, we can ask why the considerations identified by Ozar and colleagues are values in the first place. The principles of beneficence, respect for autonomy, and justice can be understood to justify or validate their correlated values, thus providing them with a normative rationale. In short, the principles indicate why a dentist *ought* to accept a particular consideration as a value in dentistry.

The methodological dispute over the ranking or prioritizing of a value or principle may also not be as significant as it initially appears. In many circumstances, the two approaches could be expected to support similar conclusions and decisions. Given that many instances of dental treatment do not risk patient life or health and that the central objective of most patients in seeking dental treatment is precisely to obtain appropriate and pain-free dental functioning, it is entirely conceivable that many clinical interactions would not pose moral conflicts regarding the two principal values in the schema offered by Ozar and colleagues.

This is not to minimize the possibility of practical disagreement between the two approaches when conflicts do emerge. For example, to anticipate the issues involved in a case that we will discuss subsequently (Case 7), what balance should dentists strike between commitment to their patients and responsibility for others who may be at risk of infectious disease from a particular patient? McCullough is willing to override patient confidentiality to protect specified others from harm,[3] whereas the lower priority Ozar and colleagues give to the dentist's consideration for public safety relative to patient autonomy seems to point in just the opposite direction.

We can also assess whether an advance prioritization method would make a practical difference in the following kind of situation.

CASE 3

J.A., a 48-year-old female patient, presented to the dentist (Dr. V.) for the first time, concerned about her lifelong struggle to maintain good dental health. J.A. indicated that she had been treated by a number of dentists over the course of her life, but has continued to require multiple fillings, root canals, and full crowns in an attempt to keep her teeth. She expresses considerable frustration, not only with the time spent with dentists, but also with the substantial expense and apparent failures of repeated dental interventions.

J.A. now has problems with her gums and comments that her previous dentist advised her that she would need extensive periodontal therapy. She has instead come to Dr. V. with a request that he extract all of her teeth and fabricate complete upper and lower dentures. Upon examination, including radiographs, periodontal evaluation, and soft tissue assessment, Dr. V. explains that complete extraction is not necessary and that J.A. can indeed save her remaining teeth.

J.A., however, continues to insist that she prefers complete dentures so that she will be "free of dental problems once and for all."

This kind of case seems to present a clear-cut instance of conflict between the value of appropriate and pain-free dental functioning or the principle of beneficence and that of respect for autonomy. Would it be resolved differently because one approach gives higher priority to patient benefit rather than patient choice? Perhaps, but perhaps not. What Dr. V. needs to find out before any action is taken is whether J.A.'s request is truly reflective of autonomous choice. That task is particularly complicated because this is their initial clinical encounter.

It may nevertheless be the case that J.A.'s request is less a well-considered choice than one born of frustration and desperation. Dr. V. needs to ensure that all relevant information about the alternatives for J.A.'s dental health and gum problems has been presented to her; more particularly, she needs to understand this information and that removing all her teeth will not guarantee, in a broad sense, lasting freedom from "dental problems." Because J.A. has mentioned the expense of repeated dental treatment, Dr. V. would do well to explore further the role this element plays in her request. If J.A. lacks insurance, for example, the expectation of continued substantial expenses may be playing a controlling influence in her preference for full dentures.

Moreover, Dr. V. needs to place J.A.'s request in the context of her past history. Why is it, for example, that J.A. has experienced chronic problems with her dentition? Is her exasperation with previous dentists and past treatments well founded, or are her problems partly attributable to neglect of dental hygiene? Adopting a practice of good hygiene may lessen, even if it does not eliminate, expectations of future dental problems. It is therefore not only J.A.'s teeth that should be the object of Dr. V.'s care, but also J.A. as a *person*. Just as J.A. needs to understand fully the implications of her choice, Dr. V. needs to seek to understand J.A. as fully as possible. That level of mutual understanding may not necessarily be achieved in the course of a single office visit, but it is vital to determining whether J.A.'s preference is autonomous or heteronomous (controlled by other persons or influences).

The central point here is that the conflict between a professional recommendation and a patient choice may dissolve if some substantial effort is made to know the patient behind the choice. Respect for patient autonomy, on any account, should encompass respect for the patient as a whole, not merely respect for a patient's will.

Having sought mutual understanding, however, it is entirely possible that J.A. will persist in her initial request, which may turn out to be well-considered, informed, and voluntary. The apparent conflict is now a real moral dilemma for Dr. V. In the scheme proposed by Ozar and colleagues, Dr. V. would need to determine whether his recommendation is consistent with the commitment to "appropriate and pain-free oral functioning," in which case it would take precedence over the value of patient autonomy, or whether it is more compatible with the "preferred practice values" of the profession and of Dr. V. himself, in which case, J.A.'s autonomy would be the primary value. While Ozar, Schiedermayer, and Siegler contend that it is unethical to "leave a patient with significantly impaired or painful oral function, even for the sake of autonomy . . . ,"[6] part of what is morally at stake in J.A.'s case is *whose* understanding of "appropriate" or "impaired functioning" should take precedence, J.A.'s or Dr. V.'s.

McCullough's method would invoke similar questions, given that beneficence encompasses an obligation to "preserve healthy teeth" against the patient's autonomous request to be rid of all her teeth. Given J.A.'s concern about costs of dental care, McCullough's analysis might devote more attention to the requirements of the principle of justice, whereas "cost" has minimal priority for Ozar and colleagues. Moreover, in the absence of a ranking schema in McCullough, Ozar and colleagues' endorsement of the priority of "appropriate and pain-free dental functioning" over autonomy is theoretically more accommodating to a paternalistic dentistry, a view that may bear on how the issue between Dr. V. and J.A. is finally decided.

It is not necessary for our purposes here to resolve either the methodological or (potential) practical disagreement. Indeed, such resolution would be premature and unfortunate, because such debates are vital to the ongoing integrity and ethos of dentistry as a moral profession. We wish instead to contribute constructively to this vibrant discussion by proposing our own account of the normative principles of dental ethics, one that seems defensible in terms of more general theories of ethics and biomedicine and, although supportable by professional ethical standards articulated by the ADA, also moves beyond and completes them.

THE PRINCIPLE OF NONMALEFICENCE

Dentists, no less than members of the other healing and caring professions, have a responsibility not to cause harm or injury to patients, an obligation that is formulated in a principle of *nonmaleficence*. The principle of nonmaleficence is a bedrock of both social and professional morality. Society as a whole and individual patients in particular give over to dentists a fiduciary power to perform procedures that provide privileged access to a part of the body in the trust that dentists will not cause them harm or injury. This principle is surely implicit in the primary value that Ozar and colleagues ascribe to procedures that do not jeopardize the life and health of patients, as well as in McCullough's principle of beneficence.

The prominent public association of a visit to the dentist's office with pain might suggest that an obligation of nonharm is irrelevant to dentistry. Of course, it is important not to reduce the practice of dentistry to "drilling, filling, and extracting." Even so, the pain or discomfort that patients do experience in undergoing certain procedures may be considered a premoral harm or an overridable harm justified by a view to the greater welfare of the patient. Nonmaleficence rules out the infliction of pain for pain's sake, and requires that dentists seek to minimize risk and unavoidable pain.

The principle of nonmaleficence may be the moral root, in whole or in part, for certain professional duties displayed in the ADA *Principles*. The requirement that "dentists shall not represent the care being rendered to their patients in a false or misleading manner"[7] draws on notions that misrepresentation and deception can result in choices that bring harm to patients, as well as on the view that patients require accurate information to make autonomous choices. The responsibility of nonmisrepresentation also entails an affirmative obligation of dentists in "keeping their knowledge and skill current,"[8] lest patients be exposed to undue levels of risk or harm as a result of dated knowledge and technical skills.

A more interesting illustration, in terms of its moral justification, is an advisory opinion regarding a professional duty of nonendangerment, one that takes on particular meaning in the context of AIDS: "A dentist who becomes ill from any disease or impaired in any way shall, with consultation and advice from a qualified physician or other authority, limit the activities of practice to those areas that do not endanger the patients or members of the dental staff."[9]

Standing by itself, the opinion reflects a concern not to create a risk of harm to others, and its rationale would thus seem to be rooted in nonmaleficence. However, the opinion comes as a specification of the ADA code of "community service," and so might be read as a qualifier on the obligation that "dentists . . . shall conduct themselves in such a manner as to maintain or elevate the esteem of the profession."[10] If the duty of nonendangerment is generated out of regard for the status of the profession rather than out of regard for patients, it is more illustrative of the guild model of dental ethics.

THE PRINCIPLE OF BENEFICENCE

It would be a bleak and minimalistic account of morality that would limit obligations merely to those of refraining from harming or endangering others. The primary moral rationale for dentistry is that quality care and specialized treatment can provide assistance and benefits to patients. The principle of patient benefit or *beneficence* encompasses obligations to prevent further harm (restoration of a carious tooth, performing a root canal, placement of a crown), remove immediate harm (extracting an abscessed tooth, for example), and promote or restore the general oral health of patients, including educational recommendations (brushing and flossing), the use of sealants, or placing orthodontic appliances to enhance proper tooth development.

Although beneficence commands universal acceptance as a normative principle in the dental ethics literature, important issues exist surrounding the sources and the scope of the principle. One question concerns whether beneficence is based on a more general duty of assistance to others in common social morality, or is dependent on the special moral commitments required by the practice of dentistry (and perhaps shared with other healing and caring professions). Some moral philosophers have argued that there is no general duty of assistance to others; the extent of our obligations is limited to refraining from harming others, except in those situations in which we voluntarily assume responsibilities to others. This approach would make the obligation to benefit patients independent of common general morality, with specific duties of aid assumed by a practitioner upon entry into the profession. The commitment to assist and benefit specific others defines the profession morally, and sets it apart from other "professed" occupations such as architecture or engineering.

Still other philosophers, such as the influential utilitarian theorist John Stuart Mill (1806-1873), have maintained that social morality does include responsibilities to render aid, but have considered these to be "imperfect duties" because we have discretion about who we may assist, how, and under what conditions. A person may be under a general duty to be charitable, for example, but he or she has discretion as to whether to be charitable toward a homeless person on the street, an organization that cares for the homeless, or an organization that promotes an altogether different social good, such as the American Heart Association or the Sierra Club.

Once having accepted patients, the discretion of dentists about providing "quality care" to those patients is minimal. The act of "profession" by a dentist to a particular patient could, on this account, be seen as transforming an imperfect duty of beneficence into a perfect duty.

Of course, dentists are not necessarily obligated to accept any and every person who requests their services. A dentist participating in a DMO, for example, is permitted to limit the number of persons under his or her treatment and care. The ADA *Principles* admonishes dentists to "exercise reasonable discretion" in patient selection, while prohibiting the denial of dental services because of the "race, creed, color, sex, or national origin" of a patient.[11] Thus, before accepting a patient, the notion of an imperfect duty seems to apply.

But just how expansive or restrictive is the "reasonable discretion" permitted dentists in decisions about refusing to accept new patients or discontinuing care of previously accepted patients? Consider the following situation.

CASE 4

Dr. H. is an associate of Dr. B. in a very successful urban practice. Most of the patients are of long standing and were part of the practice purchased by Dr. B. 5 years ago. During the last 2 years, several patients of Dr. H. revealed during recall examinations that they have developed a positive serology for the HIV antibody. In the practice to date, Dr. H. had treated one individual diagnosed with AIDS, a 28-year-old man, married, with two children, who had contracted the disease subsequent to blood transfusion after a car accident. Although all precautionary measures were followed for all patients (including disposable prophylaxis angles), Dr. B. decided that he did not wish any "high risk" patients treated in the office. He reviewed all patient records and removed charts indicating a medical history of HIV exposure or hepatitis B. Dr. B. advised Dr. H. that she could not attend these patients and that he would not do so himself. He also advised his staff to contact the patients and inform them that they would not be reappointed.

Although several layers of ethical questions are embedded in this case, we can focus on the discretion of dentists in accepting or refusing patients by considering a third account of whether a general duty of assistance exists. In this view, there is an imperfect duty in social morality that becomes an *actual* or *nondiscretionary* duty under certain conditions. A person may be obligated to assist another if the second person is in dire need, the first person can provide the aid and is a necessary source of aid (there is no alternative source), the risks of providing aid for the first person are minimal, and the benefits to the second person outweigh the possible harm to the first.

Such an account will have difficulty in supporting a view that dentists have a perfect or actual duty to accept any patient. Much dental care would not be considered a dire need, as evidenced by the many persons who voluntarily forgo it, or are involuntarily prevented from obtaining it because it is not part of their health insurance. Although a given dentist, such as Dr. B., could provide requested care, so could many other dentists, so a patient who wanted treatment could likely obtain it. With respect to not accepting new patients, then, Dr. B.'s decision does not necessarily violate these first three conditions of an actual duty to assist (we consider risk-benefit assessments shortly).

It thus appears that none of the three positions identified above—no general positive duties, positive but imperfect duties, positive and actual duties—can obligate a dentist to accept any and every patient who seeks admission to a program of dental care. The objectionable feature of Dr. B.'s decision, however, is that he has not refused just "any" patient; rather, he proposes to exclude a certain group or class of patients because of a particular characteristic; moreover, it is not clear that this characteristic, HIV + or HBV + status, necessarily impedes his capacity to deliver "quality care" to these patients, since he and his associate use similar precautions for all patients. The characteristic thus appears arbitrary from the point of view of professional dental practice.

In an advisory opinion to the code of conduct on patient selection, the ADA *Principles* affirm: "A dentist has the general obligation to provide care to those in need. A decision not to provide treatment to an individual because the individual has AIDS or is HIV seropositive, based solely on that fact, is unethical."[12] Dr. B. may well respond that his decision about excluding certain patients is not based *solely* on the fact that these patients of record are HIV +. Indeed, he has cited "high risk" as the precipitating factor in his decision; his stated rationale is not solely the presence of a medical condition, but rather of a dangerous or risky condition. He may thus contend that a decision not to accept new patients who are HIV + does not fall outside the boundaries of the "reasonable discretion" permitted by the ADA.

However, this assessment of "risk" as a rationale for denying services pertains to the *magnitude* of the risk. The *probability* of the risk of HIV or HBV transmission in the clinical setting is rather minimal, especially because in Dr. B.'s office, appropriate precautions are used in treating all patients. In this respect, the decision violates the advisory opinion's stipulation that "decisions with regard to the type of dental treatment [provided to persons with AIDS] . . . should be made on the same basis as they are made with other patients, . . . "[12] Although it would be imprudent to ignore the level of risk, it must be given some perspective.

The direct burden of Dr. B.'s decision will, of course, fall less on persons who never were his patients than on those he has instructed not to be reappointed. The proposed termination of these relationships presents additional questions about the justifiability of this decision. Although Dr. B. (or Dr. H.) most likely would not be the sole avenue of access to dental care for these patients, they could well claim the past 5 years of clinical care under this practice created expectations of a continued relationship. They are relying on responsibilities of professional beneficence implicitly enhanced by the rule of fidelity or promise-keeping. The decision to exclude them constitutes a breach of trust. Moreover, if they seek care under a new dentist who requests their previous records, questions of confidentiality will surely emerge. There are good reasons, then, to support Vincent Rogers' claim that "a dentist is ethically (and legally) bound to continue to treat or stabilize a patient undergoing dental treatment who develops AIDS or other AIDS-related conditions."[13]

As in Case 2, Dr. B.'s decision raises issues about the scope of an obligation. Unlike the patient in Case 2, however, the excluded patients do not necessarily appear to be noncompliant; indeed, for all Dr. B. knows, they have very good reasons for being his most observant patients. Thus, the decision to exclude present patients seems even harder to justify than a decision not to enroll new patients, because the establishment of a relationship itself creates moral obligations and responsibilities. Notwithstanding the risks posed to himself, his colleague, their auxiliary staff, and potentially, their families, Dr. B.'s decision appears discriminatory and in violation of principles of justice and respect for persons.

It is not our purpose to provide a comprehensive account of the ethical responsibilities of individual dentists and the profession toward HIV+ patients; an exposition of these issues can be found elsewhere in this volume (Chap. 6). Our discussion here has been intended to illustrate two points. First, the meaning and scope of the principle of beneficence in dental ethics are not completely dependent on general social morality, but rather emerge from the inherent commitments of dentistry as a moral profession and practice. Second, comprehensive dental ethics requires additional principles and rules to complement those of nonmaleficence and beneficence.

THE PRINCIPLE OF JUSTICE

As illustrated in our discussion of previous cases, it is not always possible in the practice of dentistry to avoid harm (nonmaleficence) and provide benefits (beneficence). Situations arise in which both harms and benefits are present, and the ethical consideration is how the harms and benefits are *distributed*. Who will bear the burdens and who will receive the benefits of a treatment recommendation or an institutional (or social) policy decision? Issues of fair distribution, when benefits cannot be provided without imposing some burdens or harms, are encompassed in dental ethics by the principle of justice.

The core meaning of justice is to give to other persons their due, and as indicated previously, acknowledgement of such an obligation historically has been reflected in professional statements citing the "Golden Rule" as a guide for conduct. A more current illustration of sensitivity to a dimension of justice in dental care is contained in the ADA *Principles*, which stipulate that dentists should be "caring and fair in their contact with patients."[1] This displays a professional commitment to both beneficence and justice (though without acknowledging their possible tension), and the appeal to fairness can encompass such matters as performing mutually agreed procedures, reasonable charges for professional services, or nonabandonment of patients of record.

While justice in interpersonal relations is vital to the moral practice of dentistry, Clifton Dummett has observed that historically "the dental profession has been reluctant to admit it had an ethical responsibility in reference to the larger social issues."[14] Yet, as intimated by our discussion of Case 3, many larger issues of social justice are encountered with increasing frequency by dentists, particularly with respect to access to dental care in the absence of adequate insurance coverage. There is currently no legal right to health care in general in our society, and dental care has commanded an even lower social priority. As Vincent Rogers has put it, "Dental care is viewed as an option and luxury in the United States health system. Even the federal government does not mandate dental care in either its Medicaid and Medicare programs."[15] Many private insurance programs either do not cover dental expenses, or make such coverage optional at substantial out-of-pocket expenses.

In this context, McCullough has argued that the principle of justice in dental ethics includes an individual and professional "obligation to call attention to injustice in the financing of dental care, . . ."[3] Similarly, Ozar and colleagues have asserted that "[i]n the current atmosphere of cost containment, the professional obligations of dentists regarding the equitable distribution of health care and health care resources should perhaps rank even higher" in their hierarchy of value considerations.[6] Let us consider a couple of examples to determine how dentists might balance their responsibilities to be "fair to patients" in the face of unjust financing or inequities in the distribution of resources for dental care.

CASE 5

A 14-year-old male patient presents to the dentist for the first time for care, with a chief complaint of pain. His parents, who have three other children between the ages of 7 and 10, are of modest financial means. An examination reveals gross decay in teeth nos. 2, 3, 19, and 30, and radiographic examination reveals pulpal involvement in teeth nos. 3 and 30; the dentist also is certain that excavation of teeth nos. 2 and 19 will result in pulpal exposure. Although the dentist believes that endodontic therapy would save all of the involved teeth, the cost of such care far exceeds the capacity of the state's Medicaid program, which does contain a dental benefits component for children. Alternative treatments are considered but ruled out because of costs beyond the means of the parents. The dentist feels compelled to extract all the involved teeth.

There are several levels at which the responsibilities of justice can be broached here. At the most immediate level, the dentist's decision means that both the benefits (loss of pain) and the burdens (loss of four teeth) fall on the same person, the 14-year-old patient. Financial considerations will create a life-long compromised capacity for full dental functioning. Moreover, the dentist finds his own ability to benefit this particular patient according to his professional obligation to provide "quality care" attenuated; he appears willing to opt for a course of treatment that is different from what it would be if finances were not an issue.

The question of justice is not limited to the particular choice confronting the dentist now. We need to inquire why this is the first time a 14-year-old is visiting a dental office, and how his teeth have come to be in this condition. Perhaps his parents have not instructed him sufficiently in appropriate dental hygiene; perhaps the patient himself has exacerbated the problem by continuing his childhood antipathy toward brushing his teeth. Notwithstanding these possible features, the patient's current situation speaks of inadequacies about social support for preventive dental programs and access to preventive dental care.

It is not merely this patient who might suffer from underfunded programs or lower social priorities about dental care. It is entirely possible that his siblings (among many others) are traveling the same road. What educational and preventive resources are available to them so that they can avoid having several of their teeth extracted in a few years? The circle of who bears the burdens for a low social priority for adequate dental care will gradually become larger.

The decision of the dentist to opt for extraction is a response to a bind that is not of his own making. Or is it? Decisions about treatment alternatives in dentistry differ from medical decisions in that an "acceptable" or "sanctioned" alternative may be recommended solely on the basis of economics or ability to pay. The treatment recommended is usually less than ideal and would not be considered an option for a patient with the capacity to pay for the ideal. In Case 5, the dentist possesses the skills and training to "save" the tooth, or teeth, and would do so for a similarly affected 14-year-old whose parents have the ability to pay, but may not for the patient who cannot pay for the more extensive procedure. Hence, two patients, equal in situation except ability to pay, receive different levels of care based on economics alone. Is this just? Further, does such a model of decision making exist in medicine, whose tradition of "first, do no harm" dentistry attests to embrace?

One might argue that, in extracting the offending tooth, the dentist would employ his or her skills and training for the best interest of the patient, by alleviating pain, infection, and suffering. However, the dentist also possesses the skills and training to prevent disability and dysfunction by saving the tooth, or teeth, and thereby preventing unnecessary loss of a "body part." The provision of endodontic therapy (root canal), restoration of the carious (decayed) parts of the tooth (perhaps with a post and core procedure) and then placement of a crown (complete restoration) are all costly interventions, which a practitioner can ill afford to provide to all needy patients who present with an inability to pay. Yet it can also be said that a medical practitioner, particularly in an emergency room setting, not only would not withhold, or recommend withholding, treatment that would prevent disability or a "handicapping" condition, but also would be held liable for negligence and malpractice if the decision were motivated solely on the basis of ability to pay.

The ability to propose treatment that ranges from "good" to "better" to "best" is a tradition in dentistry that is both sanctioned in its ethical code and principles of professional conduct and also accepted by the public and unquestioned by the medical tradition. Although one can argue that the ability of the dentist to maintain a viable practice and thereby serve many more patients is important, one must recognize that "similar individuals are treated dissimilarly" in the provision of service based upon economic disparities.

Determining whether such a tradition is or is not just begs several related questions. First, what are the rights to health care on the part of the patient and the duties and obligations of the dentist (or someone else) to provide that care? More importantly, what priority has society placed upon access to dental care as compared with other health services, such as medical care in an emergency room setting? The profession, from the perspective of what it sanctions ethically, and society, from the perspective of what it will accept, appear to have resolved these questions, but such practices are not immune from ethical challenge.[16]

It is difficult for dentists to fulfill what the ADA calls their "primary professional obligation" of "service to the public" if society is unwilling to commit adequate resources. Although some dentists have assumed the burden for some uncompensated care, we clearly cannot and should not rely on the exercise of the imperfect duty of charity toward a few indigent persons to resolve a far-reaching question of social justice and health care priorities. The costs of the preferred treatment for this patient are likely to be so substantial the dentist could not make this a regular practice, and if he or she did, other patients might complain of unfairness to them, because their fees are being used as a subsidy for the otherwise uncompensated care.

Justice concerns not only *what* is decided but also *who* should decide. This latter concern is what we might refer to as *procedural* justice. It is unfair and a violation of justice for persons who will assume the burdens of a decision not to have a say in that decision. The dentist in Case 5, therefore, as constrained as he is, cannot make a unilateral decision about extraction. A collaborative process is required if the person(s) making decisions are different than those who directly experience the harms or burdens of the decision. Such collaboration may well lead to alternative recommendations or choices not originally envisioned, even proposals for possible payment acceptable to the parents, the dentist, and the Medicaid administrators. Procedural justice is very much in keeping with an "interactive" model of professional dentistry, in which decision making occurs in a context of "partnership of equals."

This kind of partnership can be challenged not only when beneficence conflicts with justice (Case 5), but also when justice conflicts with the obligation to respect patient autonomy.

CASE 6

Ms. D.W., a 28-year-old woman, visited Dr. O. after performance of orthognathic surgery for a young woman whom she employed. She expressed concern about "the way my teeth look." Dr. O. attempted to inform her about the necessary surgery, but D.W. resisted, stating she didn't want to know any details, because she then "wouldn't be able to go through with it." She remained firm in her decision not to know extensive details.

D.W.'s past medical history was unremarkable and her prior dental history revealed only two small occlusal amalgams. No dental caries or periodontal disease were found. After a full diagnostic work-up, Dr. O. determined that presurgical orthodontics followed by a LeForte-I osteotomy of the maxilla with segments and bilateral osteotomies of the mandibular rami would be necessary to correct her developmental deformities.

After 10 months of presurgical orthodontics, an examination reveals that D.W. will be ready for surgery in 2 months. As Dr. O. prepares to schedule her for surgery, he believes it is necessary to talk again with D.W. about the surgery, as well as consult with D.W.'s insurance company, which will be responsible for approximately $7000 in hospital fees and $4500 in surgeon's fees.

A central issue in this case is whether, to use the language of Ozar and colleagues, D.W.'s request is for "appropriate and pain-free dental functioning," and if not, whether it is fair for *others,* the insurance contributors, to assume the burdens of paying for the surgery. Dr. O. apparently sees no dysfunctional dental development; D.W. may experience "pain" from the deformities, but it is psychic pain and suffering, not to be trivialized to be sure, but distinguishable in morally important ways from physiological pain that requires dental intervention.

Another way to put the point is that D.W.'s request is more in the realm of human desires and esthetics than in the realm of human need and ethics. She is troubled by how her teeth "look," not with their functioning. Our bodies, especially our faces and teeth, are media for self-revelation, so how we appear to others is important to self-identity. The ethical issue of justice, however, is whether one's desires and aspirations for enhanced appearance create an obligation in others to fulfill them, in this case, through insurance premiums.

Even if D.W.'s insurance company is quite willing to provide this coverage, a deeper question of justice is embedded in this case, which can be displayed through juxtaposing Cases 5 and 6. Is it fair that some receive this kind of procedure while others who have real need for necessary care undergo extractions because of limited funds and resources? Resolving this fundamental inequity is not D.W.'s responsibility or even Dr. O.'s, but there does need to be broader recognition that the existence of such an inequity affects the alternatives open to D.W. and Dr. O.

and closed to the 14-year-old boy and the dentist in Case 5.

Our culture and its philosophical and professional traditions of ethics have given much more attention to "negative rights," or rights to noninterference, such as the rule of confidentiality, than to "positive rights," or rights to assistance, such as general access to quality dental care. Critics of the ADA *Principles* have noted, for example, that its limitations on "reasonable discretion" in patient selection do not apply to denial of dental services based on indigency or inability to pay. The results of this cultural ethical imbalance are ultimately displayed in the lives of individual patients. In this respect, McCullough seems quite right to maintain that individual dentists and the profession as a whole have a justice-based obligation to draw attention to basic inequities in the structure of dental care financing and the direct implications of these inequities for millions of patients (or prospective patients).

THE PRINCIPLE OF RESPECT FOR AUTONOMY

The moral perplexities of D.W.'s case are heightened by her insistence that she not be informed of the details of the surgery. This is particularly problematic because D.W. also indicates that such knowledge would change her opinion about the surgery. Can we then say that her decision is an autonomous choice, or that, if Dr. O. performs the surgery, he has truly respected D.W.'s autonomy?

Respect for patient autonomy is a central normative principle in dental ethics, but as illustrated by both Case 3 as well as Case 6, its meaning in particular situations of choice can be very complex. Part of that complexity hinges on how attentive ethical analysis is to the "patient" as a whole as distinct from the patient's will expressed in a decision. Dentists have specialized knowledge and powers to treat diseases and conditions of the hard and soft tissues of the mouth (teeth, gingiva, etc.), but dental problems are presented by persons, embodied selves who have a social as well as health history. These persons may be very knowledgeable about dental care, they may change their minds based on the knowledge they receive, or they may not want any knowledge, as with D.W. The point to stress here is that the obligation of respect is owed to a person, not a principle.

It is therefore insufficient for dentists to simply acquiesce to requests of patients; that is really indifference and apathy masquerading as respect. Dentists have a right and a responsibility to inquire into the reasons for a patient's choices, in a relationship of equal partnership with the patient.

Respect for patient autonomy generates three basic rules in dental ethics, all of which are formulated as obligations in the ADA *Principles*. We have already noted an obligation of *veracity* or truthfulness is addressed in the *Principles* under the concept "Representation of Care": "Dentists shall not represent the care being rendered to their patients in a false or misleading manner."[7] This negative formulation does not necessarily exhaust the concept of veracity, however; the establishment of a therapeutic relationship also entails positive disclosure of information in a truthful manner in addition to avoiding misrepresentation.

This constructive element of veracity overlaps with a second obligation justified by respect for patient autonomy, the rule of obtaining *informed consent* to dental procedures. Finally, dentists have obligations of *confidentiality* respecting information disclosed by patients. We have previously examined issues of veracity (Case 1); here our analysis focuses on the rules of informed consent and confidentiality, beginning with the questions posed again by Case 6.

Informed Consent

As some authors have described it, the requirement of informed consent is "a cornerstone of moral dental practice."[17] A patient's consent to treatment can be considered valid if four conditions are met: (1) Sufficient information about a proposed treatment has been disclosed, including the risks and benefits of the treatment, of alternatives, and of no treatment; (2) the patient understands and comprehends this information; (3) the patient decides voluntarily and competently, and is not under circumstances of duress, coercion, or compromised capacity; (4) the patient authorizes the dentist to perform the procedure. Dentists should seek express consent from patients for invasive dental procedures, but in some circumstances, such as a standard office visit for routine preventive care, consent can be implied by the patient's attendance at the appointment.

The ADA *Principles* approach the idea of informed consent under the concept of "Patient Involvement": "The dentist should inform the patient of the proposed treatment, and any reasonable alternatives, in a manner that allows the patient to become involved in treatment decisions."[18] The language of "involvement" is not identical with "consent," to be sure, but it is a different approach than that reflected in "traditional dentist-patient relationships in which dental clinicians consistently made the choices of therapy for their patients."[14] The difficulty that Dr. O. confronts is that D.W. wants neither to be informed nor to be involved in the decision about her surgery. D.W. is interested solely in an outcome, not in the process, both communicative and technical, that will lead to the outcome. Indeed, although we may agree that D.W. has authorized the surgical procedure, not only is the consent not informed, but the effort to provide relevant information runs the risk that D.W. will *rescind* her authorization.

For both these reasons, Dr. O. is quite right to attempt to engage D.W. in a discussion of the procedure as the date for surgery nears. Following the ADA stipulation, he should seek to disclose the information "*in a manner* that allows the patient to become involved" (our emphasis). The manner or method of communication seems crucial to D.W.'s involvement; a recitation of risks, benefits, alternatives, possible outcomes, etc., simply will not suffice in her instance. "Determining what the patient wants to know," Eric Cassell has suggested, "may mean asking directly, indirectly, or metaphorically, or by sensing feelings."[19] This process may take time, and Dr. O. will need to do some listening; he needs to understand his patient just as she needs to understand the information he wishes to discuss. Indeed, to forgo this effort may leave Dr. O. open later to acrimonious accusations should the surgery not give D.W. precisely the outcome she wanted.

Dr. O. also needs to persist, not simply to seek informed consent but also to ensure that the consent is *authentic*. D.W. may be of two minds about the matter, as indicated by her remark that detailed knowledge would impede her willingness to have the surgery performed. D.W. may simply feel that what she doesn't know won't hurt her. Perhaps she feels the procedure will be described so technically that she won't understand the explanation, and seeks to avoid embarrassment. Alternatively, because it has been 10 months since their initial discussion, it is possible that D.W. has changed her mind about not knowing.

Whatever D.W.'s rationale for not wanting to know in the past, or her present level of interest in the information, Dr. O. has several good reasons for communicating his concerns so that both he and his patient can be assured that the choice for surgery is an authentic expression of her wishes. Finally, however, patients have a right to request nondisclosure of information, and it is an important part of respect for patient autonomy not to impose information against a patient's express wishes.[17] If D.W. continues to resist disclosure, Dr. O. should ultimately respect that choice as well.

Confidentiality

Historically, the caring professions have tended to place more emphasis on secrecy than honesty; an obligation of confidentiality is virtually universal in professional codes of ethics, whereas specific stipulations about truthfulness to patients have appeared only recently. This widespread acceptance does not mean, however, that confidentiality is an uncontroversial concept in biomedical or dental ethics. A prominent clinical ethicist, for example, has called confidentiality a "decrepit concept" because, especially with the advent of computers, so many persons can rather easily gain access to patient records.[20] Oth-

ers have examined confidentiality from the standpoint of its scope, and have questioned whether it should be considered a virtually exceptionless moral rule.

A successful clinician-patient relationship would seem to presuppose a central place for confidentiality. A patient discloses information in that relationship, of both a medical and a more personal nature, symbolizing an unveiling of the self. It has been persuasively argued in many contexts, for example, psychotherapy and HIV antibody testing, that if there is no trust that information communicated in the therapeutic relationship will not be disclosed to others, patients will not seek treatment in the first instance. The establishment of a clinician-patient relationship creates moral boundaries that excludes access by third parties and thus facilitates a process of free and candid exchange of information within the relationship. It assures patients that they will retain control over information that can be very personal and intimate.

A question that all health care professionals are facing with increasing frequency is whether some circumstances warrant breaching patient confidentiality. In the majority of circumstances, the moral dilemma is set by a conflict of nonmaleficence or justice with confidentiality, where maintaining confidentiality will impose a significant degree of risk of harm or burden on specified others outside the clinical relationship. Such a conflict, with many dimensions, is present in the following situation.

CASE 7

A 15-year-old boy presents for his regular semi-annual check-up and cleaning. The dentist knows the young man and his parents quite well because they live a few doors from her. Although the dentist finds the boy to be a likable person, she knows that he is not getting along well with his parents.

In the course of cleaning the boy's teeth, the dental hygienist has observed an ulcer in his mouth, and reported that the boy complained that it was quite painful. Upon examination, and in light of historical information provided by the patient, the dentist suspects that the ulcer is most likely syphilitic in origin.

The dentist informs the patient of his suspicion, which evokes an angry response. She indicates this is a very serious matter. If the diagnosis of syphilis is correct, the dentist is legally obligated to report him to the public health authorities, who will want to know who his contacts have been. This information increases the patient's anger, and he demands that the dentist not tell anyone about his condition. He says that if he does, his parents will be sure to find out and "all hell will break loose."

The dentist's dilemma in this case emerges because the various roles she has assumed generate conflicting duties. She is, first of all, a *friend* of the family, and that nonclinical relationship can create certain expectations about how she should act toward both the boy and his parents. She is, secondly, a *caregiver* who has been asked to use her professional skills to benefit her patient in a relationship based on confidentiality and mutual trust. Her status as a *professional*, however, also means that the dentist has civic responsibilities; fellow citizens have bestowed trust in her and the profession collectively to act, in special circumstances, on behalf of the public health.

We can also frame the dentist's dilemma in terms of her professional code of ethics. According to the ADA *Principles*, the "primary professional obligation" of a dentist "is service to the public." At the same time, "Dentists are obliged to safeguard the confidentiality of patient records. Dentists shall maintain patient records in a manner consistent with the protection of the welfare of the patient."[21] How can the dentist fulfill her professional responsibilities both to the public and to the welfare of this particular patient?

In this case, it is not clear that the dentist can fulfill her many responsibilities without some compromise, but whatever the content of her legal duties, her moral and professional obligations are certainly more extensive. The dentist must first of all be certain of the diagnosis of syphilis, and if that is verified, arrange to have the patient receive appropriate antibiotic treatment. She also needs to be sensitive to the patient's confusion and sense of betrayal. Before this visit, the patient revealed information about himself that provided the

basis for the dentist's diagnostic inference. The dentist's indication that a confirmed diagnosis of syphilis must be reported has transformed her from a confidante to an adversary in the eyes of the patient. The dentist will therefore need to rely on considerable resources of compassion and communication to re-establish the trust that the patient feels has been betrayed. Finally, although resolving the conflict between the patient and his parents is not the professional or personal responsibility of the dentist, it is important that the dentist's actions not complicate the already troubled domestic situation.

Although clinician-patient confidentiality seems universally accepted as an obligation, it is seldom recognized as an absolute obligation. That is, it can be overridden in some circumstances, provided that certain conditions are satisfied.[22] These conditions of justification include:

1. Nonmaleficence—that maintaining confidentiality would place others at unknowing risk of harm. The obligation to breach confidentiality increases according to the *severity* of the risk and the *probability* of its occurrence.

2. Effectiveness—that divulging confidential information would probably protect others from the harm. This condition reflects the interest of public health authorities in knowing about such matters as venereal diseases.

3. Last resort—that disclosure is *necessary* to protect others from harm. That is, there is no other alternative for the affected persons to learn of their risk and adopt appropriate precautions or remedies. There may be alternative avenues to communicating with the patient's contacts, including efforts by the patient or the dentist herself, although these may prove time-consuming, ineffective, and compromising.

4. Least infringement—Information communicated in confidence must be divulged to as few people as possible and only those for whom it is necessary. If the process is responsibly carried out, for example, it's not obviously clear that the patient's parents must be notified.

5. Respect for autonomy—When possible, breaching confidentiality should be

explained and justified to the person whose confidentiality is infringed. The dentist is right to insist to her patient that his condition is "a serious matter" for many people. If the dentist is going to be able to reclaim the trust of her patient, and indeed if the patient is ever going to trust medical caregivers in the future, the dentist must make clear her own personal, professional, and legal situation, and the alternatives for both her and her patient. She should seek to enlist the patient's assistance in obtaining appropriate medical care for himself and others while taking steps to safeguard against an acrimonious confrontation between the boy and his parents. What is clear is that a difficult moral dilemma such as this cannot be resolved solely on the grounds that the law requires disclosure.

ELEMENTS OF MORAL DECISION MAKING

The foregoing has illustrated how normative ethical principles may be used to clarify moral problems that emerge in the practice of dentistry and to reveal the nature and scope of dentists' moral and professional obligations. Our use of cases to illustrate how ethical principles can be applied to clinical choices has relied on an approach to moral deliberation and decision making that may be useful to structure more systematically in conclusion.[23]

Assessing the Medical and Social Context

We have stressed repeatedly that ethical conflicts emerge within clinical settings, in which the nature of the relationship and the information exchanged between the clinician and the patient is vital. Good ethics begin with good facts, and so the dentist must seek to know the patient himself or herself, and not merely the patient's set of "teeth and gums." The former calls for the clinician and patient to create a partnership, and the latter reduces the dentist to a technician. If, as in some cases we have discussed, the patient is seeing this dentist for the first time, the dentist should attempt to cultivate con-

tinuity in the relationship based on mutual trust. In a relationship of long-standing, the dentist can rely on this trust and his or her accumulated knowledge of the patient as a person if ethical conflicts arise.

Clarifying the Ethical Problem

Although every clinical encounter involves an ethical dimension, only some raise ethical problems. We need to determine what kind of conflict is present—moral weakness, moral uncertainty, moral dilemma—as well as what moral principles are embedded in the conflict. We also need to identify the nature of the choices involved, and who will make the decision. The process of clarification may itself dissolve ethical conflict; careful analysis may reveal that an apparent moral dilemma is really a question of moral uncertainty or even moral weakness.

Determining the Stakeholders

Although ethical issues in dentistry always affect two persons, several cases have illustrated how ethical choices bring many more persons into the circle of ethical concern. Decisions may affect parents or families, colleagues and assistants, unknowing third parties, public authorities, a local community, and even society as a whole. Although a dentist has a primary moral commitment to the welfare of the patient, ethical deliberation requires acknowledging the stake others may have in a decision and assessing how they will be affected by a particular choice.

Identifying Options and Alternatives

Although some moral choices in clinical dentistry inevitably involve compromise of some moral principle and value, many others may not. Ethical decision making requires imagination and creativity to discern options not originally envisioned when a conflict presents itself. In some instances, for example, Case 5 or 6, dentists should resist a forced moral choice or a belief that their hands are tied. Obtaining additional information about a patient's reasoning or values, taking the time to establish a trusting relationship, or even deferring a decision for a short time, can help both parties give more considered thought to their views, and perhaps open the way to a more mutually acceptable alternative.

Examining the Process of Decision Making

Ethical issues, we have maintained, concern not only what is decided but who decides. The literature on dental ethics seems to be adopting a middle path, rejecting a traditional model of unilateral decisions by dentists for a model that is expressed in metaphors of "collaboration," "partnership" or "interaction." This is a commendable approach inasmuch as it recognizes the right and responsibility of patient involvement in decisions regarding their dental care, without tipping towards the extreme of deference by dentists before unilateral decisions by patients. The realization of an interactive or collaborative model in clinical practice, however, will require dentists to take steps to invite involvement by patients.

Balancing Conflicting Principles and Obligations

The thoughtful scrutiny of the previous elements will help dentists, patients, and others to balance their responsibilities in the face of conflicting principles and obligations. They are also vital considerations in moral justification, when we articulate our reasons and defend our choices before various audiences—ourselves, patients, families, colleagues; indeed, all who might have a stake in the decision constitute audiences of justification.

We have not argued here for the priority of a particular principle or obligation; our approach has instead suggested that the various principles identified have equal standing or weight *in the abstract*. The practical application of a principle as the decisive moral consideration depends on the clinical context and integration of the principle with the range of elements described

previously. Thus, although respect for patient autonomy is a relevant moral consideration in every clinical encounter, our analysis has suggested both (a) the importance of clarifying that a choice is autonomous and (b) that even autonomous choices can be limited by other principles, such as nonmaleficence or justice. Moreover, a decision to compromise one obligation in the face of other obligations should be informed by the conditions for justification articulated in our discussion of confidentiality.

As Ozar, Scheidermayer, and Siegler have observed, " . . . dentistry is a profession and dentists are clinicians . . . precisely because their decisions are moral choices."[6] The choices dentists make will reflect their commitments to the moral integrity of their profession, their perceptions of the clinician-patient relationship, and their assessments of the place of dentistry in our society. It reflects a profound moral commitment to undertake caring for the needs of another person. The normative principles of dental ethics can help dentists shape their care in ways that are genuinely responsive to the needs and welfare of the persons who present themselves as patients.

DISCUSSION QUESTIONS

1. In a critical analysis of the *Principles of Ethics and Code of Professional Conduct of the American Dental Association* (January 1991), discuss those aspects which invoke: (a) a "commercial model" of dental care, (b) a "guild"-oriented model, (c) an "interactive" model.

2. Analyze the ADA *Principles* with regard to the extent to which it reflects the normative ethical principles of nonmaleficence, beneficence, justice, and respect for autonomy. How might the code be changed or modified to address the contemporary dentist-patient relationship(s)? To reflect more fully the four normative principles?

3. Based upon your understanding of the traditional medical model of duties and obligations to patients,

how does the dental profession differ from medicine? What commitments, values and principles might be shared by medicine and dentistry?

4. Beneficence is accented by paternalism, whereas the principle of respect for autonomy is accented by informed consent. Under what circumstances, if ever, might beneficence override respect for autonomy? When might respect for autonomy override beneficence?

5. In order to expand dental care for disadvantaged populations, how might the profession restructure reimbursements to permit access for more individuals?

6. Based upon your understanding of the normative principles of dental ethics, how might you resolve the following issues:

   A. Alternative treatment plans based upon ability/inability to pay.

   B. Extraction of restorable tooth (or teeth) in absence of sufficient financial resources of the patient. Remember that you possess the knowledge and skills required to save the involved dentition.

   C. A patient requests an expensive clinical procedure when you know a less expensive procedure is more appropriate, for example, repair of a functional partial prothesis versus replacement.

REFERENCES

1. Council on Ethics, Bylaws and Judicial Affairs: ADA Principles of Ethics and Code of Professional Conduct. Chicago, American Dental Association, 1991.
2. Ozar, D.T.: Three models of professionalism and professional obligation in dentistry. J. Am. Dent. Assoc., *110*:173–77, 1985.
3. McCullough, L.B.: Ethical issues in dentistry. *In* Clinical Dentistry, v. 1 (rev. ed). Edited by J.W. Hardin. Philadelphia, J.B. Lippincott, 1988.
4. Beauchamp, T.L., and Childress, J.F.: Principles of Biomedical Ethics. 3rd ed. New York, Oxford University Press, 1989.
5. Burns, C.R.: Professional codes in American dentistry. *In* Encyclopedia of Bioethics. Edited by W.T. Reich. New York, The Free Press, 1978.
6. Ozar, D.T., Schiedermayer, D.L., and Siegler, M.: Value categories in clinical dental ethics. J. Am. Dent. Assoc. *116*:366, 1988.
7. Council on Ethics, Bylaws and Judicial Affairs: ADA Principles of Ethics and Code of Professional Conduct, Section 1-J, Representation of Care. Chicago, American Dental Association, 1991.
8. Council on Ethics, Bylaws and Judicial Affairs: ADA Principles of Ethics and Code of Professional Conduct, Section 2, Education. Chicago, American Dental Association, 1991.
9. Council on Ethics, Bylaws and Judicial Affairs: ADA Principles of Ethics and Code of Professional Conduct, Section 1-C, Community Service Advisory Opinion. Chicago, American Dental Association, 1991.
10. Council on Ethics, Bylaws and Judicial Affairs: ADA Principles of Ethics and Code of Professional Conduct, Section 1-C, Community Service. Chicago, American Dental Association, 1991.
11. Council on Ethics, Bylaws and Judicial Affairs: ADA Principles of Ethics and Code of Professional Conduct, Section 1-A, Patient Selection. Chicago, American Dental Association, 1991.
12. Council on Ethics, Bylaws and Judicial Affairs: ADA Principles of Ethics and Code of Professional Conduct, Section 1-A, Patient Selection Advisory Opinion. Chicago, American Dental Association, 1991.
13. Rogers, V.C.: Dentistry, Ethics and AIDS. A Continuing Education Journal for Dentists *36*:6, 1991.
14. Dummett, C.O.: Ethical issues in dentistry. *In* Encyclopedia of Bioethics. Edited by W.T. Reich. New York, The Free Press, 1978.
15. Rogers, V.C.: Ethical considerations of appropriate versus comprehensive dental care for patients in nursing homes. J. Law Ethics Dent. *1*: 83, 1988.
16. Rogers, V.C.: Equity and justice in risk factor identification in dentistry: *In* Risk Assessment in Dentistry. Edited by J.D. Bader. Chapel Hill, University of North Carolina Dental Ecology, 1990.
17. Hirsch, A.J., and Gert, B.: Ethics in dental practice. J. Am. Dent. Assoc. *113*:599, 1986.
18. Council on Ethics, Bylaws and Judicial Affairs: ADA Principles of Ethics and Code of Professional Conduct, Section 1-L, Patient Involvement. Chicago, American Dental Association, 1991.
19. Cassell, E.: The Healer's Art: A New Approach to the Doctor-Patient Relationship. Philadelphia, J.B. Lippincott, 1976.
20. Siegler, M.: Confidentiality in medicine—A decrepit concept. N. Engl. J. Med. *307*:1518, 1982.
21. Council on Ethics, Bylaws and Judicial Affairs: ADA Principles of Ethics and Code of Professional Conduct, Section 1-B, Patient Records. Chicago, American Dental Association, 1991.
22. Childress, J.F.: The place of autonomy in bioethics. Hastings Cent. Rep. *20*:15, 1990.
23. Jennings, B., Nolan, K., Campbell, C.S., and

Donnelley, S.: New Choices, New Responsibilities: Ethical Issues in the Life Sciences. Briarcliff Manor, NY, The Hastings Center, 1990.

SUGGESTED READING

Beauchamp, T.L., and Childress, J.F.: Principles of Biomedical Ethics, 3rd ed. New York, Oxford University Press, 1989.

Beauchamp, T.L., and McCullough, L.B.: Medical Ethics: The Moral Responsibilities of Physicians. Englewood Cliffs, NJ: Prentice-Hall, Inc., 1984.

Burns, C.R.: Professional Codes in American Dentistry. *In* Encyclopedia of Bioethics. Edited by W.T. Reich. New York, The Free Press, 1978.

Faden, R., and Beauchamp, T.L.: A Theory and History of Informed Consent. New York, Oxford University Press, 1985.

The Journal of Law and Ethics in Dentistry. Edited by Pollack, B.R. Philadelphia, C.V. Mosby Co.

Chapter 3

Ethical Decision Making

Bruce D. Weinstein

SUMMARY

When you are faced with a moral problem, how should you proceed? There are many ways of answering this question, but a particularly useful way is to approach the problem *systematically*. This chapter proposes a four-step approach: (1) Gather the relevant *facts*, (2) identify the *values* that play a role, (3) generate *options* open to you, and (4) *select* an option and *justify* it. The author applies this approach to two clinical cases involving dentists faced with common ethical dilemmas. After identifying the ethical issues raised (and showing why these issues are ethical ones), he proceeds by asking what additional facts are needed. These facts include, but are not limited to, technical, social, and psychological information.

Facts are necessary but not sufficient to answer ethical questions, however. In addition to facts, values play an important role, for they give rise to *moral rules*. The author shows what values are imbedded in the cases presented, and what rules correspond to those values. The next step is to consider options open to the dentist, or in other words, to answer the question, "What *could* be done?" It is in picking an option and supporting it with reasons that put us in the position of stating what *should* be done.

Each step in the protocol builds logically on the preceding steps. Still, some steps may be easier than others; you may find it easier, for example, to gather facts than to identify values, and to generate options than to justify one. This may be because

dental education focuses on the technical aspects of dentistry, and on developing problem-solving skills rather than intellectual ones. One of the themes that emerges from this book, however, is that dentistry is not merely a technical enterprise. It is a profession, and values, especially moral values, determine what dentists ought to do in their care of patients, as well as shape what dentists actually do. The purpose of this chapter is to help you to identify some of these values, to see how they sometimes come into conflict, and to use them (along with the relevant facts) to support the choices you make. In developing such skills, you will be taking important steps toward improving patient care and doing for patients what they would want to have done for themselves.

ETHICAL DECISIONS

Consider the following scenario:

CASE 1

A patient you have never seen before presents in the clinic and asks you to remove all of her amalgam restorations. She had seen a broadcast of *60 Minutes* and read several articles suggesting that the mercury in amalgam may pose a significant health risk. Furthermore, she has multiple sclerosis (MS) and was impressed by several anecdotal accounts of spontaneous remission from the symptoms of MS. You have studied the debate carefully and understand that the best available evidence suggests that amalgam is safe and effective. You have found no scientific evidence to suggest that removing amalgams can relieve the symptoms of MS, and you know that the replacement process risks damaging the surrounding tooth structure. When you explain this to the patient, she tells you she understands, but she insists that you remove the restorations.

This case raises several questions. One might ask, for example, why the patient is adamant about having her restorations removed. This is a psychological question, because it concerns the reasons that motivate the patient to act as she does. One might also ask the economic question of how much the removal and replacement process would cost. Finally, one might ask whether you *should* remove the restorations. This is an ethical question because it concerns your conduct with respect to the rights and well-being of your patient. The purpose of this chapter is to present a method for approaching these and other ethical problems that arise in the clinical setting. I begin with a brief description of the field of ethics and the role it plays in the dental profession.

WHAT IS ETHICS AND WHAT DOES IT HAVE TO DO WITH DENTISTRY?

Ethics is the systematic study of what is right and good with respect to conduct and character. As a branch of both philosophy and theology, ethics seeks to answer two fundamental questions: (1) *What should we do?*, and (2) *Why should we do it?* As an intellectual discipline, ethics is concerned not only with making appropriate decisions but with *justifying* them. Unlike other forums for the discussion of moral issues (e.g., television talk shows, barroom debates), ethics seek to provide good reasons for our moral choices. In fact, it is the attempt to justify our actions that gives ethics its distinctive character.

Dental ethics is an application of ethical rules and principles to the practice of dentistry. To ask what a dentist should do in a particular case is to ask an ethical question, and to justify our answer we appeal to the same rules and principles that apply to persons in society generally.[1] For example, the dentist's obligation to protect patient confidentiality is merely an application of the rule that all of us have to guard carefully information that is entrusted to us. Sometimes, however, health care professionals are ethically required to assume risks not shared by laypersons, such as caring for persons with AIDS.[2] To be a professional thus involves having certain obligations not shared by nonprofessionals. To understand why this is, it is helpful to examine what it means to be a dentist, and how dentistry differs from other sorts of occupations.

Dentistry as a Moral Practice

Dentistry is a moral practice because dentists are concerned primarily with using their knowledge and skills to advance the interests of patients, and to do for patients what patients wish to have done for themselves. Unlike members of other occupations (business, for example), the dentist places the interests of others above her or his own interests. Indeed, this feature of dentistry is one of the defining characteristics of the health care professions in general. Every encounter between a dentist and a patient implicitly raises ethical issues, because a dentist may—and indeed must—ask questions about how the welfare of the patient should be promoted.

Although every encounter between dentist and patient raises ethical issues, these issues are not necessarily ethical *problems* or *dilemmas*. A situation in which two or more choices are morally justifiable, but only one is capable of being acted upon at a particular time, represents a moral dilemma.[3] A dentist who has to decide between protecting the confidentiality of a patient with syphilis and protecting society from potential harm is caught in an ethical dilemma, because there are moral reasons for justifying each of two mutually exclusive options. No moral dilemma exists when a patient provides an informed consent to have a complete set of removable dentures made and is able to pay for the dentures. However, the situation raises a moral *issue,* namely, whether the dentist ought to act in the best interests of the patient and perform the service. Moral issues are unavoidable in dentistry because of the nature of professions in general and dentistry in particular.

To ask what one should do as a dentist or hygienist is often to ask a legal question as well, but it is incorrect to *reduce* the question to a matter for the legislature or the courts to resolve. Indeed, for any legislative or judicial resolution to a problem concerning appropriate conduct, we may—and indeed should—ask, "Is the law a *good* one?," or "Was the court *right*?" It will be the assumption of this chapter that ethics, and not the law, establishes the ultimate standards for evaluating conduct.[4] Still, there is a moral obligation to obey the law, and thus ethical analyses need to take into account the relevant statutes and court decisions.

A difficult problem in ethics concerns the *source* of ethical standards. People have appealed to many sources of authority in ethics: religious texts (e.g., the Bible, the Koran), natural law, philosophical argument (reason), intuition, personal experience, governmental decree, and the free negotiations of persons within a community. Traditionally, in dentistry it has been the members of the profession who have selected its ethical norms and established codes of ethics. Because laypersons have a significant stake in the way that professionals conduct themselves, however, it is appropriate to include them in the selection of these norms.[5] Our discussion will thus be based not only on what the profession of dentistry has held to be right and good, but more broadly upon what a reasonable person with knowledge of the relevant facts might hold to be appropriate.

All moral problems have both a technical and an evaluative component. That is, the answer to the question, "What should we do?," requires technical information as well as information about values. Suppose, for example, that a 63-year-old patient states that, although she cannot pay for the dentures she claims she needs, she has a right to them. The expertise that dentists have by virtue of their scientific education and technical experience allows them to decide to what degree her *clinical* claim is justified, i.e., whether dentures would promote oral functioning. This technical expertise does not, however, confer an ability to assess the *moral* claim that the patient has a right to the treatment.[6] (The patient may be making a *legal* claim as well, because rights may be justified by an appeal to the law as well as to moral rules and principles. While it plays a role in the peaceable resolution of disputes between dentists and patients, the legal component of these issues is not considered in this chapter.) How, then, are such claims to be evaluated, if not through technical expertise? We turn next to a protocol that may help one to systematically consider ethical problems that arise in the clinical setting, or anywhere else for that matter.

STEPS IN ETHICAL DECISION MAKING (FIG. 3–1)

Suppose that your best friend calls you one evening and tells you that he or she is faced with a difficult ethical dilemma involving an intimate other. "I don't know if I should leave this relationship or try to

---

ETHICAL DECISION MAKING IN PATIENT CARE

Process

After identifying an ethical question facing you in patient care:

1. Gather the dental, medical, social, and all other clinically relevant facts of the case.
2. Identify all relevant values that play a role in the case and determine which values, if any, conflict.
3. List the options open to you. That is, answer the question, "What *could* you do?"
4. Choose the best solution from an ethical point of view, justify it, and respond to possible criticisms. That is, answer the question, "What *should* you do, and why?"

Fig. 3–1. Steps in ethical decision making.

work it out," your friend says. "Please give me some advice!" What will your response be—to make a recommendation right away, or to ask for some more information? Most people choose the latter. This is because we recognize that good moral decision making begins with getting the facts straight. Thus, the *first step* for making ethical decisions, in the clinical setting or anywhere else, is *gathering the relevant facts.*[7]

In the case presented at the beginning of the chapter, the relevant facts are that the patient appears to have made an autonomous request for amalgam removal, but she believes that the removal will help relieve her symptoms of MS. There is no scientific basis for such a belief, however.[8] At the time of this writing, it is not illegal for a dentist to remove amalgam restorations if the patient provides an informed consent to the procedure. (The concept of informed consent will be covered in greater depth in Chap. 5.) However, the American Dental Association has stated in an Advisory Opinion to its *Principles of Ethics and Code of Professional Conduct*: "[T]he removal of amalgam restorations from the non-allergic patient for the alleged purpose of removing toxic substances from the body, *when such treatment is performed solely at the recommendation or suggestion of the dentist,* is improper and unethical."[9] The ADA's statement implies that removal of amalgams is ethically permissible if initiated by the patient and, presumably, if the patient provides an informed consent to the procedure.

To resolve an ethical dilemma such as the one in this case, facts are necessary but not sufficient. Addressing moral problems differs from addressing mere technical ones in that the former involves a consideration of values as well as facts.[6] In addition to the relevant facts, an appropriate response to the question, "What should you do?," requires an account of the values that play a role in the case, and what moral guidelines or rules those values suggest. *Identifying values* is thus the *second step* of ethical analysis. Certainly one important value suggested by the case is patient autonomy, which gives rise to the moral rule, "Do for your patients what they would want to have done for themselves." Applying this rule to the present case entails that you ought to remove the amalgams, since

the patient has made such a request, and the patient has made the request autonomously.

If respect for patient self-determination were the only value that played a role in this case, you would not be faced with a moral dilemma, because it would be clear that you ought to remove the amalgams. There *are* other values, however. Chief among them is the value of avoiding harming others. As discussed in Chapter 2, this value is captured by the principle of nonmaleficence, or "do no harm." Doing what the patient asks may violate a professional value in dentistry, namely preserving and promoting oral functioning,[10] because the process of amalgam removal risks damaging hard tooth structure, the pulp, and periodontal tissue.

In addition to the two values mentioned above, respect for the profession is a third value that plays a role in the case. As mentioned in the first step, the ADA proscribes the removal of amalgams only when the removal is suggested by the dentist. Because it is the patient who has requested the procedure, you would not be violating your duty to respect professional standards (at least as those standards are articulated by the ADA) by performing the procedure after obtaining an informed consent. Still, the prevailing view among scientists and clinicians is that the mercury in amalgam does not present a risk of physical harm to patients, and its removal will not result in remission of MS. A fourth value is the dentist's conscience, which gives rise to the moral rule, "Be true to yourself." Finally, you might wish to consider whatever legal prohibitions exist. This is because there is not only a *legal* duty for professionals to obey the law, but a *moral* one as well. The last moral rule we might wish to consider, then, is, "Follow the law." As discussed in the first step, however, there is no law preventing dentists from removing amalgam restorations, provided that the patient provides an informed consent to the procedure.

We now have the makings of a genuine ethical dilemma: there appear to be good moral reasons *for* removing the amalgams (namely, your ethical obligation to respect patient autonomy), and good moral reasons *not* to do so (your obligation to do no harm, and possibly your duty to respect the professional view that there is no scientific basis for preventing physical harm by amalgam removal). What should you do, and why?

This brings us to the *third stage* of ethical analysis, *generating options*. The first option open to you is simply to remove the amalgams as the patient requests. The second option is to refuse to do so and not to give a reason, other than, "That's just not something I can do in good conscience." A third option is to present to the patient the possible risks of amalgam removal to the surrounding dentition, to explain that there is no evidence suggesting that MS can be cured by the procedure, and to suggest that there may be better ways of coping with the illness than by doing what the patient is suggesting. If the patient insists, you could then decide whether to do the procedure or not to. A fourth option is to consider referring the patient to a dentist who *will* do the procedure. Other options include replacing the amalgam restorations with either gold castings (which could last an additional 10 years), or with composite resin (which is more difficult to place and normally does not last as long as amalgam but is aesthetically more pleasing). Which one of these is best from an ethical point of view, and why?

To answer this question, we take the fourth and final step of ethical analysis, *choosing an option and justifying it*. The first option appears to realize your obligation to respect patient autonomy, but in so doing would violate your duty to protect her from harm. The second option is the moral mirror image of the first, because your duty to avoid harm would be satisfied but at the expense of the patient's having her autonomous choice respected. The third option bridges the gap between the first two by respecting the patient's autonomy *and* by allowing you to avoid harming the patient. Respect for autonomy is fulfilled by disclosing the relevant risks, benefits, and therapeutic alternatives, ensuring that the patient understands this disclosure and then consents or refuses to the treatment voluntarily; the process of obtaining informed consent or refusal suggested by option three ensures that you are doing for the patient what she would want to have done for herself. If you

choose not to perform the procedure after disclosing the above information in a way in which the patient understands it, then you are both fulfilling your obligation to do no harm *and* respecting autonomy to the extent that you have explained why you cannot do it, and why it is in her best interests not to have the procedure done.

There are good moral reasons both for referring the patient and for not doing so. Referral may be justified by the principle of respect for autonomy, because the patient would receive the treatment that she wants, and such an action would also fulfill your responsibility to be true to yourself, if you still have strong reservations about doing the procedure. However, the referral might violate your obligation to *prevent* harm to the patient, which, as explained in Chapter 2, is one of the requirements of the principle of beneficence. Deciding whether it would be ethically appropriate to refer the patient to a dentist who would remove the amalgams thus turns on how one rank–orders the competing values of respect for autonomy, beneficence and nonmaleficence.

If your obligations both to respect your patient's right of self-determination and to prevent or avoid harming the patient were absolute, then there would be no rational way to make a choice in this case, because whatever you did, you would be violating one responsibility or another. All you could do would be to make a choice on some nonrational basis (e.g., flipping a coin or going with your intuitions). There *is* a way to make a rational choice, however, if we realize that *a patient's right to self-determination is a limited right,* and it is limited by, among other considerations, the degree to which its exercise places others at risk of harm or compromises the integrity of the health care professional. For example, a patient cannot come to the office, demand that you remove all of her teeth, and *expect* that you will do so. No one has ever defended such a demanding interpretation of the principle of respect for autonomy. A patient's autonomous request to have her amalgam restorations removed does not require that the dentist respect it, because in so doing the dentist would be placing the patient at some risk, with no overriding clinical benefit, *and* the dentist may feel that he or she cannot in good conscience perform the procedure. For these reasons, option three appears to be the most defensible choice from an ethical viewpoint, recognizing that the first two options each have something to be said in their favor. In summary, it would not necessarily be *unethical* for you to perform the procedure, but it would also not be unethical for you to *refuse* to do so.[11] Avoiding harming patients is one of the reasonable limits that may be placed on the ethical principle of respect for patient autonomy.

One conclusion we may draw from this case is that turning to the law does not always help us resolve moral quandaries. It is legally permissible for a dentist to remove amalgam restorations, provided that he or she obtains an informed consent from the patient, but the dentist still may ask, "What is the *right* thing for me to do?"

The analysis also suggests that some approaches to ethical problems in the clinical setting are more ethically defensible than others, and that through ethical analysis one is able to distinguish better from worse approaches. It is sometimes the case that any option one picks will have unfortunate consequences (in this case, the patient may be extremely upset by your action), but this is not the same as saying that there are no answers to ethical problems. Indeed, the circumstances in which dentists find themselves often require *some* kind of decision or action, and thus in many instances it is impossible to avoid making moral choices. Through ethical analysis and reflection, as well as discussing the problem with others in a systematic way, one is more likely to achieve a reasoned and justifiable decision.

One might think that the process of ethical decision making is too time-consuming and complex to use in the clinical setting. Obviously, in emergent situations, the moral mandate of the dentist is to save the patient's life or prevent irreversible harm from occurring. Such situations arise relatively infrequently in dentistry, however, and for troubling ethical problems it is both prudent and ethically appropriate to take some time to reflect upon one's options and consider the best reasons for choosing some rather than others. As the second case will show, the ethical issues raised in patient care are often strikingly similar, even if the clinical details differ.

CASE 2

Ina Kirchland presents to Dr. Harold Luban's office in considerable pain and is examined between the dentist's 9:40 and 10:00 appointments. Although her teeth are generally in good condition, the first molar has been a problem for some time, and Dr. Luban has foreseen that the day would come when it would be a matter of either performing root canal therapy or removing the tooth. Now that day has come.

Ms. Kirchland is a widow, and does not have much money. She lives on her deceased husband's social security benefits, which she supplements to some extent by providing child care in her home several afternoons a week. Her resources for dental care, as for everything, are very limited, and she is often anxious about how she will make ends meet. She has no dental insurance. When Dr. Luban completes his examination of her mouth, she asks him, "What do you recommend, Dr. Luban?" Dr. Luban has several options in mind and wonders which he ought to choose.

Analysis

As we have already seen, to ask what one should or ought to do, particularly with respect to the welfare or rights of another, is to make an ethical inquiry. Let us apply the method for ethical decision making that we have just considered and try to identify the most ethical justifiable options open to Dr. Luban. Before we get to that, however, we need to consider the facts and values that play a role in the case, and all of the options that are open to the dentist.

The relevant facts of the case are that natural teeth present fewer potential problems to one's oral health than do prosthetic ones. Enamel is more durable than the various materials from which prosthetic teeth are made, and prosthetic replacements can damage adjacent natural teeth. Let us assume that Dr. Luban believes that root canal therapy would be better than an extraction.[10] However, Ms. Kirchland is of limited financial means, and if she knew that extraction were the much cheaper option, Dr. Luban is certain that she would choose that. He does not know whether she would prefer a root canal if money were not an issue, because he has not spoken with her about her values in dentistry or in general.

Even with this factual information at hand, it is not clear what Dr. Luban ought to do. This is because facts are necessary but not sufficient for answering ethical questions, as we have seen with the previous case. We now move on to the second step of our analysis by identifying the values that play a role. One value is Ms. Kirchland's right to determine what will be done for her oral health. In other words, the value of respect for her autonomy is a moral consideration in the case, and from Dr. Luban's perspective, it gives rise to the moral rule, "Do for Ms. Kirchland what she would want to have done for herself." Again, if this were the only moral consideration in the case, Dr. Luban would not be faced with an ethical dilemma; he would simply need to find out what kind of treatment she would like to have and provide it.

Other values are suggested by this case, however. A second one is Ms. Kirchland's oral health. The concept of health is a broad one and, some have argued, one that cannot itself be properly understood independently from a particular set of values.[12] We are assuming that Dr. Luban, like most dentists, values both appropriate and pain-free oral functioning as well as the preservation of natural teeth, so the moral rules that are suggested for him are, "Promote or restore appropriate and pain-free oral functioning of Ms. Kirchland's mouth," and "Attempt to preserve Ms. Kirchland's natural teeth." Notice from the *fact* that natural teeth present fewer dental problems than do artificial ones, it does not follow that they are *better*. Dr. Luban's belief that a root canal procedure is better than another procedure is based not just on the above clinical fact, but on the importance he places on appropriate oral functioning and the preservation of natural teeth. However, these values may not be shared by the patient, or at least not given the same weight as other consider-

ations. Yet another value that plays a role is respect for professional standards of care as articulated in the American Dental Association's Principles of Ethics and Code of Professional Conduct. The relevant guideline from the code requires the dentist to "inform the patient of the proposed treatment, and any reasonable alternatives, in a manner that allows the patient to become involved in treatment decisions."[9]

We are now in a position to consider the options open to Dr. Luban. One option is simply to tell Ms. Kirchland that she needs to have a root canal procedure and to do it. A second option is to mention extraction as a possibility but to pressure her to have the endodontic work done. A third option is to present the relevant information to the patient in a way that she can understand and to allow her to choose freely which procedure, if any, she would prefer. If she opts for removal of the tooth, she will be faced with having either a fixed bridge, a removable partial denture, or no replacement at all. A final option would be for Dr. Luban to refer the patient to another dentist if Ms. Kirchland chooses to have the extraction. Which option is best from an ethical point of view, and why?

Generating options is relatively easy. More difficult is to identify the most ethically appropriate options and to say what makes them so. The first option would fulfill Dr. Luban's obligation to promote Ms. Kirchland's oral health, because he understands oral health to involve appropriate and pain-free oral functioning and retaining one's own teeth. The problem with this option is that it subverts Dr. Luban's duty to respect Ms. Kirchland's autonomy, because it does not allow her to consent to the procedure with an understanding of the benefits, risks and alternatives. In choosing this option, Dr. Luban would also be failing to adhere to the professional standard of care.

Option two moves closer in the direction of respecting the patient's right of self-determination, but still is inadequate. By presenting the relevant information in such a way that the patient feels pressured to choose the root canal over the extraction, Dr. Luban has again prevented the possibility of a truly or substantially autonomous choice.[13] Only in option three does

Dr. Luban fulfill his responsibilities to respect the patient's autonomy and to act in a way consistent with the professional standard of care. One might argue that this option violates the dentist's obligation to promote the patient's oral health, because the patient may end up choosing an extraction, and in so doing would be compromising her oral health, at least with respect to having a root canal done. However, Ms. Kirchland's understanding of what constitutes her oral health may be different from Dr. Luban's (e.g., she may consider it healthier to be rid of a problem tooth than to have it in her mouth, even after endodontic treatment). What is more likely, however, is that her oral health is but one of several values that are important to her; because endodontic therapy is more expensive than an extraction, at least in the short term, she may place greater priority on keeping her finances in order. Thus, if we construe broadly Dr. Luban's obligation to promote her welfare, he would not be violating his duty of beneficence by performing the extraction, and in fact would be promoting it.

CONCLUSION

Even though the cases examined here involve different patients with different kinds of problems, the general ethical question is the same: What should the dentist do? To be more specific, the *values* that play a role in the case are the same. This chapter has suggested that being a dentist involves more than possessing certain skills or having clinical knowledge. If dentistry is understood to be a moral practice, dentists have moral obligations, including, but not limited to, promoting the welfare of patients, protecting them from harm, and respecting their right of self-determination. Still, being technically competent and respecting patients' rights are *necessary* but not *sufficient* conditions of being a good dentist. Developing the professional virtues of kindness, compassion, and a sense of justice, among others, also plays an important role in the moral life of the professional.

According to the protocol presented in this chapter, one may systematically approach ethical problems in clinical dentistry by (1) gathering the relevant *facts* pertaining to the case, (2) clarifying the *values*, (3) *generating options* open to the dentist, and finally (4) *picking an option and justifying it.* Nevertheless, ethical analysis is only a tool for the conscientious dentist. It is up to the practitioner to fulfill the moral responsibilities that give dentistry its distinctive character as a profession.

DISCUSSION QUESTIONS

1. Someone sees you carrying this book and says, "*Dental* ethics? I've heard about medical ethics, but what's an example of an ethical issue in *dentistry?*" How would you respond?

2. Sometimes we find ourselves saying, "If only I had known X, I would have made a different decision!" Although there is only so much information we can reasonably collect, what does this suggest about the importance of beginning our analysis of moral problems with getting the facts?

3. How have you typically approached ethical problems in your life? Has this approach been satisfactory? What would you like to keep, and what would you like to change, about this approach?

4. Use the protocol described in this chapter to identify and reflect upon an ethical question you have faced in the clinic. In what ways is a systematic approach to ethical problems more useful than other kinds of approaches (for example, using your intuition or asking a friend)? In what ways is it less useful?

5. Consider the following statement:
   Dentists have no moral obligations to anyone other than themselves. Dental students have to make a lot of personal sacrifices to get through dental school. By the time they graduate, they're entitled to the good life.
   Do you agree? Respond to this statement, taking into account the

points made in this chapter and the previous ones about the nature of a profession.

ACKNOWLEDGMENTS

David T. Ozar, Ph.D. prepared Case 2 and kindly allowed me to use it in this chapter. John T. Stevens, D.D.S., M.S., and Arthur E. Skidmore, D.D.S., M.S. of the West Virginia University School of Dentistry provided useful comments on an earlier version of this chapter.

REFERENCES

1. Clouser, K.D.: Bioethics. *In* Reich, W.T. (ed).: Encyclopedia of Bioethics. New York, Free Press, 1978, pp. 115–127.
2. Emmanuel E.: Do physicians have an obligation to treat patients with AIDS? N. Engl. J. Med. *318:*1686, 1988.
3. Beauchamp, T.L., and Childress, J.F.: Principles of Biomedical Ethics, ed 3. New York, Oxford University Press, 1989, pp. 4–6.
4. Callahan, J.C., ed.: Ethical Issues in Professional Life. New York, Oxford University Press, 1988.
5. Veatch, R.M.: A Theory of Medical Ethics. New York, Basic Books, 1981.
6. Veatch, R.M.: Generalization of expertise: Scientific expertise and value judgments. Hastings Center Studies *1:*29–40, 1973.
7. Ackerman, T.F., Graber, G.C., Reynolds, C.H., and Thomasma, D.C., eds.: Clinical Medical Ethics: Exploration and Assessment. Lanham, Maryland, University Press of America, 1987.
8. Thompson, C.C.: Dentistry and the multiple sclerosis patient. J. Oral Med. *41:*102, 1986.
9. American Dental Association: Principles of Ethics and Code of Professional Conduct. J. Am. Dent. Assoc. *120:*588, 1990.
10. Ozar, D.T., Schiedermayer, D.L., and Siegler, M.: Value categories for clinical ethics. J. Am. Dent. Assoc. *116:*365, 1988.
11. Odom, J.G.: Ethics and dental amalgam removal. J. Am. Dent. Assoc. *122:*69, 1991.
12. Caplan, A.L.: The concepts of health and disease. *In* R.M. Veatch, ed.: Medical Ethics: Boston, Jones & Bartlett, 1989, pp. 49–63.
13. Faden, R.R., and Beauchamp, T.L.: A History and Theory of Informed Consent. New York, Oxford University Press, 1986.

SUGGESTED READING

Books

Beauchamp, T.L.: Philosophical Ethics: An Introduction to Moral Philosophy. New York, McGraw Hill, 1982. This is an excellent introduction to the nature and methods of ethics as an intellectual discipline.

Beauchamp, T.L., and Childress, J.F.: Principles of Biomedical Ethics, ed. 3. New York, Oxford University Press, 1989. Beauchamp and Childress provide an indispensable analysis of the nature and relationship of ethical rules and principles in the context of health care.

Engelhardt, H.T., Jr.: The Foundations of Bioethics. New York, Oxford University Press, 1986. This difficult but immensely rewarding book presents a libertarian account of ethical issues in health care and is one of the few works in bioethics that can genuinely be called a classic.

Encyclopedias

Reich, W.T. (ed.): Encyclopedia of Bioethics. New York, Free Press, 1978. Although slightly outdated, this work is a standard reference source and is available in most libraries. The second edition is currently being prepared.

Journals

General Dentistry and Journal of the American Dental Association occasionally feature articles discussing ethical issues in the profession. Hastings Center Report, Journal of Clinical Ethics, Bioethics, and New England Journal of Medicine regularly feature essays on ethical issues in health care, although generally they do not pertain to dentistry directly.

Searches of the Literature

The National Reference Center for Bioethics Literature at Georgetown University runs computer searches of the literature on any topic and mails them to you at no charge. Phone toll-free 1-800-MED-ETHX.

Section II

Topical Issues

Chapter 4

The Dentist-Patient Relationship

Jeffrey P. Kahn
Thomas K. Hasegawa, Jr.

SUMMARY

The topic of this chapter, the dentist-patient relationship, begins the section devoted to various topical issues in dentistry. Chapters in the previous section challenged the reader to examine broad foundational issues in professional ethics. This chapter begins the examination and analysis of major ethical issues that relate to the profession of dentistry. The issues addressed will have different meanings for students of dentistry than for seasoned practitioners, but at the same time they should have importance for all.

The examination of the issues comprising and related to the dentist-patient relationship will help the dental professional to view the treatment of patients in a broader context than those confined to the operatory walls. How the practice of dentistry relates to the whole of health care and what components make up the relationship of people in the roles of dentist and patient are central questions worthy of study and attention.

To carry out this examination, the dentist-patient relationship is viewed first in terms of some of the models proposed both to describe the relationship and to prescribe how the relationship ought to take place. With these models as a starting point, the characteristics of the relationship between patient and provider are examined and described to advance a better understanding of the overall context of the dentist-patient relationship. Draw-

ing on the discussion of these relationships, the duties that exist between dentist and patient are enumerated, with their bases explained and analyzed. A portion of the chapter includes discussion of the limits of each duty examined, conflicts that may arise between duties, and how such conflicts may be resolved. The duties to be examined include truth-telling and promise-keeping. We conclude by considering paternalism and whether it may be justified.

DESCRIBING THE DENTIST-PATIENT RELATIONSHIP

An influential commentator on dental ethics, David Ozar, has written that there are "three models of professionalism and professional obligation in dentistry": the commercial model, the guild model, and the interactive model.[1] In the commercial model, the professional is guided to act in ways that best serve his or her commercial interests, with dental practice treated strictly as a commodity, and the dentist-patient relationship treated as primarily competitive. Therefore, decisions about dentistry as a trade and the production of it as a commodity are made according to the economic goals of creating the combination of price and demand creating the greatest overall profit. Such a free-market orientation denies any moral claim to dental services by patients beyond those for which they can pay the price set by each professional. As Ozar explains, "In this model, no one has obligations of any particular sort because he or she is a dentist."[1] Such a focus does not and cannot respect any patient's claims to dental services on any but the professional's terms, any more than a baker need respect consumers' claims to cakes on any but the baker's terms. Thus, under this model, each dentist is an independent professional with a saleable commodity, a commodity traded by the rules of the marketplace—supply, demand, and competition.

The guild model departs from the commercial model's initial premise that dental services are a commodity like any other, with the dentist acting as seller and the patient as buyer. Instead, the guild model begins from the premise that dentistry is not a business, in which independent practitioners compete with each other for "buyers;" rather, dentistry is an example of a *profession*. In such a model, the profession is of primary importance, and the professional's actions must reflect appropriate respect for it by fulfilling the duties of the role he or she plays within the profession. According to the guild model, it does make sense to speak of obligations that one has as a dentist, and those obligations are determined by the profession itself, because professionals are the ones with the relevant knowledge and skills.

The last of Ozar's models, the interactive model, views the source of decision-making power and justification for dentists' obligations and patients' claims as lying in neither free-market principles nor the profession of dentistry. The interactive model instead relies on the shared contributions of the professional as technical expert and the patient as possessor of values and preferences that must be considered in establishing the goals of therapy. In this way, what has been critically described as the "silent world" of professional and patient[2] can benefit from the insight and perspective each brings to decisions in the dental setting. Within the interactive model, the relationship between professional and patient is characterized by shared decision making, rather than competition as in the commercial model, or unilateral expertise, as in the guild model. The interactive model views the patient-professional relationship as an encounter between equals; it is a partnership formed to promote what is therapeutically best for the patient in a way consistent with patient values and goals.

These three general models are useful for describing the general nature of the relationship between dentist and patient. It is also important to consider some of the concrete obligations that dentists may have toward patients. This chapter examines some of the most important obligations that dentists have: the duties to tell the truth and to keep promises to patients. These obligations take the form of *rules* that are derived from the general ethical *principles* discussed in Chapter 2. To lay the groundwork for this discussion, we examine some of the characteristics of the dentist-patient relationship suggested by Ozar's three models. We end with an examination of the controversial topic of paternalism.

Before undertaking that discussion, however, one note of clarification. The terms "duty" and "obligation" mean an action required of an individual, based on either law or morality. These required actions can be specific to the roles individuals occupy or general societal requirements, as will be further discussed in a later section. The two terms are interchangeable, so the reader should not view "duty" as having any different connotation than "obligation."

THE BASIS OF THE DENTIST-PATIENT RELATIONSHIP

How might a dentist be motivated to act, and what are the moral implications of these motivations? We examine three bases for action: self-interest, respect for the interests of others, and respect for persons. We will then be in a better position to evaluate the obligations that dentists have toward patients.

Self-Interest

To begin, dentists may be motivated to act in ways that serve their own interest, or what philosophers call an egoistic approach. This approach is discussed generally by Beauchamp[3] and in more detail by others.[4-6] Under an egoistic approach, everyone ought to act in the ways that best serve their own interests. Conflicts may arise, however, when the interests of two people cannot both be served. Some negotiated resolution can be sought, but there is a problem of internal inconsistency in a theory that advocates acts that promote what is best for one individual while at the same time requiring him or her to advocate acts by another that are contrary to those interests. The shortcomings of egoism, then, are that it can produce conflicts of this type by its basic dictates, and that it cannot resolve conflicts between the self-interest of individuals. This sort of egoistic approach to the dentist's relationship with patients describes in large part the motivation for practicing within the commercial model identified by Ozar. Salvatore Durante summarizes this view in the following way: "He [the doctor] owes no debt to 'society' or to anyone else (specific financial loans excluded, of course)."[7]

A type of egoism that applies the commercial model is tied to the value of economic gain. When a dentist believes that his or her primary responsibility is to maximize personal profits, the dentist places his or her interests above the interests of the patient. As Durante notes, the dentist-patient relationship would, according to this view, be:

> ...essentially the same as in any other relationship between traders in a free society. A doctor offers a service, and a patient offers money, goods, or services in exchange.[7]

The discomfort many have with this type of health provider-patient relationship may be caused partly by its apparent "hard-heartedness" in placing economic considerations over patient welfare, and in the process reducing dentistry to the status of "just" another service industry.

The egoistic approach might become evident when a dentist competes for patients with other dentists in his or her referral area. Yet, in contrast to most descriptions of the commercial model, an egoistic analysis of the dentist-patient relationship would find acting out of self-interest in terms of competitive pricing not only acceptable but laudable. There are other ways that a dentist might justify doing what he or she does, however. To these we now turn.

Respect for the Interests of Others

A second basis for action might be the interests of others; in other words, the dentist might appeal to the principle of beneficence. Here the best interests of the patient, rather than the dentist, guide the decision-making process. The American Dental Association (ADA) *Principles of Ethics and Code of Professional Conduct* (1991) explains in its preamble that "[t]he ethical statements which have historically been subscribed to by the dental profession have had the benefit of the patient as their primary goal."[8] Adopting solely this approach in the dentist-patient relationship, however, runs the risk of placing the dentist in a position in which his or her technical knowledge may lead to decisions made largely by the dentist for the patient rather than by the patient aided by the dentist. Certainly, any decision regarding dental treatment and care must take relevant technical and diagnostic considerations into account. However, such considerations ought not be the sole basis for dental decision making because the dentist's knowledge of technical and diagnostic information cannot take account of the patient's individual preferences, life goals, and the like.

Dental decision making is further complicated by what Donald Sadowsky describes as the "moral dilemma of the multiple prescription in dentistry."[9] Multiple prescription refers to the myriad of materials (e.g., composite, amalgam, gold and porcelain) and techniques (e.g., fixed versus removable partial dentures, with or without dental implants) available to dentists, each having varying costs and claims of quality and effectiveness. The moral dilemma arises when the dentist is faced with recommending less than the "best" or optimal treatment, such as extraction versus endodontics/restorative treatment because the dentist understands that the patient cannot afford or does not desire optimal care. Is such a recommendation beneficent? Recommending suboptimal care may serve the best interests of the patient as they are expressed to the dentist but at the same time fail to be in the patient's best *dental* interests.

As the dilemma of the multiple prescription points out, any purely interest-regarding approach, with the guild model described by Ozar serving as a rough example,[1] does not provide an adequate account of the entirety of the dentist-patient relationship. Such an approach may treat the patient as the dental diagnosis embodied by the package of symptoms he or she presents rather than as the autonomous individual whose life is only partly that of a dental patient. This shortcoming in any interest-regarding approach can be addressed by realizing the need to respect the individual autonomy of patients, part of the dentist–patient relationship addressed next.

Respect for Persons

A third way to look at the factors motivating behavior in the dentist-patient relationship is what might be called a person-regarding approach. The person-regarding approach means viewing the relationship between dentist and patient as a relationship between persons who are autonomous equals, rather than merely viewing the relationship as being between people interacting through the roles of dentist and patient. Imbedded in such a statement is an understanding of the rights and respect persons deserve, and the roles these rights and respect play.

Any understanding of the rights and respect persons deserve must begin with the concept and value of autonomy and respect for it. Simply put, individuals who are mentally able have the right to decide what shall be done to their bodies. This concept is a longstanding one, first codified in US law in the case of *Schloendorff v. The Society of New York Hospital 1914*:

"Every human being of adult years and sound mind has a right to determine what shall be done with his own body; and a

surgeon who performs an operation without his patient's consent, commits an assault, for which he is liable in damages."[10]

This means that, whether or not the dentist agrees with the decision, a patient's wishes deserve to be respected. The value of respect for autonomy is the hallmark of a liberal, democratic society like the United States. This value was expressed by John Stuart Mill in *On Liberty*,[11] when he wrote that, unless individuals' decisions and/or actions cause harm to, or interfere with the liberty of others, the state cannot restrict their liberty. The application of this value is fundamental to understanding all aspects of the dentist-patient relationship, and is recognized in the interactive model described by Ozar.[1]

The shortcomings of being guided solely by respect for persons in the dentist-patient relationship are that the dentist may find himself or herself faced with providing unnecessary or inappropriate dental treatment so as to respect patient autonomy. Acceding to every patient demand seems inappropriate behavior for any health care professional, yet being guided solely by respect for persons seems to demand just such behavior.

Each of the three bases on which a dentist might be motivated to act on behalf of the patient gives rise to moral problems. Nevertheless, we do speak of obligations that dentists have toward patients, third parties, the profession, and society, that grow out of these bases. It is important, therefore, to consider some of the more important of these obligations, and how they might be justified, in light of the previous analysis. We turn next to a discussion of some of these obligations.

OBLIGATIONS IN THE DENTIST-PATIENT RELATIONSHIP

Having examined the various characteristics making up the relationship between dentists and their patients, the discussion can move to the duties or obligations that both dentists and patients have to each other, society, third parties, and the profession when they are interacting within the dentist-patient relationship.

The Difference Between General and Role-Specific Obligations

First, it is important to understand what is at issue when discussing duties, or obligations. All people have obligations to behave (or not behave) in certain ways, dictated by the common morality. Our duty of nonmaleficence, for example, appears to apply to all of us; everyone has a moral obligation to avoid harming others. Sometimes, however, we have obligations in virtue of the social roles we play. Parents, for example, have duties toward their children that strangers do not. One way of accounting for these role-specific duties is that children are dependent upon their parents in a way that they are not with respect to strangers. A similar kind of dependence exists when individuals seek out health care professionals in whom they necessarily entrust their welfare. Like parents, dentists have obligations in virtue of their social roles. Consider the following example:

It is 6:30 pm on Saturday, and, as usual, the dentist, Dr. Garcia, and the bank president, Ms. Jones, are running laps separately at the local junior high school track. It is April and, as is typically the case in nice weather, a few youth soccer teams are practicing. Dr. Garcia and Ms. Jones notice a group of the young men are gathered around an apparently injured player. Upon investigation, they find that the player (17 years old) has sustained a dental injury, and Dr. Garcia sees that the young man is holding his maxillary left central incisor in his hand. There is minimal bleeding and no other apparent injuries. The young man, although obviously upset at the apparent loss of his tooth, is alert and wondering what he should do. His parents are not at home, and because he just moved to town 5 months ago, he does not have a regular dentist. His teammates tell him to "throw away the tooth" and that the father driving the team that day will take him to a dentist when he returns at 9:00 pm. There are no adults present for this practice. The avulsed tooth looks intact and clean. Dr. Garcia realizes that an immediate replant is possible and that the prognosis for retaining the tooth is dependent on how quickly he acts. Ms. Jones too is concerned about the young man's welfare.

What obligations, if any, do Dr. Garcia and Ms. Jones have toward the young man? Let us assume that the principle of beneficence, which requires one to promote the welfare of others and to remove harm,[12] applies to both participants in the above drama. It is still not immediately clear what concrete duties the principle entails. It certainly would not be the case that Ms. Jones owes the same *kind* of help as the dentist to the person in need, because she does not possess the dentist's knowledge and skills. In fact, by attempting to perform a dental intervention, she might cause more harm than good, and in so doing violate her duty of nonmaleficence. Still, it may be possible for Ms. Jones to offer other forms of assistance, such as comforting the young man or calling an ambulance. If these actions do not cause a great personal burden to Ms. Jones, we may conclude that her general duty of beneficence may be fulfilled by providing them. Indeed, if she decided not to do so (say, because her workout was interrupted), we would probably hold that she has acted unethically.

Dr. Garcia, though, finds himself in quite a different situation. His professional status places him in the role of an expert in dental emergencies. Thus, for him, the principle of beneficence demands more than what is required of Ms. Jones. Like Ms. Jones, Dr. Garcia is bound by the general duty of beneficence, but he is also required to fulfill duties of beneficence that he is specially trained to perform. This means that, if Dr. Garcia merely comforted the injured athlete or called an ambulance, he would have fulfilled the general duties of beneficence but failed in his *role-specific* duties. Because Dr. Garcia is a dentist and can therefore provide the special skill needed to replant the tooth with a minimum of complications, and because the prognosis for replantation is time-dependent, the good of the young man would be best served by Dr. Garcia through immediate dental treatment at the scene.

The case of Dr. Garcia and the duties he and Ms. Jones have toward the young man who avulsed a tooth are meant to illuminate the difference between general and role-specific duties. The following sections more closely examine some of the dentist's obligations.

Duties Toward Patients

By agreeing to take part in the dentist-patient relationship, both patients and providers accept certain obligations or duties. Both accept a responsibility to disclose all information pertinent to the relationship. The provider also accepts duties to respect the patient's privacy, maintain patient confidences, and allow competent patients to make treatment decisions based on the patient's values and preferences. The duty to protect confidentiality was discussed in detail in Chapter 2. The following sections examine the other duties just mentioned, some of which are general, others of which are role-specific. We also consider whether these duties are absolute, or instead may be overridden by other obligations.

THE GENERAL DUTY OF VERACITY

Trust plays an important role in the dentist-patient relationship. Dentists maintain the trust patients place in them by fulfilling two related duties: telling their patients the truth, and disclosing the information patients need to make informed treatment decisions. We turn now to an examination of these two obligations.

Obligations to Tell the Truth. Dentists, like other health care professionals, are obligated to tell their patients the truth, but like nearly every other moral obligation, the obligation to tell the truth is not absolute. There may be cases when more good than harm will come from failing to tell the truth, and sometimes this type of balancing can be used to justify various forms of deception. For instance, the efficacy of placebos has been shown to exist, sometimes in cases when "active" agents fail to have any impact.[13,14] The use of placebos, however, requires deception for the mere possibility of effect. Thus positive effect from the use of placebos and truth-telling by the dentist are mutually exclusive. There is value in each, but both cannot exist at the same time. When is it justifiable to engage in deception? If preventing harm to a patient or promoting the patient's welfare can be achieved *only* by engaging in deception, one might believe that deception is warranted. The problem is that deception itself must be considered a harm. If the patient learns of the deception, the trust that he or she places in the dentist may be permanently eroded. A single act of deception makes it psychologically easier to deceive again, when the justification may not be so compelling. It is thus difficult to assess whether the harm that one hopes to prevent by deceiving another is greater than the harm that flows from the deception itself.

The following case illustrates this tension:

An adult male (35 years old) comments during your initial examination appointment that he is "scared of dentists," especially because his father had "cancer of the mouth." He further states that he has only had dental care in the past only when his teeth "hurt" and that the only reason he is here today is because his wife and daughter are very pleased with the care they received from you. During your review of his dental history, he states that he has used chewing tobacco since high school like most of his friends. Your oral examination reveals a 3 mm dehiscence on the facial surface of both mandibular central incisors with a characteristic corrugated appearance of the labial mucosa and vestibule, commonly seen in patients using smokeless tobacco products. Your concern is that, rather than being a white lesion, this one has an atypically "reddish" appearance, leading you to suspect a potentially cancerous growth. Your first inclination is to refer him to your colleague, an oral pathologist at a dental college in town, for a second opinion. You are concerned, however, how any news of this suspicious lesion will be received. How forthright about your concerns should you be with this fearful patient? What should you say if the patient asks "I don't have cancer, do I, doctor? I couldn't cope if I found out I have cancer."

Should you tell the patient the truth? One way to answer this question is to weigh the relative benefits and harms of disclosure. Philosophers call such calculations *utilitarian*. A dentist who considers himself or herself a utilitarian attempts to act in such a way as to provide the greatest proportion of benefit over harm. Utilitarianism as an ethical theory generally aims to maximize the utility of any situation; that is, it guides us to act in such a way as to provide the greatest proportion of benefit over harm. Notice that nowhere in this explanation is there mention of whose benefit and harm, and in fact by strict utilitarian calculus only the overall maximization of utility is at issue; the way benefits and harms are distributed is of secondary importance.

Let us consider the benefits and harms of various forms of disclosure. Telling the patient of your concerns would certainly trigger the fearful memories of his father's "cancer of the mouth." It might even cause him to leave your office without having the lesion diagnosed. Alternately, you could avoid being specific about the kind of specialist to whom the patient is being referred, thereby ensuring that the patient's fears are not (immediately) realized. This might entail telling the patient "I'm referring you to a specialist to check your gums." The inference is that the specialist is a periodontist, not an oral pathologist, and that the disease is periodontitis, not the carcinoma the dentist suspects. Note that this alternative is deceptive. The dentist could even call the oral pathologist and explain the case and the need to conduct the examination with the patient's fearful history in mind.

The benefit that such deception would yield to the patient (diagnosis of the lesion) would arguably outweigh the harms of failing to be entirely forthright—potential erosion of the patient's belief in the dentist's honesty and/or patient trust in individual dentists and the profession of dentistry as a whole when the patient eventually realizes that the specialist is a pathologist. We might further argue that being forthright would actually be more harmful than being deceptive because knowledge of the dentist's suspicions might drive the patient away from any further treatment. This rationale is what justifies the common and nearly universal practice of telling "harmless" lies,[15] such as that "we'll have to get together for lunch sometime," or that "it's been nice talking with you." Such duplicities are viewed as bringing more good than harm, and so are accepted as part of normal social interactions. Deception in the case of the fearful tobacco-chewing patient may be more harmful than the lies of everyday social interactions, but the benefits it brings arguably outweighs its harmfulness.

We ought not to ignore the option of lying outright to the patient by saying that he has nothing to worry about and that he just needs his gums checked. Such an approach, however, is morally untenable in that it fails to respect the patient's autonomy, and at the same time is likely to yield no greater benefit than the sort of deception discussed. This sort of bald lying further presumes that the dentist knows what is best for the patient, treating him paternalistically, or as a parent would treat a child (this concept is the topic of a later section of this chapter). Utilitarian calculations of the sort discussed are not the only way to determine when and if the obligation of truth-telling applies. We now examine some other approaches.

In some accounts of ethical theory, the inherent value of rules is great. Under such theories, the rule of truth-telling ought be respected even if breaking it in favor of the benefits of deception appears to yield greater overall utility. By informing the fearful patient that he ought to see a specialist about a suspicious lesion, the dentist is respecting the rule of truth-telling, but may well be sacrificing what is best for the patient. On such duty-based accounts, the value of the duty of truth-telling ought not to be calculated as a matter of its utility but rather ought to be respected due to its considered place as a duty. To explain, in duty-based theories, actions that are elevated to the status of duties achieve such status only with good cause. In the deontological (duty-based) theories typified by Kantian ethics, duties are those actions that are imperative (must be done), and are universalizable (apply to all).[16,17]

Duties like truth-telling achieve this status not for the good consequences that such actions yield, but because they honor even more basic duties such as treating individuals as ends in themselves and never as means to other ends. When multiple duties exist and are in conflict, as the duties of truth-telling and benefitting the patient seem to be in this case, the deontologist must somehow choose between them. As described, relying on the decision that yields the best consequences is not compelling in deontological approaches to ethics. How then might conflicts between duties be resolved? In one duty-based account, espoused by the philosopher W.D. Ross, situations that seem to call for conflicting actions can be resolved by intuitively balancing the rules in conflict.[18] First, Ross advocates identifying what he calls *prima facie* duties, or duties that are to be acted upon unless they conflict with an equal or stronger duty. When such conflict does occur, one's *actual* duty is determined by reasoning which action will actually bring about the greatest balance of right over wrong. The process of reasoning to determine one's actual duty is dependent on individual intuition, and thus Ross's theory is called "intuitionist" in nature. One of the shortcomings of an intuitionist approach, however, is that intuitions are subjective, thus leaving the possibility that conflicts among duties could be resolved differently by different individuals.

The focus of yet a third type of ethical theory is on moral virtue, or the qualities of character that promote good choices over the span of one's life. For all situations there are choices that reflect the range of possible actions related to a specific virtue. With respect to truth-telling, honesty is the virtue that lies between the vice of absolute deception on one end and brutal frankness on the other. In the case of the fearful patient, the dentist could choose to be deceptive by referring the patient to a specialist to check his gums, or could be brutally frank with the patient in saying that he has a suspicious lesion that may be cancer. An action that would consider the virtue of honesty could include compassionately acknowledging the patient's fears of dentistry, discussing the traumatic experience of his father's oral cancer, and explaining dentists' responsibilities to be truthful with patients so as to respect their right to know about matters of their oral health. By disclosing his concern about the suspicious lesion in this manner, the dentist would be acting virtuously. The difficulty, of course, is in knowing what constitutes virtuous action, or possessing what

Aristotle called "practical wisdom:" "Practical wisdom is a truthful rational characteristic of acting in matters involving what is good for [persons]."[19] While the most virtuous path is not always clear, continued effort is expected to eventually yield this practical wisdom. Whether achieved by viewing issues of truth-telling through a lens of utilitarian, duty-based, or virtue ethics, practical wisdom in addressing such cases should be a goal of the ethical dentist.

Whichever theory one uses to give an account of the duty of truthful disclosure, the duty itself is grounded in the patient's right to have information related to his or her care. As the case of the fearful tobacco chewer highlights, some patients wish to be shielded from certain types of information. As long as the patient is expressing this wish autonomously (i.e., voluntarily, intentionally, and with understanding), it is ethically permissible for the dentist to follow the patient's request. The moral justification for doing so is still the principle of respect for autonomy. That is, patients have a moral right to *waive* their right to know, and the dentist's obligation to respect this right may be fulfilled by establishing that the patient is making the choice freely and with an understanding of the consequences of this choice.

In some cases, it is unclear whether an individual has the capacity to make autonomous decisions. When this is the case, disclosing potentially distressing information to the patient may lead to increased confusion and further loss of the ability to act autonomously. A dentist does not have a moral duty to make truthful disclosures to a patient who lacks decision-making capacity, but he or she *does* have an obligation to make the relevant disclosures to the patient's proxy decision makers. If the patient has decision-making capacity, the dentist has no moral obligation to respect the wishes of a friend or family member to avoid being truthful with the patient; indeed, it would be unethical for the dentist to do so because it would violate the principle of respect for autonomy. The most challenging cases facing dentists involve patients of questionable decision-making capacity. For instance, if, after consultation with the dentist, the wife of the fearful tobacco-chewing patient requested that her husband not be told of his suspicious lesion, the dentist would need to assess the values of respecting (or breaking) the duty to disclose relevant dental information to the patient against the harm such disclosure (or failure to disclose) might cause. Disclosure, of course, is necessary but not sufficient to fulfill one's duties to patients or their proxy decision makers; the disclosures must be *understood*. (This is covered in more detail in Chap. 5.)

Although most of this section has focused on the dentist's duty to disclose information to patients, the patient owes similar duties to the dentist. When a patient presents himself or herself to a dentist and agrees to be treated by him or her, the patient tacitly enters into a relationship in which shared information, honesty, and trust are vital. Factors such as a medical history indicating allergic reactions to certain antibiotics is important information if the dentist is to prescribe the safest and most effective treatment to prevent infection, for example. Thus the obligations of disclosure do not belong solely to the dentist, but are shared obligations of both parties in the dentist-patient relationship.

The Duty of Promise-keeping. Promise-keeping, or fidelity, is an important part of the dentist-patient relationship, just as it is in any other interpersonal relationship. When we make a promise to someone, he or she relies on our living up to it, and often makes plans that depend on the fulfillment of that promise. The importance of keeping the promises we make is at base fundamentally the same in all relationships: When a promise is made, it is a pledge that someone trusts will be upheld. When promises are broken, the trust in a relationship dwindles and may be entirely eroded. The differences between the impact of failing to keep promises in different relationships are dependent on what is at stake when someone depends on our promises. When a friend promises to meet us for drinks after work and fails to show up, we lose faith in the friend, and we have lost out on companionship and the opportunity to have made other plans. When a dentist promises to act in ways that serve a patient's best interests and instead acts out of expedience or

convenience, he or she not only erodes a trust but also fails the patient in more serious and material ways. A further complication for professionals is that the failure to maintain fidelity undermines more than the individual patient-professional relationship and goes some way toward undermining the profession itself. For these reasons, fidelity is a key component of the dentist-patient relationship.

Consider the following case as an example of the duty of promise-keeping in the dentist-patient relationship, and how it might conflict with other role-specific and general duties:

> It is 5:00 pm on Friday, and Dr. Smith has seen his last patient. The extraction was complicated by a fractured crown, requiring the surgical removal of the root. The patient left in good spirits, biting on a gauze pack, with complete instructions on how to manage postsurgical care. Dr. Smith plans to call the patient this evening, as is routine, to assure that the patient is comfortable and stable. Dr. Smith plans to be gone this weekend and does not plan to tell his patient or to make emergency arrangements. There are many dentists in town, Dr. Smith rationalizes, and surely someone will take the call if needed.

It is difficult to justify Dr. Smith's decision to leave for the weekend without making appropriate arrangements for the patient. By agreeing to treat the patient, Dr. Smith has made an implicit promise to the patient, namely, to provide the appropriate care. Indeed, dentists, like all professionals, have duties not only to *specific* patients but to *society* generally. When one becomes a professional, one makes a contract, in a sense, with society to provide the services unique to the profession to those who need them, or to arrange for the provision of such services. This is recognized in both professional codes and the law. For example, the *ADA Code* explicitly states that "[d]entists shall be obliged to make reasonable arrangements for the emergency care of their patients of record;"[8] and at least one state's legislation speaks to the duty to treat: "A dentist shall not abandon a dental patient he [or she] has undertaken to treat."[20] Thus the duty of promise-keeping stretches beyond the relationship a dentist has with specific patients and into the larger relationship between the profession and society.

WHAT IS PATERNALISM, AND IS IT EVER JUSTIFIED?

Paternalism, as its root tells us, is to act as would a father (or in more egalitarian language, a parent). Paternalism usually takes the form of one individual acting to substitute his or her decision for that of another, under the guise of authority, and often to override the autonomous decision of another, for that person's own benefit. Objections to paternalism can be traced to eighteenth century England and John Stuart Mill's essay on political philosophy, *On Liberty*,[11] in which, as we have already mentioned, Mill argues that the state is justified in restricting individual liberty only if an individual's action poses harm to others. This is the historical benchmark for the refutation of paternalism and remains one of the hallmarks of liberal political theory and the basis for our societal presumption that individuals are free to act as they see fit.

Consider the following case:

A 29-year-old man presents at an emergency appointment with a painful tooth that has been "keeping [him] up" for the last three nights. Dr. Samuel Doe's oral examination reveals a state of general neglect, with generalized chronic gingivitis and several teeth with small occlusal and cervical caries. Surprisingly, there are no missing teeth. Tooth No. 4 has a localized cervical carious lesion, and after further clinical evaluation, the diagnosis is irreversible pulpitis with acute periradicular periodontitis caused by the caries penetrating to the pulp. Dr. Doe realizes that nonsurgical root canal therapy followed by a build-up and crown would be the preferred treatment for tooth No. 4. However, considering the patient's history of episodic dental care in the past resulting in his general state of dental neglect, the dentist decides to offer *only* extraction as his treatment plan. His reasoning is that "there is no use in discussing other alternatives because the patient obviously doesn't care about his teeth, probably couldn't afford the root canal and crown anyway, and such a discussion would probably embarrass the patient."

Dr. Doe's decision is a paradigmatic example of paternalism in dentistry because it was made without any consideration of the patient's values and preferences. It may in fact be the case that the patient would have chosen the extraction, perhaps even for the same reasons that Dr. Doe considered, but the dentist is not acting *from* this knowledge. Rather, the dentist chooses not to discover what is important to the patient. It might turn out that the patient would have preferred the root canal therapy instead; after all, he might value preserving oral functioning over saving money. The point of this example is not that Dr. Doe is *wrong* for believing that extraction is the best procedure, but that he made this determination without knowing the patient's values, and for that reason his decision was paternalistic. For the principle of respect for patient autonomy to be meaningful, treatment decisions like the one just described must be made with respect to what patients themselves prefer.

There are limits to what dentists are ethically obligated to do on behalf of their patients, however. Consider the following:

A competent adult male (55 years old) vigorously asserts during the initial examination appointment that "I'm tired of fixing these teeth. I want dentures to end these hassles once and for all!" The oral examination reveals the absence of periodontal disease and that the patient has received several small composite and amalgam restorations and three gold crowns. There is a need for the replacement of three anterior composites and one gold crown. Overall, the patient's prognosis for maintaining his teeth for a lifetime is good.

As good news about his prognosis, along with the need for some restorative care, is explained to the patient, the dentist senses continued frustration from the patient. He erupts, exclaiming "Doc, I said I want dentures—my parents have them and they are satisfied—I've saved for this now for 2 years. When can we start?"

When a patient requests a dental intervention that the dentist believes is harmful or at least not in the patient's best interests, it is important to ask why the patient is making such a request. Sometimes such requests are made because the patient's values are different than the dentist's; this may be the case with the example above. It is not paternalistic for a dentist to refuse to perform a procedure that he or she believes is not in the best interests of the patient, or that the dentist simply cannot do in good conscience. In fact, some might argue that it would be *unethical* for a dentist to perform the extraction described because the only reason for doing so is because the patient wants it, and not because it is clinically indicated. Few would deny the patient's request for full-mouth extractions and complete dentures if his oral condition included advanced periodontal disease (Type IV), rampant caries, severe malocclusion, and poor esthetics. However, removing all of the patient's teeth and fabricating complete dentures in the absence of disease bears what James Childress calls a "heavy burden of justification."[21] Even so, deciding not to do what the patient requests in this case is not paternalistic.

Another reason that patients make requests like the one above is that they do not understand the consequences of what they are asking the dentist to do and may have unrealistic expectations of the outcome. (Note that it is possible for a patient to be competent and yet to fail to understand a particular aspect of treatment; this is discussed in more detail in Chap. 5.) The problem of unrealistic expectations can often be resolved by an honest discussion with the patient.

Some scholars have made a distinction between paternalism in which clearly autonomous decisions are overridden, calling this variety "strong" paternalism, and calling paternalism in which apparently nonautonomous decisions are overridden (until such time as it can be ascertained whether the individual is competent and expressing truly autonomous desires) "weak" paternalism.[12] If the individual is deemed incompetent (or, as Odom and Bowers say in Chap. 5, if the patient lacks decision-making capacity), weak paternalism stops being paternalism at all in that the patient's expressed wishes should no longer be considered autonomous; and by the same token, if the individual is deemed competent, continued weak paternalism becomes the "strong" variety. Once deci-

sion-making capacity has been assessed, decisions for incompetent patients made by suitable proxy or decisions expressed by competent patients must both be respected or paternalism will remain.

CONCLUSION

The daily practice of dentistry places patients' beliefs and values and dentists' desires to benefit patients into potential conflict. Patients don't leave their beliefs and values at the dentist's door. Nor do dentists come to the patient-provider relationship without beliefs and values of their own. Conflicts of these beliefs and values can lead to paternalism in the dentist-patient relationship. The evolution of the *ADA Code of Ethics*[24] highlights this potential outcome. The first ADA Code (1866) contained statements that, in light of modern discussion, appear paternalistic: "His [the dentist's] manner should be firm, yet kind and sympathizing," and "[as patients] are unable to correctly estimate the character of his [the dentist's] operations, his [the dentist's] own sense of right must guarantee faithfulness in their performance." (Code of Dental Ethics. *Trans. Am. Dent. Assoc.*, 1866, pp. 403–405.) Contrast these views with the current Code regarding decision making: "The dentist should inform the patient of the proposed treatment, and any reasonable alternatives, in a manner that allows the patient to become involved in treatment decisions."[8] The evolution of the Code has incorporated the value of including the patient in the decision-making process, while continuing to value the knowledge and technical skill of the dentist. The relationship between dentists and patients will continue to evolve, and this ongoing and dynamic nature of the relationship points out the pitfalls in advocating a single model of, or approach to, the dentist-patient relationship. The interactive model posed by Ozar can best adapt to this changing nature of the dentist-patient relationship, and it, along with an understanding of the characteristics and motivations making up the relationships, will go some way toward achieving an optimal dentist-patient relationship.

DISCUSSION QUESTIONS

1. What is the value of telling the truth to patients? If a therapeutic outcome could be improved by lying to patients, would the dentist have a moral obligation to lie?
2. Which model of the dentist-patient relationship seems to best fit with your view of dentists and dentistry?
3. Is it ever justifiable for a dentist to refuse to honor a patient's wishes regarding dental care? Consider this issue in terms of both a dentist who believes it is in the best interests of a patient to undergo treatment that is refused by the patient, and in terms of a patient who requests treatment that the dentist believes is not in the patient's best interests.
4. Describe what approach you would take to one of the cases outlined in the chapter if you were (1) the dental professional; and (2) the patient.

REFERENCES

1. Ozar, D.T.: Three models of professionalism and professional obligation in dentistry. J. Am. Dent. Assoc. *110:*173, 1985.
2. Katz, J.: The Silent World of Doctor and Patient. New York, The Free Press, 1984.
3. Beauchamp, T.L.: Philosophical Ethics. New York, McGraw-Hill, 1982, pp. 56–66.
4. Baier, K.: The Moral Point of View. Ithaca, New York, Cornell University Press, 1958, Chapter 8.
5. Baumer, W.H.: Indefensible impersonal egoism. Philosophical Studies *18:*72, 1967.
6. MacIntyre, A.: Egoism and altruism. *In* Edwards, P. (ed.): The Encyclopedia of Philosophy. New York, Macmillan Company and Free Press, 1967, vol. 2, pp. 462–466.
7. Durante, S.: The fallacy and danger of "public service." J. Dent. Pract. Admin. *6:*144, 1989.
8. ADA Principles of Ethics and Code of Professional Conduct (1992), with official advisory opinions revised to January 1992.
9. Sadowsky, D.: The moral dilemmas of the multiple prescription in dentistry. J. Am. Coll. Dent. *46:*245, 1979.
10. *Schloendoff v. The Society of New York Hospital* 211 N.Y. 125, 1914.
11. Mill, J.S.: On Liberty. London, J.W. Parker, 1859.
12. Beauchamp, T.L., and Childress, J.C.: Principles of Biomedical Ethics, Third Edition. New York, Oxford University Press, 1989.
13. Brody, H.: Placebos and the Philosophy of Medicine: Clinical, Conceptual, and Ethical Issues. Chicago, University of Chicago Press, 1980, pp. 10–11.
14. Benson, H., and Epstein, M.: The placebo effect: A neglected aspect in the care of patients. JAMA *232:*1225, 1975.
15. Bok, S.: Lying: Moral Choice in Public and Private Life. London, Quartet Books, 1978.
16. Kant, I.: Foundations of the Metaphysics of Morals. Lewis White Beck, trans. Indianapolis, Bobbs-Merrill Co., Inc., 1959.
17. Acton, H.B.: Kant's Moral Philosophy. London, Macmillan & Co., Ltd., 1970.
18. Ross, W.D.: The Right and the Good. Oxford, Clarendon Press, 1930.
19. Aristotle: Nichomachean Ethics, 1140 b20.
20. Rules of the Texas State Board of Dental Examiners—Rev. 1/92, Sect. 109.121.
21. Childress, J.C.: Who Should Decide? Paternalism in Health Care. New York, Oxford University Press, 1982, p. 114.

SUGGESTED READINGS

ADA Principles of Ethics and Code of Professional Conduct (1991), with official advisory opinions revised to January 1991.

Beauchamp, T.L., and Childress, J.C.: Principles of Biomedical Ethics, 3rd ed. New York, Oxford University Press, 1989.

Benson, H., and Epstein, M.: The placebo effect: A neglected aspect in the care of patients. JAMA *232:*1225, 1975.

Bok, S.: Lying: Moral Choice in Public and Private Life. London, Quartet Books, 1978.

Brody, H.: Placebos and the Philosophy of Medicine: Clinical, Conceptual, and Ethical Issues. Chicago, University of Chicago Press, 1980.

Childress, J.C.: Who Should Decide? Paternalism in Health Care. New York, Oxford University Press, 1982.

Chiodo, G.T., and Tolle, S.W.: Doctor-patient confidentiality and the adolescent patient. J. Am. Dent. Assoc. *120:*2;126, February 1990.

Durante, S.: The fallacy and danger of "public service." J. Dent. Pract. Admin. *6:*144, 1989.

Foot, P.: The problem of abortion and the doctrine of double effect. *In* Bonnie Steinbock, ed.: Killing and Letting Die. Englewood Cliffs, NJ, Prentice-Hall, 1980, pp. 156–65.

Katz, J.: The Silent World of Doctor and Patient. New York, The Free Press, 1984.

MacIntyre, A.: Egoism and altruism. *In* Edwards, P. ed.: The Encyclopedia of Philosophy. New York, Macmillan Company and Free Press, 1967, vol. 2, pp. 462–466.

Mill, J.S.: On Liberty. London, J.W. Parker, 1859.

Ozar, D.T., Schiedermayer, D.L., and Siegler, M.: Value categories in clinical dental ethics. J. Am. Dent. Assoc. *116:*365, 1988.

Ozar, D.T.: Three models of professionalism and professional obligation in dentistry. J. Am. Dent. Assoc. *110:*173, 1985.

Sadowsky, D.: The moral dilemmas of the multiple prescription in dentistry. J. Am. Coll. Dent. *46:* 245, 1979.

Thompson, D.F.: Paternalism in medicine, law, and public policy. *In* Callahan, C., and Bok, S., editors: Ethics Teaching in Higher Education. New York, Plenum Press, 1980.

Chapter 5

Informed Consent and Refusal

John G. Odom
Donald F. Bowers

SUMMARY

Informed consent in dentistry is a patient's voluntary authorization of a dental procedure based on the patient's understanding of the relevant information provided by the dentist. It is based on the ethical principle of respect for autonomy. The high regard afforded this principle acknowledges ability of persons to comprehend knowledge, weigh alternatives, and form judgments. Encouraging and assisting patients to make treatment decisions through informed consent demonstrates respect for patient autonomy.

Respect for autonomy has only recently become an ethical standard for treatment decisions. Dentists had long appealed only to the principle of beneficence and, in so doing, often acted paternalistically. This chapter identifies several forces that influenced dentistry's recent adoption of the informed consent doctrine.

The patient's granting of informed consent for a specific treatment is the culmination of a shared decision-making process. Five factors necessary for informed consent are identified and discussed in detail: decision-making capacity, disclosure, understanding, comprehension, voluntariness, and consent. Assessing decision-making capacity to give informed consent is typically one of a practitioner's greatest concerns with respect to the process of shared decision making and informed consent. The authors describe the elements of decision-making capacity and suggestion methods for assessing such capacity.

The chapter continues with an examination of the unique circumstances associated with making decisions for those who lack decision-making capacity, including minors and some adults. Respecting patient autonomy means that patients occasionally give an informed refusal. The authors suggest a careful review of the process with the patient in order to stimulate dialogue and eliminate misunderstanding by both parties. The final topic in this chapter is a discussion of exceptions to the doctrine of informed consent.

Dentistry's growing commitment to informed consent has great potential to benefit practitioners as well as patients. The potential benefits include fulfilling doctor-patient relationships; practitioner relief from making burdensome, difficult decisions; increased patient loyalty and the esteem in which practitioners are held; and decreased probability for litigation.

INFORMED CONSENT

Decision making has long been viewed by both patients and dentists as the responsibility of the practitioner, the person who ultimately assumes the credit for doing good or the blame for doing harm. The result has been a paternalistic system in which the dentist rarely, if ever, consults the patient regarding treatment choices. The idea that the patient should play a role in decision making not only was absent from the operatory; engaging the patient in such a way might have been considered an abdication of one's professional responsibilities to make correct decisions for the patient. The profession now recognizes that the patient has an important role to play in making health care decisions. When a patient understands the relevant information about a procedure and freely consents to it, the patient has provided an *informed consent*. This chapter examines the nature and scope of this important doctrine in dental practice. It attempts to answer the following questions:

> What is the philosophical and historical basis of informed consent?
> What are the elements of informed consent?
> What are the elements of decision-making capacity, and how can decision making capacity be assessed?
> Who should make treatment decisions for patients lacking decision-making capacity?
> May patients provide an informed refusal?
> What exceptions are there to the requirement to obtain informed consent?

Philosophical and Historical Origins of Informed Consent

The moral basis for obtaining informed consent is the principle of respect for autonomy. The high regard for this principle is based on acknowledgment of and respect for rationality and cognitive abilities uniquely characteristic of the human race. To be rational is to be able to comprehend knowledge, weigh alternatives, and form judgments based on one's values and preferences. Respecting the rights of patients to participate in treatment decisions is one important way that dentists fulfill their ethical obligation to respect patient autonomy.[1–3]

Faden and Beauchamp have identified two discrete senses of informed consent.[4] The first focuses on the institutional rules and procedures that health care providers must observe in order to obtain informed consent. Frequently, this sense places exclusive importance on the information that must be disclosed to patients, and the documentation required to support the patient's consent. A second sense of informed consent emphasizes the need to engage patients in a process that is respectful of their personhood. This sense is grounded in the principle of respect for autonomy and is the focus of this chapter. The following case illustrates the differences between these two senses.

CASE 1

The Gelbachs have been patients of Dr. Leonard since they moved to this small city several years ago. Dr. Leonard was the only dentist in the locality who would provide dental care for their son, Jamie, who suffers from a spastic type of cerebral palsy. The family has been pleased with the dental care they have received from Dr. Leonard, and especially with the patience and understanding he has shown toward Jamie. In fact, the boy is very fond of Dr. Leonard and looks forward to his appointments.

A month ago, Edna Gelbach, Jamie's mother, was involved in an automobile accident. While waiting for a red light to change, her foot slipped off the brake pedal and her car bumped into the rear of the car ahead. Although the damage to the cars was minimal, the impact caused Ms. Gelbach's head to jerk forward and her mouth to strike the steering wheel. A couple of days ago, she noticed that one of her central incisors was darker than her other teeth.

After an examination, Dr. Leonard tells her that her tooth has become nonvital and that there is a sign of infection at the end of the tooth's root. He proposes that he perform endodontic treatment on the tooth, place a post and core, and restore the tooth with a porcelain jacket. Upon hearing the fee for these services, Ms. Gelbach, who does not have dental insurance, asks Dr. Leonard if there is any less expensive alternative. He says that there is not. In that case, she says, she will go ahead with the treatment and will attempt to take out a loan from the employees' credit union at her place of employment.

A few nights later, while attending a meeting of the regional chapter of the United Cerebral Palsy Foundation, she happens to have a conversation with a dentist from another city. With no motive in mind other than small talk, she describes her accident and the treatment she is to undergo. She tells the dentist that she wishes there was some less expensive alternative.

He tells her that there is; she could possibly forego the post and core and the jacket. The tooth could be treated by conventional endodontics, and the darkened crown could be bleached or a porcelain laminate could be made to cover it. Either procedure should be less expensive initially than the post and core and jacket, but there is a risk of a fracture of the crown later on, which would then require the more expensive treatment. The post and core and jacket, as proposed by her dentist, is definitely the less risky way to go.

The next day, Ms. Gelbach telephones Dr. Leonard, explains the conversation she had with the other dentist, and asks him if he would consider the alternative. She says that the family is strapped with expenses at the moment and she is willing to accept the risk rather than get further in debt. She also tells him that it is her understanding that her employer was going to offer dental insurance as an employee benefit beginning next year.

Dr. Leonard says that the alternative treatment is "poor makeshift dentistry" of which he will have no part, and furthermore, if she does not accept his treatment plan, he no longer wishes to be the Gelbachs' family dentist.

CASE 2

Oscar Loopes has been experiencing some temporomandibular discomfort recently. Some years earlier, while he was serving with the Marine Corps in Lebanon, he had two fractured premolars and an adjacent molar in a similar condition extracted by a Navy dentist. He had been "horsing around in the barracks" and had been accidentally hit in the face with a rifle butt. He served out his enlistment before having the teeth replaced, compliments of the U.S. Navy. As a civilian, he had let the situation ride because, until recently, he had experienced no discomfort and had learned to chew hard objects easily on the other side of his mouth.

After an extensive examination in which damage to the temporomandibular joint is ruled out, Dr. Clyde, his dentist, tells him that he believes that the discomfort was the result of the missing teeth, putting stress on the muscles of mastication and the ligaments, and that the situation would worsen unless he had the teeth replaced.

"It's like a couple of cog wheels that work together in a machine," the dentist explains. "If one of them has some teeth knocked out, and they continue to mesh together . . ."

". . . They won't mesh right," Oscar interrupts to finish the metaphor, "and the machine won't run true."

"Right!" Dr. Clyde responds in a complimentary tone.

"And eventually, the machine will be damaged."

Dr. Clyde affirms Oscar's comprehension of the situation and continues, "And how can we fix it, to make the wheels mesh correctly and prevent irreversible damage to the machine?"

"Replacing the missing teeth?" Oscar answers with a question.

"Right, again."

Oscar comments that it is lucky that they caught his problem in time and that he would have sought treatment much earlier if had understood the problem.

The dentist informs Oscar that his missing teeth can be replaced with either two types of partial dentures: removable or fixed. Either type of appliance would answer Oscar's needs, but he recommends the fixed appliance, which happens to be the more expensive of the two.

Oscar asks what the difference is between them.

Dr. Clyde opens a drawer in his desk and takes out two models of a dentition. One demonstrates a fixed appliance and the other a removable one. He demonstrates how the two stay in the mouth, and how one is expected to be solidly attached to some of his remaining teeth, whereas the other appliance, which can be removed, has arms that grasp some of the teeth.

"Is the fixed appliance glued to the teeth?" Oscar asks.

The dentist explains that in a sense it is; it is attached to gold crowns that are cemented over certain of his remaining teeth. To restore Oscar's mouth by the fixed method would require two separate bridges; the removable approach would require just one appliance. He shows Oscar, on a set of models of Oscar's mouth that were made earlier, how the arrangement of his remaining teeth and his bite make it relatively simple to construct two fixed partial dentures.

"Boy, it just like building a bridge over a river," Oscar, who is a civil engineer with the state highway department, observes.

Dr. Clyde congratulates Oscar on his perceptiveness and tells him that, in fact, "bridge" is a common term for the appliance.

"Do you have to grind down teeth and put caps on them for the removable appliance too?" Oscar inquires, not excited about the prospect of having his teeth subjected to the drill.

The dentist nods affirmatively and points

out on the model why it would be necessary to use crowns to alter the contour of the abutment teeth to create a pathway to seat and remove the denture. He then goes on to explain that one of the drawbacks to the other, less expensive removable partial denture is that, even with the custom-contoured abutments, clasps can be bent while the patients taking the denture out or putting it in the mouth. Sometimes partials are misplaced when they are removed, and they may be more difficult to keep clean in the mouth.

Dr. Clyde tells Oscar, "If it were my mouth, I would want the fixed appliance. No question about it."

"Me, too," Oscar agrees. "If I had the kind you can put in and take out, I would bend it up for sure and probably lose it. I am terrible with my eyeglasses. I wish they could invent a pair of glasses that you could glue to your head permanently."

"So you find it a nuisance to care for these things and are certain you want the fixed appliance. Right?" asks Dr. Clyde.

"No doubt about it. Give me something I never have to think about," Oscar answers.

The difference between Ms. Gelbach's consent and Oscar Loopes' consent illustrates the contrast between the two senses of informed consent described above. In the first case, Ms. Gelbach initially gave consent for endodontics, post and core, and a porcelain jacket and indicated she would apply for a loan to pay for the treatment. She was under no circumstances given all the information she needed to make a treatment choice consistent with her personal values and needs. Her consent to treatment was an act designed merely to satisfy the dentist's routine request for consent to treatment. Conversely, Dr. Clyde provided Oscar Loopes with all relevant information needed to make an informed decision, allowed the patient to question the alternative procedures, clarified potential outcomes of the alternative procedures, and ensured that the patient understood this information, after which the patient made a clear choice that showed consistency with his values.

What has accounted for the emphasis on patient self-determination in health care? First, the Civil Rights movement that gained momentum during the 1960s un-

doubtedly contributed to a climate that prompted individuals to assert personal rights in the medical setting. An associated development, the consumer rights movement, encouraged patients to acquire knowledge, ask questions, make comparisons, and assume greater participation in dental treatment. Dentistry's concurrent emphasis on prevention was compatible with the consumer movement, and thus patients began to expect to assume more responsibility for their dental health and to play a larger role in the operatory as well.

Laypersons were not the only ones who were responsible for this shift in decision-making authority. The public became more aware of the possibility of shared decision making with dental professionals, but greater interest in ethics was also taking place within the profession of dentistry during the 1970s and 1980s.[5] A major impetus for seeking answers through ethical inquiry was unprecedented technological progress, creating choices and dilemmas unthought of only decades before. For example, improved technology and design of dental implants and aggressive treatment of temporomandibular joint dysfunction illustrate recently developed treatments. In spite of the recent advancements in these areas, treatment does not produce certain success for all patients. Unfortunately, the failure of these treatments has the potential to result in further deterioration in oral functioning and can restrict the options for future treatment. Dentists have learned that a superficial, casual approach to informed consent is not acceptable, especially when options are complex and the outcome is not assured.

Dental professionals wisely began to re-examine fundamental principles that had guided their decision making for centuries. They questioned the previously unchallenged obligation of beneficence. If the dentist has an obligation to "do good," they wondered, is he or she the final authority on what is good? Is the dentist's duty of beneficence consistent with his or her obligation to respect patient autonomy? Are dentists who relinquish a paternalistic role abdicating professional obligations and responsibility?

Increased interest in the value of dentist-patient communication also contributed to the increased emphasis on patient autonomy. Humanistic emphasis and communication skills development initiated in the 1960s reached mainstream professionals in the 1970s and 1980s as dental schools added communication skills development to the curriculum[6] and practicing dentists enrolled in continuing education communication skills classes. When dentists developed skills in active listening and learning to understand the patient's perspective, they began to appreciate the role that patients can play in treatment decision making. The paternalistic role that dentists assumed for centuries began to be replaced by a philosophy emphasizing a covenant between the patient and practitioner and shared responsibility for treatment outcome.

It is becoming increasingly apparent that beneficence, the principle that guided treatment decision making for centuries, has been re-examined and found inadequate to meet the ethical demands of modern dentistry. The principle of respect for autonomy has not replaced beneficence, but dentistry is aware that patient autonomy can comfortably and appropriately play a role in "doing good." What is fading is the notion that the only way to provide beneficent treatment is to behave paternalistically. Although there is little documentation regarding professional attitudes on paternalistic versus patient autonomy treatment philosophies, there seems to be general agreement that dentistry is on a course leading to a standard of respect for patient autonomy. Recent empirical support for this view was provided by Odom and Messina.[7] An evaluation of ethical decision making by junior dental students showed that a majority of subjects used a decision-making process based on the principle of respect for patient autonomy. The authors concluded that patients' right to self determination was important for this population.

The following section discusses the process of shared decision making and how having all the relevant information allows a patient to make an informed choice, i.e., to give informed consent.

Shared Decision Making and Informed Consent

Applying the principle of respect for autonomy to modern dentistry means that the practitioner must allow patients to participate in decisions regarding their treatment, as well as be allowed to either consent to or refuse a proposed treatment. The literature sometimes blurs the distinction between the idea of informed consent and shared or mutual decision making. These concepts are not synonymous.[8] Shared decision making between patient (or surrogate) and practitioner is the process that lays the foundation for informed consent. Shared decision making recognizes that both the professional and the patient have something important to contribute to the clinical encounter: dentists understand the clinical aspects of a treatment decision; patients have unique values and preferences that will determine which treatments they are willing to accept. The process may be quickly brought to a conclusion or may, in the case of a difficult, complicated situation, require several conversations and negotiation to reach a solution satisfactory to both doctor and patient. Graber, Beasley, and Eaddy point out that a practitioner's request for informed consent should not come as a surprise; rather, a patient should have been gradually prepared over time through education and the development of a doctor-patient relationship that encourages honest discussion.[3]

Elements of Informed Consent

The following five conditions are necessary for obtaining an ethically sound informed consent.

First, the patient must have the capacity to make health care decisions for himself or herself. The term "competent" is sometimes used here, but competence is a legal concept, and assessments of competency can, strictly speaking, be made only by a court of law.[9] Persons are assumed to be competent unless adjudicated otherwise. For the dentist, the concept of decision-making capacity is the relevant one when obtaining informed consent for oral health interventions. According to the President's Commission for the Study of Ethical Problems in Medicine and Biomedical and Behavioral Research, decision-making capacity requires "1) possession of a set of values and goals, 2) the ability to communicate and to understand information, and 3) the ability to reason and to deliberate about one's choices."[10] Note that a person can have the capacity to make some decisions but not others. For example, a patient may have the ability to make a decision about whether or not to have root canal therapy but be unable to make broad financial decisions. Thus, decision-making capacity is *specific* to the kind of decision being made. Capacity to provide informed consent means that the patient is able to *understand* the relevant information presented to them (to be described), to *communicate* this understanding and to make a *reasoned decision* based on their *goals and values*. If a patient lacks decision-making capacity, he or she cannot make autonomous choices, and thus cannot provide an informed consent or refusal.

Second, the dentist must provide *information* regarding a proposed treatment. This is captured by the statement in the American Dental Association's *Principles of Ethics and Code of Professional Conduct,* which holds that "The dentist should inform the patient of the proposed treatment, and any reasonable alternatives, in a manner that allows the patient to become involved in treatment decisions."[11] The presentation must be thorough, truthful, and in language the patient can understand. A marriage of legal and philosophical interests in a 1972 United States court ruling reaffirmed that self-determination is the sole justification and goal of informed consent. The patient's needs for information, rather than physicians' practices, must form the basis of disclosure.[12]

What information should be included in a disclosure? In addition to an explanation of the dental problem, the dentist must inform patients of: "(a) the nature of the proposed treatment; (b) the benefits and risks of such treatment; and (c) the benefits and risks to the alternatives to treatment, including nontreatment."[13] Culver and Gert provide specific guidelines regarding the adequacy of information provided to a patient.[14] They explain that patients want benefits and risks explained in terms of the evils or harms that will likely be caused, prevented, or ameliorated by various courses of action. Culver and Gert identify the following as evils that concern patients: death, pain (both physical and psychological), disabilities (both physical and mental), and loss of freedom, opportunity, or pleasure. Although patients generally have no interest in the biochemical structure of dental materials, they care very much about pain, nausea, weakness, and loss of function. Patients want to know how likely these are to occur, how severe they may be, and how long they may last.

Dentists frequently raise concerns regarding the detail required for information disclosure. For example, how probable should a harmful result be before a patient should be informed about it? Culver and Gert provide guidance regarding this question. They suggest that the answer is a joint function of the severity of a harmful result plus the likelihood of its occurrence. As an illustration, "Any risk of death beyond a trivial risk, such as one in 10,000 or less, should be told."[14] Therefore, patients who are good operative risks for excision of oral tumors should be told of the slight risk of death associated with general anesthesia. Culver and Gert state that harmful results with low probability of occurrence need not be revealed.

The dentist has no obligation to present treatment options that he or she views as medically unacceptable or that have no scientific support. In addition, as long as no inappropriate influence is exercised, the patient has the right to know which alternative is recommended by the dentist.

The third requirement for informed consent is *comprehension.* That is, it is not enough that a patient have the *ability* to understand the relevant information presented; he or she must *actually* understand it. Many factors can interfere with a patient's comprehension, including high anxiety, fatigue, sensory deficits, and pain. It is essential that the individual fully or substantially comprehend the relevant information or a consent will not be truly informed and thus not a *valid informed consent.*

The caregiver can never be 100% certain that the patient has sufficient understanding to make an autonomous choice, but the professional can usually make a reasonable assessment of the patient's understanding.[4] This may be done by asking the patient to paraphrase the information presented to him or her.[9] Questions such as "Can you tell me what root canal therapy involves?" or directives like "Please share with me your understanding of the surgery" can provide useful information about the degree to which a patient has grasped what the dentist has disclosed. Consent for a procedure cannot be solicited and accepted as valid until patient comprehension of information has been verified.

Third, valid informed consent will be *voluntary*. No deception or coercion can accompany the process. The principle of respect for autonomy protects the individual's right to make decisions that are voluntary and intentional and are not the result of coercion, duress, or other forms of undue influence.[15] Dentists frequently wonder whether they should state their own treatment preferences or use persuasive techniques. Persuasion, defined as influence using an appeal to reason, is acceptable because it does not violate the spirit of "respect for persons" which is embodied in the concept of autonomy.

When a dentist makes an intentional effort to influence the patient to accept a particular treatment and provides sound reasons for the recommendations, the patient retains autonomy. Persuasion is acceptable when the practitioner is motivated by beneficence, that is, doing what will benefit the patient. Beauchamp notes that persuasion and education are influences, but that influence does not necessarily imply constraint, force, or compulsion. Persuasion does not deprive persons of autonomous action.[8]

In contrast to persuasion, *coercion* is unethical because it introduces a threat of harm or perhaps a bribe that makes decision making nonautonomous. The case in which Dr. Leonard threatened to terminate treatment for the Gelbach family, if Ms. Gelbach refused his proposed post and core and porcelain jacket, jeopardized dental treatment for her disabled son. This coercive statement by the dentist is clearly unethical. The son's treatment is unrelated to the decision Ms. Gelbach must make about her own treatment and has the effect forcing her to relinquish her rights to self determination.

When a dentist omits, exaggerates, or otherwise changes relevant facts such as the number of acceptable treatment alternatives available, or the risks and benefits of those alternatives, that dentist has altered the choices open to a patient, or the patient's perception of those choices. Even if this is done for benevolent (well-meaning) reasons, the dentist has violated the patient's right to have truthful information. Such a violation prevents the patient from making treatment decisions in accordance with his or her preferences and values and thus from making a voluntary choice. This breaches the dentist's obligation to respect patient self-determination, which, as we have seen, is the moral justification for informed consent. The intentional alteration of the treatment choices open to a patient, or the patient's perception of those choices, is a form of *manipulation* and is incompatible with obtaining informed consent.

The *final* requirement for informed consent is the *patient's authorization* of a dental procedure. The patient must indicate his or her consent to proceed with a particular treatment procedure. The patient who quietly listened to the disclosure and met requirements for comprehension and competence, but did not clearly state a choice, has not completed the consent process. Unless the patient is unable to speak, a smile or a nod is not sufficient evidence of authority to proceed. The patient must be encouraged to voice his or her choices or to put them in writing. If the patient is unable to communicate verbally, and if decision-making capacity is not in question, the dentist needs to establish a documented means of patient communication for the purpose of giving consent.

Some patients attempt to avoid making a decision. Being invited to participate in the decision-making process may not be appealing to an individual conditioned to assume a passive role in treatment. It may even be frightening. In addition, giving informed consent requires energy and effort from the patient, especially when the proposed procedure is complex and choices are difficult. Rather than expend energy to comprehend treatment options and outcomes as well as to make difficult choices, patients may withdraw from the process and ask the dentist to make treatment decisions for them. When the patient refuses to take responsibility for giving informed consent, the dentist should attempt to understand why this is so and to allay unrealistic fears compassionately through education.

CASE 3

Agnes Alice Suggs, age 15, is brought to the dental office by her mother and her grandmother. According to the grandmother, Ms. Hendry, the child has been complaining of a toothache in her lower jaw for several weeks, and today the pain has become unbearable. The grandmother tells Betty, the receptionist, with a wink that she wishes to have the dentist "fix the tooth so it will stop hurting."

While the grandmother is talking to Betty, Agnes Alice's mother, Elvira, a very obese woman in a flowered sack dress that has seen better days, takes a chair in the waiting room, stares at the floor, and says nothing. Meanwhile, Agnes Alice, the left side of her face obviously swollen, begins an anxious tour of the waiting room as if conducting a hurried last-minute search for something threatening or evil.

Obviously in charge, Ms. Hendry accepts the history forms from the receptionist and, sitting next to the mother, reads and completes them. She is neatly dressed in clean, faded blue jeans and a sweatshirt that tells the world, in bright pink block letters, "World's No. 1 Grandmother." Elvira, the young woman's mother, continues to stare at the floor.

Agnes Alice, neat and clean in appearance like her grandmother, also wears faded blue jeans, hers fitting considerably more snugly, and a cut-off sweatshirt that proclaims "Born to Be Wild." She stands before her mother, her whirlwind inspection completed. She announces, with tears streaming down her face, "I ain't takin' no shot. Hear?" Neither the mother nor the grandmother responds.

After checking over the history forms, Betty asks Ms. Hendry in a confidential voice if she is the child's legal guardian. She tells the receptionist she is not. "I am the Lord's guardian of her," she announces loudly enough for everyone in the waiting room to hear. "Look at that woman," she complains, "she ain't got enough sense to be a guardian to a rabbit. If she had any, she wouldn'ta had this here love child in the first place, not sure who the father is or nothing."

Betty excuses herself to find Dr. David Barnes and describes to him the recent events in the waiting room. Dr. Barnes tells his receptionist to escort the family to his private office.

In the privacy of his office, he asks the mother, who is looking down and drooling on her dirty white sneakers, if she is Agnes Alice's mother and legal guardian and if she understands what is going on. Not looking up, the mother tells the dentist that it doesn't matter.

"It's her jaw what hurts, it's what her wants, not what me want," Elvira mumbles.

"I ain't takin' no shot. Hear?" Agnes Alice pipes in, holding her jaw.

"See," Ms. Hendry points out to the dentist, "I told you she ain't got no sense." There is a distinct odor of alcohol on the older woman's breath.

Dr. Barnes asks Ms. Hendry if Elvira has been found to be legally incompetent. The grandmother explains that she has purposely avoided courts since she helped birth Agnes Alice in their own home "to stay clear of them prying social workers" in the hospital. She feared that a judge would take Agnes Alice away from both of them and place her in a foster home. She says that, if it were not for her devotion to keeping the three of them together, "this precious child woulda been brung up by strangers."

The dentist explains to the grandmother and mother that he cannot treat the child unless the mother or a legal guardian signs the form. Otherwise, he would be in jeopardy with the law.

"You mean you're going to let this sweet child suffer?" Ms. Hendry asks in disbelief. "Listen, Doc, I'll take the responsibility. Why if it's money," she says, pulling a 100-dollar bill from her pocket and putting it on Dr. Barnes desk, "take this, and if it ain't enough, I'll get more. There ain't nothing I wouldn't do for this love child."

"It's her jaw what hurts," Elvira repeats, "it's what her wants, not what me want."

"I ain't takin' no shot, you jackass." Agnes Alice snarls.

This case raises several issues regarding informed consent. In addition to the problem of managing an uncooperative, hostile adolescent in apparent pain, each of the three individuals presents characteristics associated with lack of decisional capacity to give informed consent. The identified patient is a minor, the mother appears to be mentally incapacitated, and the grandmother may be decisionally impaired because of alcohol consumption.

What is the dentist's responsibility to Agnes Alice? Can he ethically refuse to treat this young woman? Can any of the three females give informed consent? If not, could an exception to the informed consent doctrine be made on the basis of a dental emergency? Should the dentist attempt to determine decisional capacity for either the grandmother or the mother? What approach can he use to determine capacity? Is Agnes Alice's refusal of treatment an informed refusal? If Agnes Alice can be persuaded to consent to treatment, is the consent of a minor sufficient to proceed with treatment? What form of persuasion would be appropriate to use for Agnes Alice?

The following sections on capacity, surrogate decision making, informed refusal, and exceptions to informed consent requirements provide insight and guidance for answering these questions.

DECISION-MAKING CAPACITY

If a patient has decision-making capacity with respect to making choices about his or her health care, the patient is capable of providing an informed consent or refusal. If the patient does not have this capacity, he or she cannot provide such consent or refusal, and another person must make the relevant decisions. Decision-making capacity, then, is a threshold concept that determines the person with whom the dentist should attempt to negotiate in an effort to provide oral health care. Because it is such an important concept, it is worth exploring in detail.

First, a patient's ability to *understand* information presented by the dentist requires not only cognitive and conceptual skills, such as the ability to process information presented by the dentist about various treatment options, but imaginative skills as well.[16] That is, a patient should be able to envision to a reasonable degree what various dental conditions might be like. A patient must also be able to *communicate* this understanding, so the patient should have sufficiently developed linguistic skills and an ability to interact with the dentist by asking questions or requesting clarification. Without such ability, the dentist will be unable to determine whether the patient has adequate understanding.

The second requirement for capacity is an awareness of and stability of personal *goals and values* regarding one's health and well-being. The patient must have a conception of what is important in his or her life and how personal values affect his or her sense of well being. In addition, the values held by the patient must be relatively stable over time. A strongly expressed conviction regarding the outcome of temporomandibular joint surgery is invalid if the patient changes his or her mind on the way to the operating room.

Third, capacity also requires the ability to reach an independent decision by comparing one's goals and values with the advantages and disadvantages of the proposed treatment alternatives. This requirement implies skills in *reasoning and deliberation*. The patient must be able to rely upon short-term memory, use probability, make inferences, and reach a conclusion. In short, the process demands complex cognitive skills. Referrals to psychologists and psychiatrists for evaluation of capacity typically focus on the array of cognitive skills and operations necessary to deliberate and make a decision. For example, an overall I.Q. score is generally of little value in evaluating decision-making capacity to make a specific decision, but measures of short-term memory or the ability to make inferences (if I choose X, Y will happen) supply meaningful data regarding a patient's ability to perform the requisite cognitive tasks.

There is some debate in the literature about whether the standard for decision-making capacity should vary in accordance with the risk of the proposed treatment.[16,17] Those who argue against this view hold that the standard does not vary with risk per se. Rather, they claim, the standard varies with the complexity of the decision, and the complexity of the decision can be correlated with risk. Thus, both views might agree that a decision to use gold rather than amalgam in a simple restoration calls for a low standard of decision-making capacity, whereas a patient choosing from a variety of potentially disfiguring treatments for oral cancer should be held to a higher standard. However, proponents of a risk-related standard would attribute the difference in standards to a difference in the *level of risk*, and critics would attribute the difference in standards to a difference in the *level of understanding and reasoning* which a patient must have to make each of the two decisions.

In some situations, the two views can have different implications. Suppose, say, a tooth extraction is low-risk and will clearly benefit a demented elderly patient, and a failure to have the tooth extracted is likely to result in substantial harm to the patient. Those who favor a risk-related standard might claim that the patient has capacity if she accepts the procedure, but lacks capacity if she refuses it. Critics would hold that a decision between the two options requires a certain level of understanding and reasoning no matter which option is chosen. They would argue that it is therefore mistaken to say that the patient has decision-making capacity if she assents to the recommended low-risk option but lacks capacity if she refuses it. Whatever the outcome of this debate, however, dentists are fully capable of evaluating decision-making capacity in all but the most perplexing cases. In cases that are questionable or in which the dentist feels uncertain about capacity, it is appropriate to arrange a referral to a psychiatrist or psychologist for further evaluation or a second opinion.

Some of the most difficult situations arise when the patient appears to meet capacity requirements but proceeds to make a decision that the dentist feels is questionable or harmful. When this occurs, the dentist must review the information and explanations given the patient and be certain that a patient's questionable decision is not attributable to misinformation or incomplete information. The dentist should attempt to understand the patient's

reasoning process and the motivation for the patient's decision by asking questions like, "Help me understand how you arrived at this decision," or "What important things in your life led to your choice?" If the patient's answers reveal evidence of diminished capacity, the practitioner can choose to seek a second opinion of capacity or to seek a surrogate decision maker.

Sometimes a patient with decision-making capacity makes an irrational choice, i.e., one that is not in accordance with the patient's own values and goals.[18] The principle of respect for autonomy requires the dentist to assist the patient in understanding that the treatment the patient requests will not enable him or her to achieve stated objectives. There are limits to this principle, however, and if a patient insists on such treatment, a dentist is not ethically obligated to provide treatment that is irrational. Note that "irrational" here does not refer to a request for treatment that the dentist believes to be harmful (because this would turn on the dentist's values and preferences), but rather to a request that would not realize the patient's own values.

Surrogate Decision Making

The moral principle of respect for autonomy requires dental personnel to seek informed consent from the patient before proceeding with treatment. However, some patients are not capable or are not willing to participate in the process leading to consent. In addition to minors, adults occasionally lack the capacity to make treatment decisions for themselves. Persons in this latter category include, but are not limited to, those cognitive deficits stemming from dementing illnesses.[19] Pain, anxiety, and extreme passivity can also diminish a patient's decision-making capacity. Sometimes it is not possible to remove the obstacles to shared decision making between dentist and patient, but this does not remove the dentist's ethical responsibility to respect patient self-determination. What should a dentist in such a situation do?

When the patient is judged unable to make a treatment decision for him or herself, the introduction of third parties into the informed consent procedure becomes a necessity. The fact that the patient is unable to comprehend and appreciate the nature and necessity of treatment does not eliminate the necessity for informed consent. When the patient lacks decision-making capacity, the dentist must obtain informed consent from a surrogate decision maker. The best surrogate decision maker is one who knows the patient's values and preferences well, and this is usually, although not necessarily, the spouse, partner, parent, sibling, or child (not necessarily in that order). To avoid confusion with consent authorization by the patient, consent by a surrogate is called "proxy consent."

Sometimes a patient makes arrangements for care and decision making before losing decision-making capacity. The patient may execute an advance directive in the form of a living will, a written document specifying what kinds of treatment the patient would prefer when he or she is terminally ill or in a persistent vegetative state.[20] Another form of advance directive, the medical power of attorney, allows the patient to appoint a representative to make health care decisions for him or her when the patient loses decision-making capacity. As of this writing, most states have statutes recognizing the living will, and about half have statutes recognizing the medical power of attorney.

The ethical argument favoring advance directives most commonly rests on the position that a patient's right to self-determination does not end with the loss of decision-making capacity.[21] Wettle has observed that, although there has been a great deal of attention on advance directives in medicine, advance directives have received little attention in dentistry.[15] One reason for dentistry's lack of attention to advance directives may be the propensity of some advance directives to focus on procedures rather than on the underlying values that support decisions.[21] Directives that address the patient's preferences regarding life-sustaining treatment, such as cardiopulmonary resuscitation or artificial nutrition and hydration rarely provide guidance for dental treatment. However, if a patient makes it clear that he or she values being substantially free of pain even above having all of his or her natural teeth,

the dentist is in a better position to do for the patient what he or she would have wanted done.

Once a family member, friend, or attorney accepts the role of surrogate decision maker, two standards are available for guiding each decision in lieu of specific directives left by the patient: (A) substituted judgment, or (B) the best-interests standard. In the former, the surrogate attempts to duplicate the decision that the patient would have made had he or she been capable. Surrogates using substituted judgment rely on memories of previous conversations with the patient, or patterns of behavior suggesting what kinds of treatments the patient would have preferred. In lieu of such evidence, the surrogate is left with no choice but to consider what would be in the patient's best interest. Because the goal of proxy consent or refusal is to realize what patients would have wanted were they able to make a choice themselves, the ideal situation for the dentist is to be able to negotiate with the patient directly. For patients lacking decision-making capacity who have not left specific directives for their care, a surrogate's substituted judgment is a next-best effort to realize patient self-determination. The best-interests standard should be employed only when even a substituted judgment cannot be made.

The 1990 Patient Self-Determination Act has called attention to a movement advocating the use of advance directives. However, a 1990 study by High indicates that elderly persons tend to reject making formal advance directives regarding medical care and prefer instead to rely on informal methods of substitute decision making by trusted family members.[22] High reported that his subjects had some aversion to and procrastination about writing directives and formally appointing proxies. They preferred the use of informal arrangements with family members to make decisions for them. In addition, High's studies provide evidence showing that elderly persons may prefer the more paternalistic best interests standard to substituted judgment. As awareness is raised regarding the benefits of advance directives and appointment of proxies, public support for these documents may increase.

Minors

Children and youth under age 18 have traditionally been considered unable to play a major role in treatment decision making. Exceptions have generally included medical treatment for substance abuse or sexually related problems, medical conditions that may go untreated if young people are required to inform their parents. Additional exceptions are made if the person under 18 is married, a parent, or presents other evidence of social and financial independence.

Many children of school age have sufficient linguistic capacity to provide informed consent. According to Piaget's theories of cognitive development, most adolescents aged 14 to 16 have developed complex cognitive skills such as the ability to reason deductively and to weigh various treatment alternatives.[23] However, the development of stable aims and values may not occur until late adolescence or early adulthood, and the capacity to make some treatment decisions requires the ability to reach an accord between future consequences of current treatment and values that may change in the intervening years. In summary, value instability can be a serious handicap when minors wish to make informed choices. Decision-making capacity issues should be raised when a minor makes treatment choices that would produce questionable long-term results.

Although the practitioner may wish to honor the principle of respect for persons and allow minors with sufficiently developed cognitive skills to make treatment decisions, it must be remembered that most minors are not truly autonomous. They are not able to choose freely because they are subject to the outside influence of parents. Parents exert strong influence, particularly when financial considerations affect treatment choice. Even if an adolescent with decision-making capacity is sufficiently liberated from parental influence to express views contrary to those of the parents, the parents' obligation to finance the treatment typically limits adolescent autonomy. Dentists should take advantage of every opportunity to appropriately engage all minors in discussions of treatment. Each such positive doctor-patient interaction strengthens the relationship, provides patient education, and fosters the skills necessary for future opportunities to give informed consent.

INFORMED REFUSAL

Discussions of informed consent rarely address the topic of informed refusal. However, an acceptance of the principle of respect for patient autonomy requires the practitioner to respect the patient choices that are contrary to the practitioner's recommendations. Both informed consent and informed refusal are based on the ethical principle of respect for autonomy. Respecting patients' right to self-determination sometimes means allowing the patient to refuse to have a procedure performed, even if the dentist believes that the procedure would be in the patient's best interest.

Practitioners should not view refusal as a personal affront or an indication of lack of respect or trust. Neither should dentists take the position that an informed refusal is license for the professional to abrogate responsibility for the patient. Keeping in mind that the practitioner is never obligated to provide treatment that he or she judges inadequate or inferior, the dentist nevertheless must enter the process of shared decision making with the knowledge that patients do not always agree with the practitioner. Applebaum et al. note that autonomy does not mean doing whatever one might want to do, and that patients' rights to make medical decisions should not be thought of as allowing patients to have whatever medical care they wish.[24]

Rosoff reminds us that the refusal of patients with decision-making capacity must be honored whether the refusal is based on doubts that the proposed procedure will be successful, a concern about the results of the procedure, a lack of confidence in the provider, a religious belief, or even a mere whim.[25] One might argue that a dentist is within his or her rights to accept a patient's refusal, properly document the decision, and make no further effort to pursue the matter. However, refusals usually raise some of the same questions generated when patient decision-making capacity is questioned. In fact, patient decision-making capacity is rarely questioned when the patient gives informed consent, but is questioned frequently when the patient refuses to give informed consent!

When a patient refuses a procedure that the dentist believes is beneficial, several questions should be considered: Was the dentist's explanation complete and clearly given in language the patient could understand? Did the patient have adequate time to ask questions and evaluate the consequences of treatment and nontreatment? Is the patient withholding information, e.g., financial considerations, that affects the decision? Most importantly, why is the patient refusing the treatment? Dentists have an ethical obligation to review the process of obtaining informed consent and eliminate any questions that jeopardize its legitimacy. A careful review of the process that stimulates dialogue and eliminates misunderstanding by either practitioner or patient typically leads to a treatment decision that is acceptable to both participants in the process, or in other words, a truly shared decision that respects the patient's needs, values, and especially his or her autonomy.

EXCEPTIONS TO INFORMED CONSENT REQUIREMENTS

An emergency situation, one in which there is imminent danger of irreparable harm or loss of life to a patient without decision-making capacity (e.g., a patient who is unconscious, a minor, or experiencing delirium tremens), is the major exception to the necessity for obtaining informed consent before treatment. Even in an emergency, reasonable attempts should be made to obtain consent from an appropriate surrogate.

Therapeutic privilege is another traditional justification for not obtaining consent. The concept of therapeutic privilege is based on a belief that, in rare circumstances, disclosure can be contraindicated for medical reasons. As an illustration, psychological damage is one of the contraindications traditionally identified as a justification for overriding consent requirements. However, therapeutic privilege is a paternalistic notion with significant potential for abuse, and its use is properly and strongly contested.

The bioethics literature occasionally lists one additional exception to the requirement that dentists must obtain informed consent.[14,26] Practitioners occasionally encounter patients who have, for one reason or another, a strong aversion to hearing the details regarding proposed dental treatment. A practitioner cannot force a patient to listen to the information required to give informed consent. Although some ethicists disagree, a dentist may use discretion regarding whether or not to treat an uninformed patient under these circumstances. Some authors contend that a health care provider has no obligation to pursue the matter if a patient expresses the desire not to be informed.[14,26] It must be remembered that dentists have no moral duty, except in emergencies, to treat patients who have not given an informed consent.[27]

The issue of the patient who is too passive to give informed consent or who prefers to avoid hearing information necessary for giving valid consent can generally be avoided through development of a constructive, trusting doctor-patient relationship. As mentioned previously in this chapter, a request for informed consent should never come as a surprise. It should be the culmination of one or more discussions in which the patient is actively engaged. The dentist who makes a conscious effort to make patient education part of every dental visit and who elicits patient questions and concerns rarely encounters a patient who insists on making uninformed treatment choices.

When all efforts to engage a patient in the decision-making process fail, the dentist must make a decision to treat the patient, to insist on a surrogate decision maker, or to refuse treatment. The decision should be based, in part, on the potential risks of harm if the proposed treatment is either completed or denied. For example, a treatment accompanied by high risk of harm should not be delivered without consent by a surrogate. On the other hand, a treatment with little risk of harm may be performed at the dentist's discretion.

CONCLUSION

The paternalistic notion that the doctor has not only a right, but an obligation, to make all treatment decisions has been rejected by the dental profession. It has been replaced with a standard of care based on the moral principle of respect for patient autonomy. The slow but certain movement from reliance on a paternalistic model of treatment decision making to a model based on patient autonomy has been observed during the past two decades. Most ethicists would agree that the informed consent approach to treatment choice is now the standard in both bioethical and dental literature.

Implementation of the shared decision-making process and obtaining informed consent or refusal from each patient requires many dentists to relinquish a long held commitment to paternalistic decision making. It also requires both willingness to spend the time necessary to engage in shared decision making and willingness to develop the requisite communication skills. Awareness and acceptance of the moral importance of informed consent has steadily grown during the past two decades.

The dental profession has much to gain from granting patients greater autonomy in making treatment decisions. First, practitioners and the profession can receive gratification from adhering to the highest standards of ethical conduct. Second, the individual practitioner and the profession profit from an enhanced image based on demonstrated respect for patients. Third, although shared decision making can be time-consuming, many practitioners find person satisfaction and fulfillment through engaging in more meaningful interaction with patients. Fourth, patients typically appreciate the opportunity to develop a positive doctor-patient relationship and to make their own decisions. Fifth, it has been proposed that shared decision making fosters patient loyalty to a practitioner and reduces the probability of litigation. Finally, practitioners are relieved of the burdensome responsibility of making difficult treatment choices for patients. Implementing the patient autonomy model requires the dentist to assist others in making the difficult choices, and not assume total responsibility.

In summary, not only is obtaining informed consent consistent with practicing dentistry according to the highest ethical standards, but implementing the shared decision-making process in the operatory can generate beneficial results for both practitioners and patients.

CASE FOR DISCUSSION

Is it possible for the dentist to obtain an informed consent in the following case? Why or why not? What could be done to facilitate the process?

Bonita Graham, a 28-year-old legal secretary, learns to her dismay at the conclusion of her regular annual dental recall appointment that she has "developed cavities," her first, on the occlusal surfaces of the left maxillary and mandibular molars. Although dismayed, she is not surprised. Since she quit smoking about 16 months earlier, she had developed the habit of holding a lemon drop between the two teeth while preparing correspondence or taking dictation. Furthermore, she had recently experienced some sensitivity in the mandibular tooth when it came in contact with the candy.

Dr. Delgado carefully explains to her the necessity of removing the decay, as well as the process, and the need to restore the resultant preparation. He tells her that there are three restorative materials from which to choose: silver amalgam, cast gold, and a composite resin material. He discusses the three materials, attempting to point out the advantages and disadvantages of each.

He tells her that the resin restorations would be tooth-colored but that the extent of the preparations following the removal of the decay would place the margins of the restorations under the heavy cusps of the opposing teeth, possibly leading to a failure of the restoration at its margins. Gold restorations, although not tooth-colored, would withstand the forces of the opposing teeth. However, one-surface gold inlays are often difficult to retain, and may be dislodged by sticky foods. Amalgam restorations, although not tooth-colored, would resist chewing forces and not be dislodged. Amalgam would be his choice.

Without hesitation, Ms. Graham said, "Gold sounds expensive, so I want the resin."

Dr. Delgado was perplexed at the quick decision as well as the rejection of his recommendation. Ms. Graham appeared to be making an informed refusal of preferred treatment.

Rather than proceed with her choice, the dentist asked, "What factors led to your decision to rule out the amalgam?"

Ms. Graham quietly answered, "My sister has multiple sclerosis, and I don't want it too."

Dr. Delgado asked her to explain what she meant. "Isn't amalgam that mercury stuff that they said causes multiple sclerosis and arthritis on the '60 Minutes' show?" she asks.

"Yes," he says, "that's the material they bashed."

"Well, then," she declares, "I don't want that. I want the tooth-colored material instead."

"So you fell for that '60 Minutes' stuff too. Why, the scientists shot that nonsense down; there are a number of studies that show that silver amalgam is safe; they had a big national conference last summer and said amalgam was safe. It was in the newspapers."

Ms. Graham looked embarrassed, and apologized to the dentist.

"No need for apologies. That report needlessly upset a lot of folks, and you have special reason to worry. Why don't I give you some articles to read about mercury amalgam, and we'll reschedule your appointment so you can think about your decision."

DISCUSSION QUESTIONS

1. Write a brief case scenario and indicate whether informed consent has been given. Review each of the elements of informed consent to demonstrate how you arrived at your conclusion.

2. Dr. Newsome is at a local dental society meeting where the issues of patients' rights and informed consent are being discussed. Dr. Newsome becomes incensed and argues that the patients don't have all the rights, and that she refuses to abdicate her responsibilities to patients by letting them make treatment decisions. "After all," she says, "it is the dentist who has the knowledge and skill to make treatment decisions." You are one of Dr. Newsome's dental colleagues. How would you respond to her argument?

3. Write a dental case situation in which the patient's capacity to make a decision is in question. Using criteria identified in this chapter, analyze your case in a manner that will allow you to determine the patient's "capacity," and the actions you would take based on your decision.

4. Under what conditions is it appropriate for a surrogate decision maker to become involved in the dental treatment process? Explain the "best interests" standard and the "substituted judgment" standard for surrogate decision making.

ACKNOWLEDGMENT

The authors wish to thank Mark R. Wicclair for his kind contribution to this chapter.

REFERENCES

1. Beauchamp, T.L., and Childress, J.: Principles of Biomedical Ethics. Third edition. New York, Oxford University Press, 1983.
2. Odom, J.G., and Morris, W.O.: The autonomy of the practitioner. J. Dent. Pract. Admin. 6:12, 1989.
3. Graber, G.C., Beasley, A.D., and Eaddy, J.A.: Ethical Analysis of Clinical Medicine. Baltimore, Urban and Schwarzenberg, 1985.
4. Faden, R.R., and Beauchamp, T.L.: A History and Theory of Informed Consent. New York: Oxford University Press, 1986.
5. Odom, J.G.: Formal ethics instruction in dental education. J. Dent. Educ. 46:553, 1982.
6. Wittemann, J., and Odom, J.: Current Research On/In Dental Behavioral Sciences. Presented at the Annual Meeting of the American Psychological Association, September, 1976.
7. Odom, J.G., and Messina, M.: Treatment decision making: student choices of autonomy versus paternalism. J. Law. Ethics Dent. 4:12, 1991.
8. Beauchamp, T.L.: Informed consent. In Medical Ethics. Edited by Robert M. Veatch. Boston, Jones and Bartlett, 1991.

9. Lo, B. Assessing decision-making capacity. Law, Medicine and Health Care *18*:193, 1990.
10. President's Commission for the Study of Ethical Problems in Biomedical and Behavioral Research: Making Health Care Decisions: The Ethical and Legal Implications of Informed Consent in the Patient-Practitioner Relationship. Washington, Government Printing Office, 1982. Quotation appears on p. 57.
11. American Dental Association: Principles of ethics and code of professional conduct. J. Am. Dent. Assoc. *120*:588, 1990.
12. *Canterbury v. Spence.* 464 F.2nd:783,784 (D.C.Circuit 1972).
13. Bailey, B.L.: Informed consent in dentistry. J. Am. Dent. Assoc. *110*:709, 1985.
14. Culver, C.M., and Gert, B.: Ethical issues in oncology. Psych. Med. *5*:389, 1987.
15. Wettle, T.: Ethical issues in geriatric dentistry. Gerodontology *6*:73, 1987.
16. Wicclair, M.R. Patient decision-making capacity and risk. Bioethics *5*:91, 1991.
17. Brock, D.W., and Buchanan, A.E. Deciding for Others: The Ethics of Surrogate Decision Making. Cambridge, Cambridge University Press, 1989.
18. Brock, D.W., and Wartman, S.A. When competent patients make irrational choices. N. Engl. J. Med. *322*:1595, 1990.
19. Shuman, S.K.: Ethics and the patient with dementia. J. Am. Dent. Assoc. *119*:747, 1989.
20. Annas, G.J. The health care proxy and the living will. N. Engl. J. Med. *324*:1210, 1991.
21. Tupper, E.: Advance directives and the patient self-determination act. SHHV Student Bulletin *2*:2, 1991.
22. High, D.M.: Who will make health care decisions for me when I can't? J. Aging Health *2*:291, 1990.
23. Rosen, H.: The Development of Sociomoral Knowledge: A Cognitive-Structural Approach. New York, Columbia University Press, 1980.
24. Applebaum, P.S., Lidz, C.W., and Meisel, J.D.: Informed Consent: Legal Theory and Clinical Practice. New York, Oxford University Press, 1987.
25. Rosoff, A.J.: Informed Consent: A Guide for Health Care Providers. Rockville, MD, Aspen Systems Corporation, 1981.
26. Hirsch, A.C., and Gert, B.: Ethics in dental practice. J. Am. Dent. Assoc. *113*:599, 1986.
27. Foley, H.T., and Dornette, W.H.: Consent and informed consent. *In* Dornett's Legal Issues in Anesthesia Practice. Philadelphia, F.A. Davis Company, 1991.

Chapter 6

HIV Infection in Dentistry: Ethical and Legal Issues

Gordon G. Keyes
Mary Ellen Waithe

SUMMARY

This chapter discusses the core ethical and legal issues presented by HIV infection in the clinical-dental setting. The discussion is organized around two central moral viewpoints in the dentist-patient relationship: first, professional obligations and responses to the (potentially) HIV-infected dental patient; and second, the responsibilities of (potentially) HIV-infected dentists to their patients. In several respects, the chapter builds on the analyses of other ethical and legal concepts that play a role in the dentist-patient relationship. These include the principles of respect for autonomy, beneficence, nonmaleficence, and care, and rules regarding informed consent, confidentiality, and truth-telling. These rules and principles are discussed in the specific context of HIV infection.

Here, more perhaps than in any area of dental ethics, the dentist must look to a range of sources for guidance concerning his or her professional rights and responsibilities. Ethical standards have been set by organized medicine through codes of professional associations (such as the ADA) and by policy statements of state medical and dental societies. These standards, codes and policies partly reflect and partly interpret and apply the aforementioned principles and duties in the context of professional practice. The Centers for Disease Control have taken a very proactive stance on both infection control procedures and HIV testing, issuing a number of recommended guidelines. The past decade has also seen rapid growth in the law's response to the acquired immune deficiency syndrome (AIDS) epidemic. Increasingly, statutes have been enacted and regulations adopted (primarily at the state level) to govern such questions as HIV reporting, confidentiality, warning of third parties, and the use of infection control procedures. Several state licensing boards have adopted formal standards for professional conduct which carry the force of law. The courts have provided considerable guidance in a myriad of judicial opinions rendered over the years. Thus, both statutory and case law partially reflect and interpret ethical principles and duties in the context of professional practice. Additionally, more basic constitutional principles, such as the right to privacy, may be articulated in the context of health care and provide the foundation for expanding the application of moral principles such as autonomy.

It is important to recognize here that the law and professional codes set only minimum standards of professional conduct. Health care professionals who fail to meet these standards risk not only lawsuits from patients, but also professional discipline and possible loss of license and employment. At the same time, it should be emphasized that in determining a health care professional's legal duty of care, courts often look to professional codes and statements of professional associations as evidence of the customary and accepted standard to which professionals should be held.[1] Moreover, legal and ethical principles articulated in nonmedical areas of law are subject to application in medical areas. Thus, for example, the recognition of a constitutional right to privacy in birth control had its origin in dissenting opinions to cases affecting fishing and meat-packing in the 1800s![2] Cases such as *Tarasoff v. Regents of University of California* explored the relationship between the duties to protect patient confidentiality and to prevent harm to others. Dental professionals should seek to remain informed, on a continuing basis, of professional code and legal developments at the state and national levels, as well as of philosophical analyses of professional ethics issues in what most certainly will be a rapidly evolving area. The analysis here draws upon these various sources to present an ethical and legal perspective on issues surrounding HIV-infection in dentistry. The discussion stresses key issues and emerging consensus, but is not intended to compass the current landscape of legal developments or professional statements.

HIV INFECTION IN DENTISTRY

The first decade of the AIDS epidemic has transformed our health care system. The HIV virus (first identified in 1983 under a different name), which causes a spectrum of illnesses that terminate in AIDS, raises new and critical challenges for the health care professions, policy makers and the public. Of the many questions we now confront, perhaps the greatest professional and public concerns in recent years have focused on medical, ethical, legal, and public health responses to the possibility of transmission of HIV infection in the clinical setting.

Concerns for patient safety when undergoing treatment by an HIV-positive physician or dentist were first raised in a meaningful way in the literature in 1988.[3,4] Previously, thoughts that the patient could acquire HIV from an infected surgeon or dentist were not generally taken seriously. Neither the American Dental Association (ADA) nor the American Association of Dental Schools felt it necessary to adopt a definite position on whether or not HIV-positive dentists or dental students should perform invasive procedures. The common wisdom in the late 1980s was that the risk of disease transmission from doctor to patient was either too remote to warrant consideration or that there was no risk at all. In contrast, there was considerable discussion at that time about the probability that a dentist could acquire HIV from an infected patient in the course of providing care. Although the professional literature during this period discussed why simultaneous denial of the risk of transmission from dentist to patient was illogical,[5] there was no significant discussion in the lay press about HIV transmission from doctor to patient.

Universal Precautions and Exposure-Prone Procedures

Fear of acquiring HIV disease emerged among dental practitioners as soon as the viral etiology and mode of transmission of the disease was understood.[6] Because blood was the primary body fluid that could potentially transmit infection in the health care setting, the fear issue focused not only on surgeons and dentists, but also with paramedics and others exposed to blood.[7] The call for HIV testing of patients, especially patients undergoing major surgery, has not gone away because some doctors feel that they will be extra careful if they know the patient is HIV-positive. The efficacy, from a safety point of view, of this attitude has not been established. In dentistry, a spectrum of methods was suggested, intended to aid the practitioner's determination of when universal precautions guidelines issued by the Centers for Disease Control in 1983 should be followed.[7] These guidelines for infection control were reiterated specifically for dental practice by the U.S. Department of Health and Human Services in 1986,[8] and again in 1987 by the Centers for Disease Control for use with all patients.[9] The guidelines were called "Universal Precautions." Universal precautions call, at a minimum, for the use of gloves, masks, and protective eyewear, for the sterilization of instruments and intraoral devices, and for disinfection of surfaces in the dental operatory. Use of fluid-resistant gowns is suggested, but not mandated, for dental procedures. These recommendations were current as of early 1992, but may be amended at any time. The CDC guidelines are now widely accepted throughout dental practice; however, their utilization is to be credited in part to the Occupational Safety and Health Act. The Occupational Safety and Health Administration (OSHA) has the authority to enforce the use of universal precautions in any dental office in which there is a nonproprietary employee.

Before the detection in 1984 of HIV in saliva,[10] universal precautions were called for only when exposure to blood, semen, or vaginal secretions was possible.[11] The original precautions did not apply to saliva per se, because the titre of HIV in saliva is so low.[12] These precautions were, nevertheless, recommended for dental procedures because saliva is often mixed with nearly undetectable amounts of blood.[9] Generally speaking, universal precautions were advocated for any dental procedure, whether or not it was invasive. Because contact with saliva was almost inevitable in dental practice, the invasiveness of the procedure was not the triggering consideration in dentistry as it was in medical practice.

THE DUTY TO TREAT

Does the dentist, by virtue of his or her role as a health care professional, have a duty to treat a patient with AIDS or HIV infection? Conversely, does the dentist have the right to refuse to treat a patient on the ground of the patient's HIV status? The fundamental question of the duty to treat may be framed as a question of a legal right to treatment, as a question of the interpretation of the requirements of professional codes enunciating a duty to treat, or as a question about the philosophical foundation of those duties addressed by laws, judicial decisions and professional codes.

The Legal Right to Receive Dental Care

In the early years of the AIDS epidemic, it was widely debated whether or not those who were HIV-positive enjoyed the protection of state or federal antidiscrimination laws. They would be protected by antidiscrimination laws if AIDS or the HIV-positive condition were considered a handicap. The Rehabilitation Act of 1973 was the major federal legislation that protected the rights of the handicapped.[13] It applied only to employers or institutions that contract with the federal government or have received federal funding. The Supreme Court decision of *School Board of Nassau County v. Arline* made it clear that infectious disease could be a handicapping condition under the Rehabilitation Act.[14] After this decision, lower federal courts were more explicit in stating that the various stages of HIV infection qualified as handicapping conditions and, thus, those infected had some measure of protection from discrimination, including denial of medical care.[15]

In the years since the *Arline* decision, significant protection of the rights of HIV-positive persons has developed at the state level. All states have antidiscrimination laws that are similar to the Rehabilitation Act.[16] Thus, denial of dental or medical care can result in lawsuits in state courts if the state recognized AIDS as a handicapping condition. Some states have done this through statutory amendment or court decision.[17] In addition, some states have passed laws that specifically make it unlawful to deny medical and dental care to those infected with HIV.[18]

On July 26, 1990, the Americans with Disabilities Act was signed into law.[19] This additional federal source of law is very similar to the Rehabilitation Act. The Act also affords protection from discrimination for those who are HIV-positive. Unlike the Rehabilitation Act, however, the Americans with Disabilities Act applies to private employers. Thus, private dental offices, whether or not they receive federal funds, come into the sweep of this new federal antidiscrimination law. It goes a long way toward filling the gaps in protections offered under the Rehabilitation Act. Many millions of disabled (HIV-positive) individuals who would not be protected by the Rehabilitation Act are covered by the Americans with Disabilities Act. The broad body of federal and state law leaves no doubt about the legal obligations to provide health care to HIV-positive patients. As compelling as these laws are, it is equally important to know of the ethical mandates promulgated by the various health profession organizations.

Although some early statements of professional organizations were equivocal, and others were slow to respond, many health care professional groups, including for example the American Medical Association, the American Dental Association, the CDC, and numerous commentators, now stand firmly behind the principle that health care professionals have a duty to treat patients with AIDS or HIV infection, and that patients should not be denied care solely on the basis of their HIV status. As stated in the ADA Code, Advisory Opinion on Patient Selection:

> A dentist has the general obligation to provide care to those in need. A decision not to provide treatment to an individual because the individual has AIDS or is HIV seropositive, based solely on the fact, is unethical. Decisions with regard to the type of dental treatment provided or referrals made or suggested, in such instances, should be made on the same basis as they are made with other patients, that is, whether the individual dentist believes he or she has the need of another's skills, knowledge, equipment or experience and whether the dentist believes, after consultation with the patient's physician if appropriate, the patient's health status would be significantly compromised by the provision of dental treatment.[20]

The American Dental Association's Principles of Ethics makes it clear that dentists have an ethical obligation to treat AIDS patients.[21] Some states have codes of ethics that are similar to the ADA's, and failure to abide by such ethical codes may lead to license revocation by state dental boards. This may be more costly to the dentist than the monetary damages incurred from violation of federal or state laws.

Today, there is no question that both laws and codes affirm that dentists have a duty to treat HIV-positive patients. Although this duty is understood, it is accepted with reluctance by many dentists and other health care practitioners who honestly question whether this is an absolute or only a *prima facie* duty. (We review this distinction shortly.) There appears to be a widespread assumption among professionals that professional behavior is ethical if it is not expressly contravened by a code of ethics or by law. We do not know where this assumption originates, but it appears to be based on a view that a law or a code of ethics is the *source* of an ethical duty, rather than a sometimes confusing and usually incomplete report of consensus among practitioners. Codes tend to be treated by practitioners as though they were a list of regulations; indeed the provisions of a code are often written that way. But ethical duties are derived from ethical principles and values that are inherent in the values of the profession, in the system of law, and in the society itself. The natural tendency to treat a code as a "laundry list" of "no-no's" rather than as a description of values and principles to which the profession is committed often leads practitioners to engage in superficial analysis of the nature of their ethical obligations. It is important therefore to recognize the interrelatedness of laws governing professional practice, professional association codes of ethics, and the philosophical foundations of professional ethics. One might consider, therefore, whether the legal duty to treat is a case of bad law, and whether the professional code obligation to treat is a misguided echo of bad law. One might also ask whether both law and code turn out to be inconsistent with the very philosophical principles they are intended to apply and interpret.

Many practitioners honestly inquire: when a conflict of duty arises between the duty to treat and the right to preserve one's own health and life, which, morally speaking, is the more compelling? Ultimately, the sources of ethical obligations are the general ethical principles and values that at once form the foundations of constitutional law and codes of professional responsibility. What is important to recognize is that laws and codes not only have common sources in ethical principles like freedom, justice, and self-determination, but at best, laws and codes reflect formal interpretations and applications of those principles in response to concrete historical situations. Thus, the Civil Rights Act reflected an application and interpretation of principles of freedom and justice in response to growing public outcry against inherently oppressive and unjust conditions. Likewise, the Patient Self-Determination Act reflects a response of law to growing public concern that the health care community ignores choices to forego treatment made by autonomous, competent, but dying adults. An understanding of moral principles and their potential interpretation and application in clinical situations helps professionals make morally defensible decisions in hard cases in which law and professional codes have not yet addressed the ethical issues, or have inadequately addressed them. Principles such as justice require that individuals obey just laws and meet their contractual obligations, including obligations to keep their promises. In a society in which individuals are free to choose their professional affiliations, and in which through licensure and other requirements, states protect the welfare of the public, licensed practitioners have a *prima facie* duty to obey licensing laws. (*Prima facie* means "at first glance," and as authors of previous chapters have noted, someone who has a *prima facie* duty to do something must so act unless there are overriding, serious, compelling moral reasons not to do so.) When a duty is freely chosen, self-interest is rarely acknowledged as an overriding, serious, compelling moral reason for failing to meet one's duty. In addition, there is a *prima facie* duty to fulfill the legitimate expectations of the society regarding professional practice. Traditionally and historically, at least since the third century B.C.,[22] this has included a duty to provide care for a patient in need. The practitioner may be excused from that duty when the practitioner is disabled, when there is a conflicting duty to care for someone in greater need, when the professional lacks particular expertise and arrangements have been made for another to provide more expert care, and

perhaps in other circumstances. The duty, therefore, is not absolute, but is a *prima facie* duty. However, given the requirements of justice and the purely voluntary nature of professional practice, it appears that there are few morally defensible reasons for refusing to treat. Particularly when it is considered in light of the precautions discussed earlier in this chapter for reducing risk of transmission of HIV, the decision to become or to remain a member of the health care professions appears to incur a duty to treat.

This question was most articulately addressed by Emanuel,[23] who based his conclusions on an analysis of the doctor-patient relationship as a professional rather than a commercial relationship:

> The objective of a commercial enterprise is the pursuit of wealth; the objective of the medical profession is devotion to a moral ideal—in particular, healing the sick and rendering the ill healthy and well.... When a person joins the profession, he or she professes a commitment to these ideals and accepts the obligation to serve the sick. It is the profession that is chosen. The obligation is neither chosen or transferable; it is constitutive of the professional activity.[23]

Emanuel recites some familiar exceptions to this obligation: lack of expertise and excessive patient load (excepting emergency care). Further,

> In fulfilling the obligation to treat persons with AIDS, physicians are expected to accept some personal risk, since risk is in the nature of work with sick people who have communicable diseases ... such as hepatitis and tuberculosis.... In this respect, medicine is no different from other occupations in which one is expected to accept some personal risk in pursuit of one's aim.... Taking such risks is part of joining the profession and affirming its objective to help the needy.[23]

The "ordinary risk" that a doctor faces of contracting a communicable disease is greater than the "ordinary risk" faced by patients that they will contract a communicable disease in the normal course of events. The doctor's "ordinary risk" then is greater than the usual "ordinary risk." Emanuel explores the *prima facie* nature of of the duty to treat and how that duty is limited when there is excessive risk of death to the professional. Excessive risk must therefore be understood not merely as greater than the ordinary patient's "ordinary risk," but as greater than the ordinary doctor's "ordinary risk." After identifying the risk of death in the course of the practice of medical specialties (12% per year for orthopedic surgeons serving a patient population at San Francisco General Hospital believed to be at high risk for HIV seropositivity; 1% per year for Emergency Department Surgeons; 0.5% per year for internists), Emanuel compares those risk levels to the (relatively low) risk of death in other dangerous professions such as firefighting (0.2 to 0.5% per year) and to the (comparatively high) risk of those serving in the military during wartime (under 3% during the Vietnam War). He concludes that:

> The risk [1% per year] taken by surgeons in the emergency department is high and probably bordering on the excessive.[23]

Lesser risks, particularly those equivalent to other known risk professions such as firefighting, must be considered usual, nonexcessive risks. Practitioners who are not at excessive risk for contracting HIV (for example, internists) voluntarily assume as a duty, in consequence of joining the profession, a specific obligation to care for patients with AIDS. Competing duties to other patients or to the practitioner's family members do not override this duty in the absence of excessive risks: "Identifying competing duties does not itself determine which one has a greater claim."[23]

What if some practitioners refuse to provide care to those in need? John Arras argues that, in our society, there is not a two-tiered health care profession, one tier consisting of practitioners committed to treating the sick and another consisting of those committed to treating only patients who pose less than the ordinary risk to the practitioner. All practitioners enter into the same social contract with society and assume a duty to treat. Exempting oneself from that duty violates the very nature of the contract with society that was voluntarily entered into by the professional.

Furthermore, Arras argues, it places an unfair burden on one's colleagues:

> . . . a duty to treat one's colleagues fairly will prove that exempting oneself from treating HIV patients will only increase the burden on others who are willing to do so, increasing their risk.[24]

Confidentiality

There is an inherent conflict between patients' interests in confidentiality and the public's interest in protection from infectious diseases. On the one hand, HIV-positive individuals risk discrimination in such fundamental areas of life as employment, housing, and insurance coverage, as well as social stigmatization, with disclosure of HIV-positive status. This is particularly true of those in known high-risk groups, such as gay men and intravenous drug users. On the other hand, disclosure of HIV status in statistical form is essential to the public's interest in epidemiologic study of the disease, whereas disclosure of named HIV positive patients makes possible contact tracing and partner notification by public health authorities and caregivers. Inadequate confidentiality protections threaten to discourage HIV-infected individuals from early presentation to the health care system for testing, treatment, and care. This contributes not only to the spread of the disease but also to morbidity and mortality in already infected but undiagnosed patients. As with the duty to treat, the duty to respect patient confidentiality is reflected in law and professional codes, and has its foundations in moral theory.

Maintaining appropriate confidentiality of patient information is a well-established legal duty grounded in the fiduciary nature of the health care professional-patient relationship. Legislation has been adopted nationwide to govern confidentiality, disclosure, and other issues relating to AIDS and HIV information.[25] These statutes interpret the moral duty of confidentiality in light of competing principles of justice, beneficence, and protection of third parties from harm. Thus, they address specific questions such as reporting of known or suspected AIDS cases to public health authorities. In many states, legislative enactments allow (but do not require) a dentist to warn third parties.[26] In some states, statutes and/or case law impose a duty to warn third parties of potential harm. *Tarasoff v. Regents of University of California* provides the framework for this duty.[27] In this case, the California Supreme Court held a psychotherapist liable for failing to warn a named third party (a woman who had dated a student who was in therapy) of death threats made by a patient. Once the doctor had reason to believe that a particular third party was at risk of harm by the actions of his or her patient, the duty to warn arose. The *Tarasoff* principle has the force of legal precedent in only a few states. However, the *Tarasoff* case articulated the way in which conflicts between duties of confidentiality and protecting the lives of third parties was to be resolved by health care providers. Therefore it may at any time become law in other states through statutory enactment or judicial decision.

Professional codes also identify a duty of confidentiality. As articulated in the ADA Code, "[d]entists are obligated to safeguard the confidentiality of patient records."[28] Similar rules of confidentiality (sometimes more expansively stated) are shared by the spectrum of health care professions as a core duty of the professional-patient relationship. From the patient's point of view, he or she has a right to expect, when entering into a dentist-patient relationship, that information revealed or knowledge obtained in the context of that relationship will be held in confidence. (As discussed subsequently, there are some important exceptions to this rule.)

Both legal and professional code-based duties of confidentiality have their foundation in philosophical traditions. Duties of confidentiality rest on the principle of respect for patient autonomy, especially as autonomy relates to privacy or control of personal information. Virtue-based and duty-based moral philosophies hold that it is important to fulfill one's promises. They have, as a consequence, the view that fidelity to the promise of confidentiality, whether implicit or explicit, is inherent in the forming of a dentist-patient relationship. Absent assurance that dentists can be trusted not to reveal certain personal information to others, patients would likely be reluctant to fully disclose relevant information about their medical condition, personal behaviors and concerns, thereby compromising the dentist's ability to render needed care.[29] Despite antidiscrimination laws, disclosure of a positive HIV test result to third parties may have morally indefensible consequences. For a patient, disclosure could mean loss of insurance, loss of ability to pay for needed care, and loss of employment, as well as the lost support of established social networks.

Although duties of confidentiality comprise a core element of the dentist-patient relationship, the duty of confidentiality is a *prima facie* duty rather than an absolute duty. Again, this means that we must not disclose patient confidential information unless there are serious, compelling overriding moral reasons not to do so. For example, when your irate, intoxicated neighbor demands to know where your deer rifle is, moral philosophers, except for perhaps Immanuel Kant, would agree that you are not obligated to tell the truth. Why not? Because the duty to tell the truth conflicts with the duty to do no harm to others (nonmaleficence), and you have every reason to believe that your neighbor is likely to harm someone. When duties conflict, we must prioritize them, and act according to the higher-order duty. In this hypothetical case, we must act according to the duty to prevent harm to others. The Tarasoff case mentioned previously held just such a view. It held that, even though neither the law nor the American Psychiatric Association Professional Code explicitly stated circumstances under which the duty of confidentiality was overridden by a competing duty, the practitioner should have realized that when the life of a third party was at risk, patient confidentiality was a less compelling moral duty.

There is another type of situation in which there is an exception to a *prima facie* duty: when the patient explicitly permits disclosure, or, as when consulting with colleagues (who are themselves also bound by confidentiality), the duty is extended to third parties. Thus, relevant information may be disclosed to another dentist or medical professional when needed to render appropriate patient care. In such situations, confidentiality is not violated by the disclosure; rather, the duty of confidentiality extends to others. The practitioner therefore has the responsibility of explaining the nature and scope of this duty to coprofessionals as well as to nonprofessional support staff. This is true, however, only in states having laws that allow extending to others the duty of confidentiality. In the absence of such laws, the dentist is wise never to breach confidentiality.

THE HIV-INFECTED DENTIST OR DENTAL PROFESSIONAL

The question of the invasiveness of the procedure has become important in dentistry, not because it signals the need for universal precautions, but, in recent years, because of the possible restrictions that should be placed on HIV-positive practitioners. In early July of 1990, the media was awash with stories of Kimberly Bergalis, the first person thought to have acquired HIV from Dr. David J. Acer, and in fact from any health care worker. Not only did she become nationally recognized, but the dental profession was thrust into the developing debate over the rights and responsibilities of HIV-positive health care workers in the provision of patient care. The earliest public statements from the ADA concerning the alleged transmission of the HIV virus were both skeptical and defensive.

On July 27, 1990, the CDC discussed the possible HIV transmission to Ms. Bergalis.[30] The CDC concluded that the facts of the case were "consistent" with a transmission to the patient from her dentist in the course of extracting impacted third molars. Although another source of infection (such as from another patient) could not be definitely excluded, the most convincing evidence supporting the transmission, which the ADA and other scientists ultimately were forced to accept, was polymerase chain reaction determination of DNA sequences of the virus from the dentist and Ms. Bergalis. This analysis revealed sufficient similarities between the viral isolates of the dentist and the patient to allow a qualified conclusion that Dr. Acer was the source of Ms. Bergalis' infection. The exact mode of transmission has not been determined as of this writing.

On January 18, 1991, the CDC updated the initial report of the Bergalis case.[31] A reported study of Dr. Acer's other dental patients revealed that four additional patients were HIV-positive, and only one of them had identifiable personal risk factors for acquiring HIV. It was likely, therefore, that three other patients have been infected in the course of invasive dental procedures. Several weeks later, on February 4, 1991, the ADA developed an interim policy statement recommending that those who perform such procedures, and who are HIV-positive, either stop performing such procedures or inform the patient of his or her HIV status.[32]

Over the next 6 months, the previously dormant issue of practice restrictions on HIV-positive dentists who perform invasive procedures, as well as the issue of disclosure of practitioner HIV status and the patient's right to know, became one of the leading topics of debate in the AIDS arena. Although it was recognized that the possibility of professional-patient transmission in the general practice population was remote, the reality of transmission by Dr. Acer and the ethical dilemmas posed by the risk of transmission, however remote, could no longer be ignored. A vigorous and widespread debate developed over whether or not HIV-positive practitioners should continue to perform invasive procedures, and whether patient notification of practitioner's seropositivity is warranted. This debate has received widespread media attention, with countless stories of the Bergalis case and debates over the relative rights and responsibilities of patient and doctor.

Although the risk of HIV transmission in the clinical setting is still widely recognized as a remote possibility, public concern over the demonstrated transfer of infection has forced the health care professions to examine seriously an issue that was willingly dismissed just a short time previously. Kimberly Bergalis died on December 8, 1991.[33] Perhaps the most enduring legacy of her tragic experience is the heightened awareness of the ethical, legal, social, and personal issues that surround the HIV-positive practitioner (and, to a lesser extent, the HIV-positive patient). These issues are now at the fore of public and professional debate; there is widespread recognition that we must address these challenging issues in a straightforward and open fashion.

The Risk of HIV Transmission in the Health Care Setting

The ethical and legal debate concerning HIV-positive health care workers and patients turns on the degree to which such persons present a *risk* of infection to others. Risk assessment is not strictly a technical judgment because values and psychological predispositions as well as epidemiological factors play a role in deciding whether a particular act represents a risk worth taking. There is also disagreement about which facts are relevant in assessing risks. Even if it is agreed, for example, that the risk of HIV transmission to a patient from a dentist who observes universal precautions is close to zero, some may believe that the risk is to be avoided at all costs because the personal consequences of HIV infection are severe. Others might compare the risk of HIV infection in such a circumstance to the risk of being killed in an automobile and argue that the latter is more likely but does not prevent them from driving to the dentist's office. They would conclude, therefore, that it would be inconsistent for them to drive a car but refuse to be treated by a dentist with HIV. How, then, can we make responsible decisions and establish sound public policy, given the variance of our values, psychological states, and what we consider to be relevant to the debate?

The American Medical Association's amicus brief in the *Arline* decision is helpful in addressing this problem.[34] It advised the courts and other decision makers to consider: (1) the nature of the risk (how the disease is transmitted), (2) the duration of the risk (how long the carrier is infectious), (3) the severity of the risk (the potential harm to third parties), and (4) the probability that the disease will be transmitted. If these are indeed the factors that ought to be considered in framing the discussion, then it might be justified to restrict the activities of HIV-positive health care workers, not because viral transmission is likely, but because the impact to the person infected is catastrophic. The court in *Estate of William Behringer, M.D. v. The Medical Center at Princeton, N.J.* followed this line of reasoning in supporting a hospital that barred an HIV-positive surgeon from performing surgery. The court held that any risk of transmission of HIV was too great, given the magnitude of the outcome.[35]

What do we know of the actual risk of HIV transmission in the clinical setting? As of this writing, it is generally accepted that the risk of a dentist acquiring HIV from an infected patient is very low.[36] The CDC determined that, even if a dentist experienced a needle-stick through a glove that resulted in blood contact with a known HIV-positive patient, the risk of the dentist acquiring HIV from that single exposure was less than 0.5%.[37] This means that the odds are that it takes 200 needle-stick blood transfers with an HIV seropositive patient before a dentist will contract HIV, because HIV does not easily transfer through small amounts of blood. In its assessment of such risks, the American Dental Association adopts a similar figure of 0.3%.[38]

The CDC and ADA have reached different conclusions, however, regarding the risk of HIV transmission from dentist to patient. Both calculations are extremely low, though they differ by a factor of ten: the CDC calculates the risk to be $3.8 \times 10-[6]$ in absolute numbers, which leads the CDC to estimate that no more than 100 patients in the United States are likely to be infected over a 9-year period.[38] The ADA calculates the risk to be $2.1 \times 10-[7]$, so that no more than 7 patients over a 9-year period are likely to become infected.[38]

The CDC had originally defined invasiveness to mean the surgical entry to tissues ... for cutting or removal of oral tissues, including tooth structure.[38] In July 1991, a shift in terminology used by the CDC occurred with the use of a new term, "exposure-prone." This addition to the CDC terminology was intended to assist the profession in more accurately identifying which procedures allowed the possibility of blood transmission from an infected health care worker to a patient. Potential restrictions on doctors were to be accurately tailored to those procedures in which the patient was at some palpable risk for acquiring the disease. The ADA declined to assist the CDC in the formulation of a list of exposure-prone procedures and, as of this writing, the CDC has abandoned the idea.[39]

Whatever model one uses to make risk assessments, it appears likely that HIV transmission is a rare event in the clinical setting. However, deciding what dentists owe their patients requires an appreciation for the *consequences* of infection, and not just a quantification of the risk of transmission. With this in mind, we now consider whether the doctrine of informed consent requires disclosure of the dentist's HIV status.

Informed Consent and Disclosure of the Dentist's HIV Status

Must HIV-positive dentists inform their patients of their infection? This question arises only when the practitioner performs exposure-prone procedures because it is only under such circumstances that any risk of transmission of HIV to patient could occur. It must be remembered that the HIV-infected dentist is both a health professional, with fiduciary responsibilities owed to the patient, and a patient, with his or her own rights of privacy. His or her professional responsibilities to patients appear to be in direct conflict with his or her individual, personal rights. Although the transmission of HIV from dentist to patient is rare, the risk is likely to increase over time because of the delay in determining seropositivity.[5] Informing the patient of the practitioner's HIV status and providing the patient with the option of removing himself or herself from the relationship reduces that patient's risk of contracting HIV. However, even a widespread disclosure among HIV-positive dentists would produce at best a negligible decrement in the rate of HIV transmission in the general population. Why, then, might one argue that dentists have an obligation to make such disclosures?

The reason is that the patient engages the dentist as a professional, not as a private individual and not as a commercial service provider. The most compelling and articulate argument for this view is also founded on an analysis of the doctor-patient relationship. As mentioned, the patient assumes no risk greater than the "ordinary risk" of contracting HIV in the normal course of daily life. When the patient enters into a relationship with a health care professional, the patient does *not* thereby accept a greater-than-ordinary risk of death. In our discussion of practitioner risk, we noted that Emanuel had identified internists as having a 0.5% risk of contracting HIV from a needle-stick with a known HIV-seropositive patient.[23] We had also noted that the CDC had estimated the same level of risk for a general dentist. We suggested that these be considered "ordinary professional risks." Here, in the discussion of what level of risk the patient assumes, we wish to suggest that the "ordinary risk" that a patient assumes is not greater than that assumed in ordinary life. We assume, without further argument, that periodic treatment by an internist and by a dentist is part of ordinary life. Therefore, the risk that the patient accepts in ordinary life of contracting HIV, includes the risk of transmission from an internist or from a dentist, *both of whom are assumed to practice their professions in a manner consistent with current standards of practice for their respective professions.* The most relevant feature of the doctor-patient relationship is that the doctor has a duty to do no harm (nonmaleficence), and has a duty, grounded in the social contract nature of professional licensure, to respect patient autonomy. Nonmaleficence requires, at a minimum, that no bodily harm be done to the patient that is not outweighed by the good done. In some interpretations, it can also mean that the doctor may do no harm to the patient's interests *as those interests are defined by the patient.* (This latter interpretation partly supports arguments in favor of living wills and other advance directives.) Even if the duty to do no harm is not so widely interpreted, the duty to respect patient autonomy generally obligates the doctor to respect the patient's interests *as those interests are defined by the patient*. Thus, the duty to respect patient autonomy also obligates the doctor to obtain informed consent from the patient to proposed courses of treatment. Informed consent requires that the patient be given the opportunity to consider all relevant factors, including risk factors and likely benefits of treatment. The dentist must adhere to the ethical duty to do no harm as well as to the ethical principle of respect for patient autonomy, and must put the patient's interests first. It is a well-established legal principle that a health care provider has an ethical duty to provide care and to promote patient self-determination only to those with whom she or he has an established relationship. It is when the dentist has established such a relationship with another that his or her responsibilities to inform the patient of any increase in risk greater than that which the patient ordinarily assumes (however slight that increase may be) supersedes his or her personal rights to privacy.

Such an obligation is not owed to another when the dentist acts as a private person. (This is not, of course, to suggest that, in his or her personal life, the dentist does not have other duties: toward spouse, etc. But *those* duties are acquired in virtue of *those* other relationships, and not in virtue of his or her professional status as a dentist.)

Patient consent to treatment is a fundamental component of the doctor-patient relationship. The legal doctrine of informed consent recognizes that, within the doctor-patient relationship, the patient is autonomous and free to decide the best therapy. Informed consent in many states focuses on patient assessment of the risks and benefits inherent to a medical procedure. Informed consent also may involve considering qualifications of the provider, such as experience in performing the procedure.[40] Full philosophical and legal theories of informed consent have been articulated and summarized elsewhere.[41] The essential components of those theories closely correspond to standard legal doctrines. In the following paragraphs, we focus on only one component of informed

consent, the standard of adequate disclosure. Who is best suited to determine what information is needed for the patient's consent to be genuinely informed? Is HIV status likely to be part of that required information?

There are two primary legal standards of disclosure: the physician standard and the reasonable-patient standard. In a leading case on informed consent, *Canterbury v. Spence*, the District of Columbia Circuit discussed both standards and found that the reasonable-patient standard better supports patient autonomy. The court stated:

> In our view, the patient's right of self-decision shapes the boundaries of the duty to reveal. That right can be effectively exercised only if the patient possesses enough information to enable an intelligent choice. The scope of the physician's communications to the patient, then, must be measured by the patient's need, and that need is the information material to the decision.[42]

The *Canterbury* court reasoned, as have many others, that patients are best informed of the risks of a procedure when they are told what a reasonable, prudent patient in a similar situation would want to know. The physician standard, on the other hand, mandates disclosure of risks according to customary medical practice.

The reasonable-patient standard requires the physician to disclose all the facts "material" to the patient's ability to make an informed decision. The *Canterbury* case addressed the issue of materiality:

> [A] risk is thus material when a reasonable person, in what the physician knows or should know to be the patient's position, would be likely to attach significance to the risk or cluster of risks in deciding whether to forego the proposed therapy.[42]

Important to our discussion is the court's statement that a "very small chance of death or serious disablement may well be significant." Under the reasonable-patient standard, the clinician's HIV-positive status is most likely to be significant to the patient. Requiring HIV-positive healthcare providers to inform patients of their infection would therefore appear to be a requirement under the *Canterbury* decision.

Faden and Beauchamp articulate a third standard of disclosure, the "subjective" standard.[41] Here, the health-care provider discloses information to a patient that *this particular patient*, and not some hypothetical "reasonable person," would consider important. The risk, however small, of contracting an incurable, fatal disease is a consideration that can be considered important only by the person bearing the risk. The patient, and only the patient, can determine how to fit that risk into an assessment of all the factors involved in the proposed treatment. With this "subjective" standard, practitioner homosexuality per se, like shoe size, would probably not be material to the patient. However, if the practitioner engages in at-risk behavior (e.g., nonmonogamous, unprotected intercourse with a partner who engages in at-risk behavior), this may very well, like HIV seropositivity, be significant to the patient, and would on that account require disclosure.

Restricting HIV-Positive Dentists

It is impossible to know how many HIV-positive health-care workers have had their professional activities restricted based on patient safety or institutional liability concerns. A few noted cases have been widely discussed and have resulted in legal action. Sound legal precedent is minimal as of this writing. It is to be remembered that the cases mentioned in the following paragraphs serve as legal precedents only in the jurisdictions in which they were decided. Nevertheless, they provide an early glimpse of judicial thinking on this aspect of HIV infection in dentistry.

The first case of interest to the dental profession, and especially dental students, *John Doe v. Washington University* involved an HIV-positive student at the University of Washington at St. Louis School of Dentistry. The student filed suit against the school in 1988 when he was dismissed from the School because he was found to be HIV-positive. The suit was based on section 504 of the Rehabilitation Act of 1973. In short, the student claimed that it was discriminatory for the school to dismiss him based on a handicapping condition,

i.e., being HIV-positive. The dental school's concern, and basis for the dismissal, was patient safety. It would not allow the student to perform invasive procedures, the performance of which was critical to completion of the curriculum. Both sides of the dispute appreciated the importance of federal handicap laws, but interpreted those laws differently. The court's decision continued the tradition of judicial deference to academic decisions made in good faith.

In late 1991, the U.S. District Court for the Eastern District of Missouri decided in favor of the dental school.[43] The Court made note of CDC guidelines concerning HIV-positive workers who perform invasive procedures, and the chances that an inexperienced student would cut himself in the course of such procedures. Although recognizing the value of barriers in preventing disease transmission, the Court relied on CDC statements that gloves could not prevent penetrating injuries to the student's hands. The Bergalis case also informed the Court's opinion on the efficacy of barrier techniques under certain circumstances. The school's actions were upheld because it acted with deliberation and based its decision on sound ethical, legal, and academic principles.

A similar situation arose at the Medical College of Georgia School of Dentistry. An HIV-positive dental student was removed from school because of patient safety concerns. This case did not result in litigation, but is instructive because it reveals a constructive approach to resolving a difficult situation. The approach the dental school took and an analysis of its actions are available to the interested reader.[44,45]

Finally, in *Estate of William Behringer, M.D. v. The Medical Center at Princeton* (mentioned previously), an HIV-positive ENT physician had his hospital privileges revoked. The hospital medical and dental staff took this action after the physician's illness led to the diagnosis of HIV disease. In a suit decided in 1991, the trial level court ruled that the hospital should take reasonable steps to eliminate "any" risk of transmission of HIV to the physician's patients. The court acknowledged that although the surgeon could invoke the force of discrimination laws, based on his handicapped status, he was not otherwise qualified to hold his staff privileges because of the risk of transmitting disease. The notion of informing the patient of the doctor's HIV status was also supported in this decision. Because *Behringer* was a trial court decision, it has little or no precedential value. It is under appeal and, if upheld, will become a more significant legal force.

These judicial decisions are legally prescriptive in other jurisdictions only to a very small extent. Various professional organizations are free to provide guidance to practitioners until such time as legal precedent on restricting the activities of HIV-positive dentists becomes pervasive. Even then, professional organizations and practitioners may choose to establish and follow ethical and policy guidelines which vary from legal prescriptions. Often (but not always), laws are changed in the face of ethical beliefs that are widely held by conscientious professionals. To the extent (if any) that restrictions on HIV-positive health care workers have been legally enforced because of emotion and lack of informed reason, the ethical and policy positions advocated by professional organizations will, over time, have a corrective effect.

It was mentioned previously that the ADA interim policy on the HIV-infected dentists required restraint from performing invasive procedures or obtaining informed consent from the patient. In October, 1991 the House of Delegates to the ADA Adopted Resolution 84H, which no longer advocates informing the patient of a dentist's seropositive status. The relevant portion of the resolution reads:

> All HIV-seropositive dental health care workers who perform procedures viewed to have identifiable risk should practice only under the evaluation and monitoring of their personal physician and/or under recommendations of public health officials, expert review panels, or in compliance with institutional policies. HIV infection alone does not justify the limiting of professional duties, or automatically mandate disclosure, unless the dental health care worker poses a risk of transmitting infection through non-compliance with universal precautions, lack of infection control competence, or presents signs of functional impairment.[46]

As a practical matter, the new position adopted by the ADA avoids the issue of what procedures are invasive or exposure prone and leaves that determination to local expert review panels. This position appears to violate the ethical duty to respect patient autonomy. As we understand this resolution, disclosure to patients may be appropriately required in three situations: noncompliance with universal precautions, lack of infection control competence, and function impairment. One cannot avoid the conclusion that the ADA's position is that informing the patient because of a dentist's fiduciary responsibilities or because the patient has the moral or legal right to know is neither a requirement of the ADA's professional code of ethics nor a desirable dental public health policy consideration.

In contrast to the position taken by the ADA, the CDC guidelines more clearly state that HIV-positive practitioners who perform exposure-prone procedures should be restricted from such procedures unless an expert panel advises under what circumstances, if any, such procedures may be performed.[47] Additionally, disclosure to patients is clearly recommended.

It may be instructive at this point to note the different status of ADA and CDC recommendations. The ADA is a professional society whose members include many, but not all, of the dentists who hold professional practice licenses. Individual states, in determining licensure requirements, have accepted standards of practice and of professional curricula proposed by the ADA. ADA standards are therefore advisory only. State licensing boards, state health departments, and other arms of government are free to accept, modify, or reject them. The recommendations have legal significance only as advisory opinions in malpractice suits and in nonjudicial licensure revocation proceedings. The CDC solicits professional opinions from associations such as the ADA in formulating its own recommendations. CDC recommendations are made to the National Institutes of Health (NIH) (as well as directly to the practice community) for the purpose of assisting the NIH in obtaining scientific consensus from public health, epidemiological, medical, and other scientific organizations. That consensus represents the highest state of current collective scientific wisdom: a knowledge base to which professionals and professional associations alike aspire and which they claim, in their professional codes, to draw on and apply in practice. That consensus is disseminated to the appropriate health care professions and to the affected and at-risk populations. In addition, the consensus based on CDC recommendations become standards for enforcement agencies such as OSHA. It appears to be inconsistent with its own professed ideals for the ADA to reject scientific consensus in favor of a putative professional right to privacy.

These variable policy considerations and guidelines, along with the lack of solid legal prescriptions, reflect the moral, ethical, and legal tensions that presently exist in the area of the relative rights and obligations of doctor and patient. Tensions that may exist between professional codes on the one hand and science, ethics and law on the other, will persist until the data gathered following widespread practitioner experience lead the ADA to the same logical conclusion regarding practitioner disclosure of HIV status to which case law and scientific and moral theory now point, namely that disclosure is required. Tragically, it may be that only when the long-term epidemiological data confirm that concealment of dentists' HIV seropositivity contributed to the spread of HIV, that the professional association will reinstate its earlier position that HIV seropositivity must be disclosed to patients.

We reject the analogy of the ADA Associate General Counsel regarding the risk that a patient would seroconvert from an HIV-infected dentist:

> . . . one could postulate that the risk is similar to that of seropositive chefs and other food handlers who anonymously remain on the job while infectious; there is no guarantee they will never cut a hand while handling food that goes to a customer.[48]

Although we do not encourage HIV-positive food handlers to infect their customers, a chef or cafeteria worker has an occupational, but not a *professional*, relationship to the consumer. Absent are equal

duties of nonmaleficence, or obligations of care, obtaining informed consent, and other responsibilities that are the hallmarks of professional relationships. It may be argued that only duties to refrain from those acts prohibited by the criminal law, civil code, and health and safety codes constrain members of the service occupations. For these and other reasons, the suggestion that the cases are analogous is rejected. Although the risk of infection may be comparable, surely dentists reject the suggestion that their relationship with, and ethical duties toward, patients is analogous to that of the roast beef carver toward diners on the sandwich line!

To summarize, there are good reasons to believe that an HIV-positive practitioner has a duty to disclose to patients his or her HIV status: First, there is a scientific consensus that a small risk of HIV transmission from dentist to patient exists. Second, under the "reasonable person" standard of the informed consent doctrine, healthcare providers have an obligation to provide any information to the patient that is material to making an informed choice, as determined by what a reasonable person would consider material. Third, the duty to obtain informed consent is not overridden by autonomy rights to privacy because those rights exist *outside* the professional relationship, *not inside it* when the otherwise private information materially affects a patient's ability to make an informed choice. Fourth, the fiduciary nature of the doctor-patient relationship, as well as the moral duty of nonmaleficence, require disclosure.

Finally, according to a "subjective" standard of disclosure of informed consent, a patient is entitled to information that *he or she*, and not some hypothetical "reasonable person," would consider important, so it would be up to the health-care provider to determine if the patient would consider such information significant. The provider may accomplish this by having an honest discussion about the patient's preferences and values. This may be the most important consequence of such a standard, as Faden and Beauchamp note:

> Professionals would do well to end their traditional preoccupation with disclosure and instead ask questions, elicit the con-

cerns and interests of the patient . . . and establish a climate that encourages the patient . . . to ask questions. This is the most promising course to ensure that the patient . . . will receive information that is personally material—that is, the kind of description that will permit the . . . patient, on the basis of his or her values, desires, and beliefs, to act with substantial autonomy.[41]

HIV Testing of Dentists and Dental Students

The preceding discussion suggests some measure of legal support for the position that HIV-positive health care workers should not perform exposure-prone procedures. It has been suggested that this, in turn, provides the rationale for routine HIV testing of such workers. By "routine testing," it is meant that whole groups of people are systematically tested for HIV either without their consent or as a condition of their employment. In respect to testing the general population, legal and ethical concerns for privacy, confidentiality, freedom from unreasonable search and seizure, and the very limited means through which the virus can be transmitted provide little basis for adopting this position on either legal or public policy grounds. Nevertheless, routine screening and immunization for other communicable diseases (when available) is widely practiced in public schools and is supported by state legislation. For example, tuberculosis screening is routinely performed on immigrants and school-age children. Immunization against a variety of communicable diseases that historically have resulted in high morbidity and mortality rates for children is almost universally practiced in the United States. Nevertheless, because HIV is much more difficult to transmit than, for example, tuberculosis, requiring routine HIV testing of nonpractitioner populations is generally considered an unacceptable response to such concerns. However, as we have seen, the *John Doe v. Washington University* and *Behringer* cases have held that dental schools and hospitals may restrict professional practice in the face of legitimate concerns for patient safety. Many dental schools now require

proof of hepatitis-B immunity from students before the clinical years. In view of these developments, is it reasonable to require routine HIV testing of health care practitioners?

Anyone who attempts to determine the HIV status of another must demonstrate a need to know. Routine unconsented-to screening of *patients* has traditionally been rejected on the basis of their confidentiality needs outweighing a doctor's need to know. Universal precautions have been considered sufficient protection from disease transmission, so that a doctor's concern for his or her well-being is not enough to counter the privacy and confidentiality needs of the patient. However, the converse is not necessarily true. As discussed previously in this chapter, the professional relationship between a patient and a doctor is not a symmetrical one. The doctor, by virtue of voluntarily choosing to enter a profession, owes certain duties to protect the patient from harm. The patient, who has not taken a professional oath that obligates him or her to assume risks, does not owe similar duties to the doctor. On that account, the patient may justifiably seek to avoid any risk of infection that is greater than that patient would face in everyday life, including, for example, risks faced when visiting an internist.

As a general matter, before a school or other agency can require routine testing of dentists, a sufficient and defensible need to know must be demonstrated, and this need must be based on the professional duties owed by the practitioner to the patient and which the institution has a fiduciary responsibility to enforce. Individuals targeted for routine testing have defeated such attempts when they invoke protective rights to privacy and to freedom from unreasonable search and seizure. The protection of these individual rights is considered superior to an institution's need to know. This is most often the case when the institution has no clear reason to think that nondisclosure of HIV status will violate the duties that the institution, through its practitioners, owes to its patients. The following cases illustrate how the conflict between a practitioner's rights to privacy and to freedom from unreasonable search and seizure has been weighed by the courts in an attempt to balance those rights against the patient's right to protection from harm.

In the late 1980s, a dispute arose between the administrators of a state home for the mentally impaired and the employees of the home.[49] There was concern that the residents of the home (some of whom had a habit of biting people) might contract HIV if they bit an employee who was unknowingly HIV-positive. No employee was known to be or suspected of being HIV-positive. Central to resolving this dispute was the fact that the safety of the clients, although of legitimate concern, was overshadowed by the constitutional rights of the employees to be free from unreasonable searches or seizures, i.e., the forced submission to a blood test. The rights of the employees were found to be superior to the safety interests of the clients *because no case was known of a person acquiring HIV from a bite*. There was no medical basis for such a mode of transmission. This case, *Glover v. Eastern Nebraska Community Office of Retardation* (1989), illustrates a common legal approach to problems in that, when interests compete, the one more justified, given the facts and law, prevails. This outcome suggests that, when there is no reason to believe that, in the course of rendering professional care, the patient will undergo exposure-prone procedures, unconsenting testing of practitioners will not be allowed. Because there was no evidence that HIV could be transmitted through biting, *there was no material risk to patients that HIV could be contracted* if a patient bit a provider during the course of receiving professional care. Therefore, the provider's right to be free from unreasonable search and seizure was not overridden by a conflicting moral/fiduciary duty to protect patients from harm. The care rendered was not "exposure-prone," and therefore no risk of harm to patients existed.

A different outcome may result when there is reasonable belief that HIV *can* be transmitted in the course of rendering professional care. In a 1990 case, *Leckelt v. Board of Commissions of Hospital District No. 1*, a nurse, whose lover was a patient in the hospital suffering from AIDS, was thought by hospital administration to be HIV-positive.[50] The nurse performed invasive procedures and, in the interest of patient safety, was asked to reveal the results of a previously administered HIV test. Upon his refusal, the nurse was fired. He lost the discrimination suit brought against the hospital because it was felt that proper patient management and proper protection for the nurse himself could not be provided unless the hospital had all the relevant information it needed. Because the nurse performed invasive procedures and it was clear that the chances for HIV positivity were high, requiring the test was seen to be a *reasonable* search and seizure and a *warranted* invasion of privacy. The nurse's rights against unreasonable search and seizure were overridden by the duty to protect patients from harm, *once a material risk of HIV-seropositivity and therefore harm was demonstrated*.

A variation on this rationale was demonstrated in *Anonymous Firemen v. Willoughby, Ohio* (1991). In this case city firefighters and paramedics were forced to undergo routine testing because they themselves, were at higher than ordinary professional risk for acquiring HIV in the course of rendering professional care.[51] Because they had an increased chance of becoming HIV-positive, they had an increased chance of transmitting HIV to others during emergency medical care. In that event, it could be argued that patients who sought emergency services would nonconsentually be placed at a higher-than-ordinary risk of contracting HIV. Although no one firefighter or paramedic was suspected of being HIV-positive, as a group they were more likely to be so than the general public. Mandatory testing was upheld.

Taken together, these three cases reveal a possible judicial trend toward mandatory HIV testing of health care professionals when there is a reasonable belief that, in the course of a professional's rendering professional care, patients will be placed at a higher-than-ordinary risk of contracting HIV. Mandatory HIV testing will most likely be upheld by the courts when there is good reason to believe that two factors are present: (1) when there is a material risk of transmission because of the performance of exposure-prone procedures and

(2) when a practitioner, either because of professional practice or through personal disclosure of high-risk activities, is at a higher-than-ordinary professional risk for being HIV-positive. It is not possible at this point to determine whether future courts will follow *Glover v. Eastern Nebraska Community Office of Retardation* in requiring only a demonstration that the practitioner engages in exposure-prone procedures, or will follow *Leckelt v. Board of Commissions of Hospital District No. 1* and *Anonymous Firemen v. Willoughby, Ohio* and require in addition a demonstration that the practitioner engages in high-risk activities before overriding constitutional rights to freedom from unreasonable searches and seizures and to privacy.

From an ethical point of view, addressing the issue of mandatory HIV testing of the general population requires society to balance its obligation to respect individual autonomy with its duty to promote or protect the welfare of all.[52] Because current screening protocols yield both false-positive and negative results, the efficacy of widespread HIV screening of the general population arguably is not sufficient to warrant an intrusion on individual liberty. Obtaining informed consent before testing, with confidentiality safeguards, allows individuals to act for the benefit of society while keeping autonomy interests largely intact. However, because practitioners *do* but patients *do not* have a duty to accept higher-than-ordinary risk of contracting communicable diseases, the same conclusions may not apply to all health care practitioners. This is especially true when factors are present that tend to place patients at a higher-than-ordinary risk of contracting HIV than they would have, for example, in ordinary life, including the ordinary risk that would be faced when visiting an internist.

CONCLUSION

Dentistry has played a central role in shaping the ethical and legal aspects of HIV infection. This disease has revolutionized the profession's approach to infection control, and has forced an analysis of the relative responsibilities and rights of dentist and patient. As is the case with other issues in dental ethics, the moral rights and responsibilities that one posits for dentists are grounded in the model of the dentist-patient relationship one holds. If the relationship is viewed as a purely commercial one, the dentist is free to limit the provision of services to those who pose a risk to the dentist that does not exceed the "ordinary person" risk. Thus, the dentist assumes no greater risk in the business setting than is assumed by ordinary persons in everyday life. The commercial dentist is not morally obligated to provide treatment for HIV-infected patients, need not disclose HIV seropositivity to the dental customer, and may decline to be screened for HIV, even if he or she, by virtue of occupational procedures or personal activities, is at increased risk for HIV seropositivity.

If one views dentistry as a profession, however, it makes sense to speak of an obligation to treat those who are HIV-positive. The dentist accepts a level of risk that is greater than that of the "ordinary person," but that is not greater than that of the "ordinary professional." This duty to accept risk is therefore limited by the concept of "excessive risk" as determined by the frequency and degree of invasive procedures and the risk factors of the patient population served. On this professional model, it can be argued, the dentist whose risk factor for HIV seropositivity exceeds that of the "ordinary professional" by virtue of either professional procedures or personal activities, voluntarily submits to HIV screening and discloses seropositivity to prospective patients. In contrast to the commercial model of dentistry, the dentist as professional is trusted by the patient and accordingly places the welfare of the patient above his or her personal interests. The dentist, according to this model, acknowledges both the moral and fiduciary nature of the patient relationship, and accepts the consequent duties. In American society, dentistry is considered a profession, although there are numerous commercial aspects to it. It is not a commercial enterprise with some professional aura attached to it. The dentist who accepts the privileges granted by professional licensure, while covertly practicing as a commercial service provider, secretly infiltrates a two-tiered system of practice that unjustly increases the burdens and risks borne by other dentists.

HIV infection in dentistry raises fundamental questions about what it means to be a good dentist or patient. To answer these questions, we turn to both the law, which establishes minimum standards of conduct, and moral reflection, which provides the basis of much law. For those practitioners who do not take the initiative to engage in moral inquiry, peer review committees and dental society ethics committees are often the first to alert (and possibly sanction) errant dentists. Dentists and students who take the time to grapple with these issues from a moral perspective will more readily assume the responsibilities to, and live up to the expectations of, a society that accepts nothing less than the high standards of ethics and professionalism it has licensed dentists to exemplify.

DISCUSSION QUESTIONS AND SAMPLE CASES

1. Discuss the nature of the doctor-patient relationship and how HIV infection has forced an examination of it.
2. Discuss the concepts "ordinary risk," "ordinary professional risk," "higher-than-ordinary professional risk," and "material risk." Who decides what risks should be taken into consideration when consenting to care by an HIV-seropositive provider? What factors, taken together, "quantify" health care providers' risk?
3. Under what circumstances is mandatory HIV testing of health care workers most likely to be morally and legally justified? Explain why.
4. What is the legal basis for a dentist's requirement to treat HIV-positive patients? Are the legal requirements the same as those that might be expected from an ethical analysis of the same question?
5. What are the nature and extent of moral and legal requirement to protect patient confidentiality in the dentist-patient relationship?
6. Should the duty to protect confidentiality prevent a dentist from warning an unknowing woman that her husband is HIV-positive and does not want to reveal that fact to her or follow safe sex practices?

CASE 1

Bill is 25 years old and has gone to the dentist on a regular basis for most of his life. Until very recently, his periodontal structures have been very good. Recently, however, his general dentist has discovered that Bill's periodontal condition has deteriorated rapidly. The situation has become so bad that Bill's dentist decides to refer him to a periodontist. At Bill's first appointment with the periodontist, the progressive nature of the periodontal background is confirmed. The periodontist also notices bilateral white plaques on the tongue, which she confidently feels represent hairy leukoplakia (a cardinal sign, along with severe periodontal disease, of HIV disease). The periodontist takes the usual health history, but does not elicit any response suggesting systemic disease. Bill does not suggest that he has engaged in any of the known risk behaviors for contraction of the HIV virus. Nonetheless, the periodontist strongly suspects that Bill is HIV-positive and is at least beginning to show symptoms of disease. Bill is clearly in need of reconstructive surgery. Although she is always careful to wear a mask and gloves and to sterilize instruments for each patient, as recommended by the CDC and the local dental board, she is concerned about the risk of exposure to the HIV virus. The periodontist decides to call the general dentist to discuss Bill's case.

DISCUSSION QUESTIONS FOR CASE 1

1. What are the periodontist's ethical obligations to treat Bill for his periodontal condition? What are her legal obligations?
2. Was it appropriate or inappropriate for Bill's general dentist to make the referral?
3. May the periodontist ask Bill to have an HIV test? If he refuses, can she insist that he have the test? On what basis may such a test be medically justified?

4. To whom may the general dentist or the periodontist disclose his or her belief that Bill is HIV-positive? What is the basis for the duty of confidentiality? In what circumstances, and on what basis, may this information be disclosed?

5. What obligations does the periodontist have to warn others with whom Bill may come in contact, such as sexual partners, that Bill is HIV-infectious?

CASE 2

In Case 1, assume that Bill is not HIV-positive, and does not exhibit the symptoms of hairy leukoplakia or any other symptoms of HIV disease. However, in preparation for scheduled hip replacement surgery, the periodontist has had her blood tested, including the HIV test. She has recently learned the test results, and knows that she herself is HIV-positive. This news was quite a shock, because, other than occasional pain and discomfort in the hip, she has been feeling fine and has shown no signs or symptoms of HIV disease.

DISCUSSION QUESTIONS FOR CASE 2

1. Does the periodontist have an ethical obligation to inform Bill of her HIV status? Does she have a legal obligation?

2. Should the periodontist refer Bill to another periodontist?

3. Should the periodontist withdraw from all patient care? Perhaps just from performing invasive procedures?

4. What obligations does the periodontist have to inform the state dental board of her HIV status?

5. Would your answer to any of these questions be different if the periodontist were exhibiting the physical symptoms of AIDS? What if she were suffering from an AIDS-related neuropsychological disorder?

REFERENCES

1. Annas, G.: Not saints, but healers: The legal duties of health care professionals in the AIDS epidemic. Am. J. Public Health *78*:844, 1988.

2. *Barron v. Mayor and City of Baltimore* 32 US243, 1833, and In re Slaughter-House Cases 83 US 36, 1872.

3. Keyes, G.: HIV-positive dental students and faculty: Their right to provide care in light of federal constitutional and antidiscrimination laws. J. Law and Ethics in Dentistry *1*:199, 1988.

4. Gostin, L.: HIV-infected physicians and the practice of seriously invasive procedures. Hastings Center Report *19*:32, 1989.

5. Waithe, M.E.: AIDS and dentistry: Conflicting rights and the public's health. Biomed. Ethics Rev. 141, 1988.

6. Centers for Disease Control: Acquired immunodeficiency syndrome (AIDS): Precautions for health care workers and allied professionals. M.M.W.R. *32*:450, 1983.

7. Barr, C.E., and Marder, M.Z.: AIDS: A Guide for Dental Practice. Chicago, Quintessence Publishing Co., 1987.

8. U.S. Department of Health and Human Services, Public Health Service: Recommended infection-control practices for dentistry. M.M.W.R. *35*:15, 1986.

9. Centers for Disease Control: M.M.W.R. *36*:25 (Supp.), 1987.

10. Groopman, J.F., et al. HTLV-III in saliva of people with AIDS-related complex. Science *226*: 444, 1984.

11. Centers for Disease Control. M.M.W.R. *37*:24, 1988.

12. Ho, D.D., et al.: Infrequency of isolation of HTLV-III virus from saliva in AIDS. N. Engl. J. Med. *31*:1606, 1985.

13. Rehabilitation Act of 1973, Pub. L. No. 93-112, 96 Stat. 355 (codified as amended at 29 USC Secs. 701-756), 1987.

14. *Nassau County v. Arline*, 480 U.S. 273, 1987.

15. *Chalk v. U.S. District Court*, 840 F. 2d 701 (9th Cir.), 1988.

16. West Virginia Human Rights Act, Code section 5-11-2 et seq. (example).

17. *Benjamin R. v. Orkin Exterminating Co., Inc.*, 390 S.E. 2d 814 (West Virginia), 1990 (example).

18. West Virginia Code section 16-3C-1 et seq. (example).

19. Pub. L. No. 101-336, 104 STAT. 327 (42 USC section 12102) (1990).

20. American Dental Association: ADA Principles of Ethics and Code of Professional Conduct, Section 1-A, Advisory Opinion (as revised to January 1991).

21. ADA Principles of Ethics and Code of Professional Conduct at 2, January 1990.

22. Letter, Theano to Eukleides, the Doctor. *In* Waithe, M.E. (ed): A History of Women Philosophers, Volume 1, Ancient Women Philosophers. Dordrecht and Boston: Martinus Nijhoff/Kluwer, 1987, pp. 53–54.

23. Emanuel, E.J.: Do physicians have an obligation to treat patients with AIDS? N. Engl. J. Med. *318*:1686, 1988.

24. Arras, J. The fragile web of responsibility: AIDS and the duty to treat. Hastings Center Report *18*:10, 1988.

25. West Virginia Code section 16-3C-3 (a) (4) (example).

26. West Virginia Code section 16-3C-3 (e) (example).
27. *Tarasoff v. Regents of University of California*, 551 P. 2d 334, 1976.
28. ADA Code, Principle 1-B.
29. Beauchamp, T., and Childress, J.: Principles of Biomedical Ethics. 3rd ed. New York, Oxford Univ. Press, 1989, pp. 329–335.
30. Centers for Disease Control: M.M.W.R. *39*:29, 1990.
31. Centers For Disease Control: M.M.W.R. *40*:2, 1991.
32. ADA Adopts Interim Policy on HIV-Infected Dentists. ADA News *22*:3, February 4, 1991.
33. Kimberly Bergalis is Dead at 23; Symbol of Debate Over AIDS Tests. New York Times, 9 December 1991.
34. *School Board of Nassau County v. Arline*, 480 U.S. at 288.
35. *Estate of William Behringer, M.D. v. The Medical Center at Princeton, N.J.* Super, (docket #L88-2250) Superior Court of N.J., Law Division, Mercer County.
36. Klein, R.S., et al.: Low occupational risk of human immunodeficiency virus infection among dental professionals. N. Engl. J. Med. *318*:86, 1988.
37. Centers for Disease Control: M.M.W.R. *38*:S-6, 1989.
38. Neidle, E.: Estimates of the Risk of Endemic Transmission of Hepatitis B Virus and Human Immunodeficiency Virus to Patients by the Percutaneous Route During Invasive Surgical and Dental Procedures. American Dental Association, Feb. 21, 1991.
39. McCann, D.: CDC hears ADA, others oppose lists. ADA News *22*:1, 7, 1991.
40. *Hales v. Pittman*, 576 P. 2d 493, 1978.
41. Faden, R.R., and Beauchamp, T.L.: A History of Theory of Informed Consent. New York and Oxford, Oxford University Press, 1986.
42. *Canterbury v. Spence*, 464 F. 2d 772 (D.C. Cir.), 1972.
43. *John Doe v. Washington University*, WL 264858 (E.D. Mo.), 1991.
44. Comer, R.W., Myers, D.R., et al.: Management considerations for an HIV-positive dental student. J. Dent. Educ. *54*:187, 1991.
45. Weinstein, B.D., and Keyes, G.G.: Management Considerations for an HIV-Positive Dental Student; Ethical and Legal Commentary. J. Dent. Educ. *55*:238, 1991.
46. Actions of the American Dental Association House of Delegates, adopted October 1991 regarding HIV/AIDS issues, p. 5.
47. Gostin, L.: CDC Guidelines on HIV or HBV-Positive Health Care Professionals Performing Exposure-Prone Invasive Procedures. Law Med. Health Care *19*:140, 1991.
48. Logan, M.K.: The HIV-infected dental professional: A challenge to law, ethics, and the dental profession. J. Dent. Pract. Admin. *6*:162, 1989.
49. *Glover v. Eastern Nebraska Community Office of Retardation*, 867 F. 2d 461 (8th Cir.), 1989.
50. *Leckelt v. Board of Commissions of Hospital District*, No. 1, 714 F. Supp 1377 (ED La 1989), Affirmed, 909 F. 2d 820 (5th Cir.), 1990.
51. *Anonymous Firemen v. Willoughby, Ohio*, WL 270600 (N.D. Ohio), 1991.
52. O'Brien, M.: Mandatory HIV antibody testing policies: An ethical analysis. Bioethics *3*:273, 1989.

Chapter 7

Professional Responsibilities Toward Incompetent or Chemically Dependent Colleagues

Lisa S. Parker
Jeffrey Hollway

SUMMARY

In this chapter, we explore the circumstances and ethical values that do not merely justify, but require, that dentists blow the whistle on colleagues' misconduct. We discuss intraprofessional and external mechanisms for reporting, investigating, and disciplining professional misconduct and consider the role played by professional loyalty and other ethical values in decisions to utilize these mechanisms.

To place in context the importance of peer review of dental care and the important role played by the individual dentist in ensuring the effectiveness of peer review mechanisms, we first consider the nature of dentistry as a profession, as well as the nature of the relationship among dental colleagues and the consequent responsibilities of dentists to ensure the quality of their colleagues' professional conduct. We then articulate three basic options which members of the dental team have available to them when confronted with what they believe to be a case of poor quality care or chemical dependency. These options include: (1) doing nothing, (2) initiating some form of personal dialogue with the involved practitioner, and (3) contacting a third party within the profession.

In the balance of the chapter, we explore these three options both in relation to patient care cases and the profession's code of ethics. Although no one is likely to argue that the first option, to do nothing, is acceptable behavior, a long-term observer of the profession's actual behavior might conclude that this has indeed been the preferred option, particularly with regard to early signs of chemical dependency or patient care that is debatably (rather than clearly) substandard. On the other hand, understanding the relationship among dentists as a collegial one seems to support the second option of personal intervention. Although the personal intervention approach is sometimes successful, we argue that the third option, responsible intraprofessional whistle blowing, offers the greatest promise of achieving the goals of professional self-regulation.

In our second section, we consider a case of substandard care in light of the provisions of and deficiencies in the ADA's *Code of Ethics*. We stress the importance of establishing standards of conduct and consider the relative merits of engaging in personal intervention or intraprofessional whistle blowing when one discovers substandard care. In our third section, we discuss the ethical grounds for reporting, to both patients and peers, misconduct and inferior care. We also discuss different conceptions on whistle blowing and their relationship to professional responsibility.

In our fourth and fifth sections, we consider the profession's response to chemically dependent dentists and the obligation of dentists to blow the whistle on their substance-abusing colleagues. We suggest that the profession might model its peer review mechanisms concerning poor quality care after the mechanisms that it has developed to address the problems of chemically impaired dentists.

DENTISTRY'S PRIVILEGE AND RESPONSIBILITY OF SELF-REGULATION

Dentistry as a profession is largely self-regulating. Of course, a profession is, after all, identified with and by the group of individuals who engage in particular professional practices. So it is the individual members of the dental profession, acting individually and collectively, who establish, preserve, and inculcate in new members professional standards of conduct. Dentists are thus not only responsible for adhering to a prescribed standard of conduct, but they prescribe that standard to themselves.

One reason that professions traditionally have been left to regulate themselves is that professional activities employ specialized knowledge and skills not usually possessed by those outside of the profession. Not knowing what the professionals themselves know, regulators outside of the dental profession would be hard pressed to establish standards of conduct, performance, or care for practicing professionals. Another reason why the professions have been self-regulating reflects the economic, social, and political power typically wielded by members; as people in powerful and prestigious social positions, professionals traditionally have demanded and have been allowed substantial latitude in establishing the standards of their professional conduct.

Professionals themselves control the dissemination of their specialized knowledge and the perpetuation of their prestigious professional social role. Dentists go to

professional schools, receive professional licenses, and typically belong to professional associations. These aspects of professionalism help to establish, preserve, and instill in new members the professional mores and standards of conduct characteristic of dentistry. If these standards of conduct are set sufficiently high, e.g., if they demand that dentists behave ethically and use state-of-the-art techniques, these self-regulatory mechanisms can operate to benefit both the profession and the public which it serves. If, on the other hand, the standards are not sufficiently high or are not stringently enforced, self-regulation can establish and perpetuate a professional conspiracy of silence, shoddy professional practices, and poor patient care.

The relationship among professionals is traditionally highly collegial rather than hierarchical. Colleagues deem themselves to be equals in sharing the rights and responsibilities bestowed in virtue of their membership in the group and their pursuit of the group's common goals. Thus, even in settings in which individual dentists are not self employed (e.g., universities, corporations, large clinics, or prisons), they are still the equal colleagues of dentists in and outside of that setting, and policing of the individual dentist's conduct to ensure that it is ethical and competent is left not only to the dentist's own conscience, but also to that of his or her colleagues.

Because of this collegial relationship, the requirement that dentists regulate their own professional conduct presents a special conflict. Most basically, to be a professional is to be a member of the profession. Membership implies a sense of belonging and a sense of loyalty to both the whole and the other individuals who comprise the whole. Establishing standards of conduct contributes to the unity of the profession, but enforcing them, identifying departures from them, and applying sanctions to those who transgress against them can emphasize value differences, generate conflict, create disunity, and undermine professional's sense of identity with the whole. Some of those who rightfully fulfill their responsibility to enforce the standards of professional conduct nevertheless feel that they are disloyal in doing so. Blowing the whistle on a colleague effectively creates a hypothetical hierarchy wherein the whistle blower, who both represents and enforces the professional standards, stands above the alleged wrongdoer. In the context of collegial, nonhierarchial professional relationships, this stance is not easily adopted by the whistleblower, nor has it been easily accepted by many who witness the whistle blower's action. Whistle blowers have been considered professional dissenters or deviants.[1] (This sense of violating collegiality can be exacerbated when subordinates expose their supervisors.)

An unwillingness to extend themselves for the good of their colleague, their profession, and the public they serve—sometimes rationalized by a misguided sense of loyalty or supported by fear of reprisals—has led some dentists to shirk their professional responsibility and to do nothing when confronted with substandard care. Of the three basic courses of action open to those confronting substandard care—(1) doing nothing, (2) personal intervention, and (3) intraprofessional whistleblowing—doing nothing is clearly the least justifiable. The choice to do nothing has traditionally been rationalized by arguing, for example, that the involved party is nearing retirement, is under temporary domestic stress, or is overworked. In such cases, or so the rationalization goes, to raise questions about the practitioner's impairment either is unnecessary (because the concerns are obvious) or might exacerbate the problems (for example, by increasing stress). The option of doing nothing, however, leaves both the public, the profession, and the individual professional at risk. Doing nothing is thus almost never the correct choice.

Understanding the relationship among dentists as a collegial one seems to support pursuing the course of personal intervention. This collegial approach of learning more about the circumstances leading to an apparent lack of quality and offering personal assistance is now probably the prevailing practice in the profession and is a practice which, like other collegial aspects of the profession, is inculcated in new members by dental education and literature. Although this approach is sometimes successful in persuading a practitioner to seek help with chemical dependency or stress or to improve his or her standard of patient care, personal intervention more often leads to denial behaviors, a list of "excuses," unfulfilled promises to retrain or rehabilitate, and sometimes a failure of genuine communication and the severing of personal and professional relationships, which become strained beyond repair by the confrontation. We therefore argue that the path of personal intervention not only is the most personally demanding, but also presents the greatest risk of personal damage and professional disintegration. Sometimes it works to protect the public and rescue the impaired or incompetent professional and a stronger collegial bond results, but more often than not, this approach achieves none of these goals effectively.

The third option, responsible intraprofessional whistle blowing, offers the greatest promise of achieving the goals of professional self-regulation. It is clearly the choice in cases of chemical dependency, wherein a degree of interpersonal skill and the ability both to fend off the dependent person's usual defensive responses and to monitor his or her progress in rehabilitation have been recognized not merely as desirable, but as necessary. The profession has recognized that when intraprofessional channels are established for reporting, counseling, and monitoring chemically impaired dentists, everyone wins. The whistle blower's identity is reasonably protected, the impaired professional is offered a temporary "safe haven" in which his or her problems can be addressed away from the public's eye, and the public is protected from the risks of treatment by an impaired practitioner. The counselor, as a supportive third party, can help the dependent professional while keeping in mind the public's and the profession's interest in the provision of quality dental care.

It is not clear, however, that whistle blowing has, at least until now, had the same positive effect on situations in which poor quality care is the issue. Although the process of rehabilitation has had documented success,[2] there are no established programs of retraining for professionals who provide substandard care. Although it shares with dependency intervention programs the goals of protecting the public and preserving the standards of the profession, the peer review process often functions punitively, rather than supportively, with respect to the individual dentist whose patient care is deficient. Consideration of the following case in light of the profession's guidelines for handling misconduct highlights the need to revise the existing peer review process. Nevertheless, when confronted with professional misconduct, using intraprofessional whistle blowing mechanisms is superior to either doing nothing or accepting the risks to both oneself and the public of pursuing personal intervention alone.

COLLEAGUES, COMPETENCE, AND THE ADA CODE

To guide dentists' conduct in pursuit of their professional goals—indeed, to shape those goals—the Council on Ethics, Bylaws, and Judicial Affairs of the American Dental Association (ADA) adopted its *Principles of Ethics and Code of Professional Conduct*, hereinafter referred to as the ADA Code, which codifies the principles of conduct and shared goals to which those practicing in the profession have historically subscribed.[3]

Although rules and principles do not tell the whole story about the ethics of a profession, examining the basic ethical principles adopted by any culture provides clues about that culture's values and about how members of that culture resolve ethical problems and regard members who act unethically. Just as basic principles of dentistry allow for alternate treatment plans, the basic rules and principles of ethical conduct provide a framework for ethical decisionmaking. In ethics, as in treatment planning, guidelines suggest which facts must be ascertained, what of value is at stake, and which of several possible courses of action should be ruled out from the outset as being unacceptable. Consider the following case and the guidance offered by the ADA Code.

CASE 1

Just over 3 years ago, Dr. Boley began practicing general dentistry in a community of 10 dentists. One of them, Dr. Leeds, has been in practice in the community for over 30 years and treats many of the older residents, who are very loyal to him as one of the "old-timers." During one of Dr. Leeds' infrequent absences, Ms. Wentworth, a long-time patient of Dr. Leeds, visited Dr. Boley for emergency treatment, which involved dental work recently completed by Dr. Leeds. Ms. Wentworth presented the sixth unsatisfactory case of Dr. Leeds' work that Dr. Boley had observed during the past two years. In Ms. Wentworth's case, an infected root tip had been left close to the sinus following an extraction and caused her considerable pain. After Dr. Boley recommended that the operation site be opened to remove the root tip, Ms. Wentworth questioned Dr. Boley about why Dr. Leeds had not removed the root tip at the time of the initial operation. She also asked about the quality of Dr. Leeds' care in general.

It had been apparent to Dr. Boley for some time that Dr. Leeds had not kept up with the latest advances in dentistry and that both his technical ability and his clinical judgment were slipping. Ms. Wentworth, for example, suffered from advanced periodontal disease and needed replacement of almost all restorations. Ms. Wentworth reported to Dr. Boley, however, that Dr. Leeds had recently told her that she required no additional dental care. What should Dr. Boley do? How should she respond to Ms. Wentworth's inquiries?[4]

Suppose that Dr. Boley turned to the ADA Code for guidance. The Code's first principle states that "the dentist's primary professional obligation shall be service to the public. The competent and timely delivery of quality care within the bounds of the clinical circumstances presented by the patient, with due consideration being given to the needs and desires of the patient, shall be the most important aspect of that obligation."[3] (Note that the Code does not limit the dentist's primary obligation to his or her own patients, but states that service to the public is the dentist's primary obligation. Some argue that dentistry is undergoing a transformation from a private practice orientation to a public health model of providing professional services.[5]

The task of applying general rules and principles in particular cases is not easy because they do not always require the same conduct in each case. The statement of the primary professional obligation shared by all dentists, for example, acknowledges that what the individual dentist must actually do to fulfill this obligation differs from case to case depending on the patient's clinical circumstances, needs, and desires. Indeed rules are usually too general to yield by themselves a correct course of action in a particular case. In the first principle, for example, the value-laden terms "competent," "timely," and "quality" are not defined. Yet, to fulfill their primary professional obligation, dentists must determine the standard of care owed members of the public. Dr. Boley, for example, must be able to determine what constitutes competent and quality care to decide whether Dr. Leeds has breached that standard.

In addition to these difficulties, two or more rules can offer conflicting guidance with respect to a particular case. Indeed, if Dr. Boley reads further in the ADA Code, such a conflict becomes apparent. The ADA Code's section entitled "Justifiable Criticism" imposes obligations that may conflict with the Code's first principle. The section states that:

> . . . dentists shall be obliged to report to the appropriate reviewing agency as determined by the local component or constituent society instances of gross or continual faulty treatment by other dentists.
>
> Patients should be informed of their present oral health status without disparaging comment about prior service.
>
> Dentists issuing a public statement with respect to the profession shall have a reasonable basis to believe that the comments made are true.[3]

The Code's advisory opinion on this section further qualifies the dentist's obligations:

> A dentist's duty to the public imposes a responsibility to report instances of gross or continual faulty treatment. However, the heading of this section is 'Justifiable Criticism.' Therefore, when informing a patient of the status of his oral health, the dentist should exercise care that the comments made are justifiable. For example, a difference of opinion as to preferred treatment should not be communicated to the patient in a manner which would imply mistreatment. There will necessarily be cases where it will be difficult to determine whether the comments made are justifiable. Therefore, this section is phrased to address the discretion of dentists and advises against disparaging statements against another dentist. However, it should be noted that where comments are made which are obviously not supportable and therefore unjustified, such comments can be the basis for the institution of a disciplinary proceeding against the dentist making such statements.

Dr. Boley would be justified in feeling a bit confused about the ADA Code's advice. Although the Code clearly states that her primary obligation is to the public, the Code does not seem to authorize her to respond to Ms. Wentworth's inquiries with critical comments about the work of her colleague. Nevertheless, such an honest response would be, as far as Dr. Boley can reasonably determine, in the patient's best interests. Moreover, in order to avoid offering disparaging remarks about Dr. Leeds' work, Dr. Boley would have to deceive Ms. Wentworth either with blatant lies or by purposely misleading her. Dr. Boley could, one supposes, simply refuse to answer Ms. Wentworth's questions. Such silence would be likely to create mistrust and hostility, and do little to improve the patient's oral health, which would be neither in the patient's nor the profession's interest. Respect for Ms. Wentworth as an autonomous individual, as well as concern for her welfare, should prompt Dr. Boley to answer her questions honestly.

Indeed, another section of the Code admonishes dentists "to elevate the esteem of the profession.[3] Engaging in a conspiratorial silence about substandard dental care would surely lower the esteem of the profession by justifying public mistrust. If one of the reasons why dentistry is self-regulating is that dentists possess specialized knowledge, which the public cannot be expected to have, dentistry has a special trust or duty to use that knowledge for the public's benefit and, contrary to the Code's provisions, to share that knowledge when it is in the public's interest or when particular patients, acting in a reasonable manner, seek to know it.

Because this is the sixth case of substandard care among Dr. Leeds' patients that she has seen, Dr. Boley would be justified in reporting Dr. Leeds to the appropriate reviewing agency as determined by the local component or constituent society. Surely six instances of substandard care constitute evidence of continual faulty treatment, which, according to the ADA Code, justifies peer review. Or do they? If Dr. Leeds has been in practice for over 30 years, he probably has treated more than 6000 patients (based on his seeing 25 patients per day and working 48 weeks per year). Dr. Boley has only seen 6 cases out of approximately 6000 patients (0.10%). Does she have enough evidence to establish a pattern of misconduct or substandard care? Moreover, what if this sixth case were instead the only one that she had witnessed? Does leaving an infected root tip near the sinus constitute grossly faulty care?

Moreover, with respect to her diagnosis of advanced periodontal disease and the need for restoration replacement, could Dr. Boley and Dr. Leeds simply have "a difference of opinion as to preferred treatment," which therefore should not, according to the Code, be communicated to the patient in a manner which would imply mistreatment? Even if periodontal disease and the need for restoration replacement are so routinely diagnosed today that the failure to do so does constitute negligence, not just a mere difference of opinion, a judgment is sometimes needed for treatments that fall on the borderline between routine or standard treatments and those that are experimental or state of the art. The ADA Code does not provide specific guidance in determining what to do in these borderline cases.

In fact, between the "gross or continual faulty treatment" mentioned in the Code's "Justifiable Criticism" section and the competent quality care that it is the dentist's primary obligation to provide, there is a vast grey area of conduct and dental practice which is neither of good quality nor

grossly or continually faulty. What is the responsible dentist supposed to do about a colleague's substandard, but not grossly or continually faulty, conduct or treatment? The existence of a grey area in which a rule does not clearly apply does not suggest that this is an opportunity to ignore the demands of ethics. When the "letter of the law" does not clearly address the issue at hand, one looks to the "spirit of the law" for guidance in specific cases or in drafting more specific guidelines.

Although some state dental societies amplify or augment the ADA Code, in the absence of more specific guidelines, dentists must use their discretion and rely upon the fundamental ethical values that inform their practice and their professional code.[6] Unfortunately, because of the Code's emphasis upon avoidance of unjustified criticism, a rather cynical interpretation of the spirit of the ADA Code might suggest that Dr. Boley should place the protection of the profession's and a professional's image over the protection of and service to the public.[7] This view, however, is not only incompatible with dentistry's primary goal, but is ultimately incompatible with dentistry's self-image as a profession worthy of respect and of the privilege to regulate the conduct of its own members. The overriding, guiding spirit of the ADA Code lies in its statement of dentistry's primary obligation to serve the public and promote public health. Substandard conduct or treatment, even if not gross or continually faulty, does not promote the public's health, and hence fails to serve dentistry's goal. Therefore, dentists with knowledge of substandard treatment cannot justifiably do nothing, and although personal intervention is an option, it is often an ineffective one. Thus, dentists seem to be ethically charged with reporting all substandard conduct or treatment to local bodies for review.

Moreover, the spirit or underlying ethical values of the ADA Code dictate that, contrary to provisions in the Code's "Justifiable Criticism" section, dentists in situations such as Dr. Boley's are obligated to bring substandard treatment to the attention of the colleague's patient (e.g., Ms. Wentworth). Informing patients that they have been inappropriately treated promotes their welfare and their autonomy by enabling them to seek other opinions and to avoid their former practitioner in the future and by placing them in a better position to evaluate the quality of their future dental care.

The Code correctly states that justifiable differences of opinion—cases in which one could be justified in holding either of two opposing opinions—should be conveyed in a way that does not imply that one of the treatment options constitutes mistreatment. On the other hand, when mistreatment has occurred or might reasonably be expected to occur in the future, the patient has a right—grounded in his or her autonomy—to know it. A dentist who has knowledge of past or potential future mistreatment has an obligation—grounded in the professional obligation to promote the public's dental health—to inform the patient. Moreover, in the case of prior treatment that was indeed grossly faulty, patients have the legal and moral right to seek legal redress and monetary compensation. When mistreatment is detected, those dentists who do not inform the mistreated patient (1) prevent the patient from choosing to exercise legally guaranteed rights, (2) fail to prevent future harm by failing to educate the patient about both substandard care and the particular dentist, i.e., breach a duty of beneficence to prevent harm, and (3) fail to respect the patient's desire know about and right to control what happens to his or her body.

Thus, Dr. Boley should explain to Ms. Wentworth that she believes that her current difficulty is the result of an infected root tip having been mistakenly left near her sinus during her previous extraction. Dr. Boley should focus her professional criticisms on the procedure that was performed and avoid personal criticisms of the person (Dr. Leeds) who performed it, but contrary to the apparent provisions of the ADA Code, Dr. Boley should inform Ms. Wentworth that her current condition is likely to have been caused by prior inappropriate treatment.

All criticism of colleague's work should be offered constructively with the intermediate goal of finding avenues for remedying deficiencies and for avoiding future instances of misconduct. In this spirit, Dr.

Boley may choose to inform her colleague, Dr. Leeds, of her findings of his substandard treatment and of the steps she will take (or has taken) both to inform professional authorities and to inform Ms. Wentworth of the problem and reestablish her dental health. By informing Dr. Leeds, Dr. Boley would evidence her respect for him as a colleague who, she may presume, would want to know of his mistakes in order to correct them. According to the prevailing practice in dentistry, except in unusual circumstances, Dr. Boley should discuss Ms. Wentworth's mistreatment with Dr. Leeds before taking any other steps, such as reporting his substandard treatment to local authorities. (If, for example, illegal actions are involved or she has reason to think that Dr. Leeds might take steps to cover up evidence of his negligence, Dr. Boley would be justified in not telling him of her discoveries or her actions in reporting them.) According to the rationale underlying this prevailing practice, if Dr. Leeds did not respond to these personal efforts to remedy his professional deficiencies and the substandard dentistry continued, then and only then should Dr. Boley carry her concerns, together with any substantiating evidence to the local dental society for its investigation.

This personal intervention approach unfortunately assumes that Dr. Boley will be in a position to monitor Dr. Leeds' future professional conduct. It places a great practical and ethical burden on Dr. Boley; she must first assess Dr. Leeds' sincerity in desiring to correct his conduct and then his success in doing so. Therefore, we argue that it is far more appropriate and efficacious for Dr. Boley to leave this responsibility to those bodies charged with this function. Although speaking to Dr. Leeds first does respect his autonomy (by allowing him to correct his conduct himself), it may not best serve either the patient's welfare or the profession's interest in its efficacious and autonomous regulation. According to our argument, Dr. Boley should report Dr. Leeds' substandard treatment of Ms. Wentworth to the local dental society for peer review and should monitor their review to ascertain that an investigation was indeed implemented and, if appropriate, that disciplinary action taken. Disciplinary action can range from reprimand to the suspension or loss of one's license to practice.

Indeed, Dr. Boley should have taken action when the first of the six of Dr. Leeds' patients presented evidence of his substandard care. While it may seem harsh not to allow "just one mistake," Dr. Boley would, in fact, have had no way of knowing whether the first case that she witnessed was indeed the result of Dr. Leeds' first or only mistake. In fact, no one person can know whether a single case of wrongdoing, misconduct, negligence, or substandard treatment is actually a single isolated case, or whether it is part of a pattern of such incidents. Thus we argue that all cases of misconduct or substandard treatment should be reported to a local peer review board so that a centralized database of reported infractions could be maintained and thereby better justify reporting to appropriate regulatory authorities those practitioners who show evidence of continued or seriously substandard dentistry. Ideally, local peer review groups, charged with a supportive and constructively corrective role, not a punitive one, should be established and should be the body to which dentists in Dr. Boley's position could first turn. If implicated practitioners, like Dr. Leeds, did not respond to retraining or to other efforts to protect their patient's welfare, or if their substandard practices persisted, they could be reported to regional or state review boards for additional intervention efforts and possible disciplinary action. Because of difficulties with the personal intervention approach, in the absence of this ideal two-tiered (first supportive, then potentially punitive) system, dentists have an obligation to report substandard care to existing professional bodies.

WHISTLE BLOWING AS A PROFESSIONAL RESPONSIBILITY

The obligation to blow the whistle on professional misconduct is thus a very stringent one grounded in the ethical values of nonmaleficence, which requires that dentists avoid harming patients, and of beneficence, which requires that dentists promote and prevent harm to the public's dental health. It is also grounded in concern for the autonomy of both dental patients and the dental profession. Patients have a right to control and consent to what happens to their bodies. Their right to know if something adverse has been perpetrated on them and their moral and legal right to seek redress in such cases is based on recognition of their autonomy. The profession's right to autonomy or self-rule (based on the Greek *autos* or self and *nomos* or rule) is not an absolute right, but a socially granted one that may be overridden by other rights and important interests. If the profession's attempt at self-rule conflicts with its overriding goal of fulfilling the public's interest in receiving quality dental care, then the profession must give precedence to the interests of the public's health.

Therefore, in its title this chapter refers to "professional responsibility" rather than "whistle blowing," a term which is often used in literature on the responsibilities of professionals. The former term has consistently positive connotations, while the latter has various interpretations and, accordingly, has met with varying degrees of approbation. Some accounts of handling professional misconduct distinguish, for example, between legitimate and illegitimate whistle blowing. The so-called illegitimate whistle blower raises allegations of misconduct to further his or her own interests, perhaps vindictively, or acts irresponsibly by raising the allegations without having sufficient evidence to support his or her charges. Dentists need not be *certain* that their allegations are true, but their suspicions must be sufficiently well founded that further investigation is clearly warranted. Moreover, they should blow the whistle on alleged misconduct to protect public health and to preserve patient and professional autonomy, not to attract patients, gain publicity, damage a colleague's reputation, settle a vendetta, or resolve a difference of opinion. Legitimate whistle blowing is thus an act of professional responsibility. "Illegitimate whistle blowing," whether intentional or negligent, is not a response to misconduct; it is itself a type of professional misconduct. In referring to "whistle blowing," this chapter, therefore, refers to legitimate whistle blowing, i.e., to an act of professional responsibility.

In addition, some use a narrower definition of whistleblowing to distinguish it from other means of reporting professional misconduct.[8] According to this narrower view, a whistle blower is one who circumvents the profession's prescribed channels of self-regulatory authority by "going public" (e.g., talking to the press) or "going outside" (e.g., by reporting to a governmental agency). One might appropriately go public or outside the profession with one's concerns if indeed one had already pursued internal means of addressing misconduct to no avail, or if one had good reason to believe that pursuing such channels would be both unproductive and seriously detrimental to one's professional standing. To avoid the necessity of going public, the ADA Code provides for various internal levels of redress: "If a satisfactory decision cannot be reached [at a local level], the question should be referred on appeal to the constituent society and the Council on Ethics, Bylaws and Judicial Affairs of the American Dental Association."[3] If, for example, Dr. Boley felt that her concerns about Dr. Leeds' competence to practice would not be taken seriously at the local level by her colleagues in her small, tightly knit professional community, and if she feared reprisals, she could report her findings of Dr. Leeds' mistreatment directly to state or national levels of the profession. Only if she did not receive satisfactory response at those levels (or did not receive one in a sufficiently timely manner to avoid preventable serious harm) would Dr. Boley be justified in going public with her concerns. Whistle blowing in the sense of going outside of the profession is thus an ethically appropriate response to the inadequacies of internal self-regulatory mechanisms.

In understanding whistle blowing as an act of professional responsibility, this chapter does not limit the term "whistle blowing" to only those cases in which the responsible dentist goes outside the profession. Quite importantly, we urge that professional responsibility demands adequate internal channels of responsibility

and authority to investigate, correct, and discipline alleged misconduct. These channels are established through professional organizations, but should also be established within clinical practices and other institutional settings (e.g., universities and companies) where dentists carry out their professional activities.

For cases involving chemically impaired dentists, a network of supportive, nonpunitive, intraprofessional channels have already been established. These bodies may serve as models for establishing similar mechanisms for dealing with poor quality dental care not involving chemical dependency.

WHISTLE BLOWING AND THE CHEMICALLY DEPENDENT PRACTITIONER

Practicing dentistry while impaired through chemical dependency constitutes a clear case of unacceptable professional conduct. The New York State Board for Dentistry, for example, specifically defines the act of "practicing the profession while the ability to practice is impaired by alcohol, drugs, physical or mental disability" as grounds for discipline. Furthermore, even the state of "being habitually drunk or dependent on the habitual use of narcotics, barbiturates, amphetamines, hallucinogens or similar drugs" is viewed as requiring disciplinary action.[6] These regulatory statements, when combined with ethical obligations grounded in beneficence and nonmaleficence, or when combined with the ADA Code's provisions for justifiable criticism, obligate those having reasonable knowledge that a dental practitioner is a substance abuser to take some type of action.

Historically, alcohol and drug dependency have been looked upon as resulting from a lack of self-control caused by moral weakness in one's character. Scientific research, however, continues to show that such psychopathologic dependency is the consequence, not of moral deficit, but of a biogenetic disease in which there is a strong interplay between heredity and environment.[9] Although some still deny this evidence, in general, therapy has replaced moral judgment. Perhaps for this reason, the ADA at the national level aggressively promotes educational and referral programs to assist the recovery of chemically dependent dental professionals.

The First National Conference on Alcohol and Chemical Dependency was held in 1985, and in 1986 the ADA formally recognized "chemical dependency as a disease entity that affects all of society" and, as a result of this view, committed itself to "assist the chemically dependent member of the dental family toward recovery from the disease by education, information and referral."[10] The ADA Council on Dental Practice formed the Advisory Committee on Chemical Dependency Issues to serve as a clearing house for information and treatment resources for impaired dentists and to assist state and local dental societies in implementing their own impaired dentists programs. As of 1988, the ADA could identify 45 state and 47 local dental societies that had active chemical dependency assistance programs.[9] The backbone of these programs consists of volunteer dentists (some of whom have themselves suffered from chemical dependency) who have a committed interest in helping their suffering colleagues. Typically, these programs are nonjudgmental, nonpunitive and therapeutically oriented.[2]

Chemical dependency among dentists is a fairly prevalent problem. Alcohol is most commonly abused, and cross-dependency—the combination of other drugs with alcohol—is not uncommon.[10] After alcohol, tranquilizers have been rated by dentists as the most serious drug risk, followed by stimulants and nitrous oxide.[11] In a recent survey of Michigan dentists, 48% of 370 respondents indicated that they were aware of a colleague with an obvious chemical dependency problem.[11] Based on the national estimate that 10% of the general population is chemically dependent, the Council on Dental Practice has projected that at least 18,000 United States dentists are at risk for alcoholism and other drug dependencies.[9] It is not unreasonable, however, to assume that this figure should actually be projected as being higher for dentists, who often view themselves as operating within a stressful work environment marked by a demanding workload, threat of malpractice, difficult patient relations, high social expectations of their work performance, limited immediate rewards, and a lack of peer support.[11,12] Dentists who have been identified as having a drug dependency problem often are described as having a "type A" personality: they are hard-working, highly competitive, and achievement-oriented, with little balance between their professional and private lives, a condition often intensified by their feeling of being under continual economic pressure.[2]

In addition, the majority of dentists practice alone or with only one associate.[11] Because there is little opportunity to share daily experience and frustrations with professional peers, the isolated dentist may be tempted to turn to alcohol or other drugs to relieve tension. Solo practitioners operate in an environment wherein they have free and easy access to prescription drugs with minimal chance of being observed by colleagues. Moreover, impaired dentists become adept at masking their dependency and conveying an appearance of normal functioning.[11] As noted by Ercell Miller, former member of the ADA Advisory Committee on Chemical Dependency Issues, "the last things to go in addiction are learned skills,"[13] thus allowing the impaired practitioner to perform dental procedures with some semblance of normality. The dentist's typically isolated work environment affords a greater opportunity to escape the early detection of substance abuse. Moreover, those who do work with the dentist, and who thus may be in the best position to detect a dependency problem in its earlier stages, often rely on the dentist for their livelihood and therefore remain silent. In addition, hygienists, who work most closely with dentists, have traditionally been female, whereas dentists have traditionally been male. Issues of gender and power intertwine with concerns about financial dependence to further deter the identification of impaired dentists. Unfortunately, those close to the impaired dentist often enable the disease to progress until it is the patient who recognizes the problem and takes action that could indeed result in the suspension or revocation of the dentist's license to practice.[14]

Personal denial and rationalization, strong components of the chemical dependency syndrome, are intensified by professional indoctrination and social expectations. Beginning in dental education, dentists are geared toward perfectionism, a professional self-image which is reinforced by the public's perception of dentists' infallibility.[11] Therefore, until some catastrophic event shakes them into the reality of their problem, dentists often delude themselves that they remain in control and can cease their substance abuse at anytime. Even then, there is a reluctance to admit to their addiction and to seek recovery for fear that this will mean the automatic loss of their dental license.

Because the chemically dependent dentist in most instances is not capable of acknowledging and stopping his or her addiction alone, a special burden to intervene falls on those with whom he or she has direct contact in the work environment. A random sample survey of Michigan dentists showed that common tactics taken by dentists when encountering a chemically dependent colleague were to: (1) personally try to help, (2) urge the dentist to seek counseling, (3) avoid the dentist, or (4) report the afflicted dentist to the local dental society or state licensing board.[11] The majority of the 177 dentists who responded to the survey felt that peer intervention was justified to assist a troubled colleague, to protect patient welfare, and to maintain quality standards of the profession.[11] Friendship and commitment to an afflicted associate can compel one to act out of "tough loyalty," whereby one acts in ways that may appear disloyal—for example, reporting the associate to local professional societies—but which actually reflect a heightened sense of loyalty and concern for the welfare of the afflicted colleague.[15]

Out of respect for an impaired professional's autonomy, a work associate may first try an informal approach and initiate a personal discussion to persuade the afflicted colleague to seek recovery assistance. Although this personal intervention alerts the dentist that his or her abusive behavior has become observable and gives him or her an opportunity to take corrective action, such one-to-one efforts unfortunately tend to be ineffective. A perceived confrontation often sparks defensiveness and hostility toward the accuser who, if a subordinate, could be exposed to job termination or other retaliatory actions. Moreover, unless the individual colleague takes the burden upon himself or herself, direct personal intervention also does not afford the opportunity to monitor the impaired professional's success in recovering from his or her dependency problem. Respect for the profession's autonomy and concomitant privilege to self-regulate—as well as the overriding concern for the efficacious prevention of harm—should instead prompt the concerned colleague to seek intervention assistance through intraprofessional channels specifically established to assist and to monitor impaired dentists.

For those who know of, or strongly suspect, a dentist with a substance abuse problem, advice hotlines are commonly available to contact state or local peer assistance programs involving direct intervention and referral. Anyone using these helplines to seek assistance for an impaired dentist is guaranteed confidentiality and anonymity. This promise of confidentiality and anonymity is offered to decrease the likelihood of any retaliatory action being taken against those who contact the dental society on behalf of a chemically dependent dentist. The acceptance of "anonymous tips," however, increases the opportunity for injustice to be done to innocent practitioners, particularly in a constrained economic climate where competition for patients may motivate malicious tactics. Unfortunately, it is not inconceivable that an unscrupulous professional would wrongly point an accusing finger toward a professional peer for personal gain or that a disgruntled office staff member would use this mechanism for retaliatory purposes. The moral responsibility for the accuracy of reports must lie with those who report an addicted associate. Thus some mechanism of accountability should be instituted to deter and to discipline those who would bring frivolous or malicious accusations.

Once the peer assistance program is contacted, typically, a small group of specially trained intervention team members

conduct a fact-finding investigation to determine if a problem does in fact exist.
Should a problem be evident, they meet
with the impaired dentist to encourage
him or her to enter treatment before unavoidable problems arise with state licensing authorities. These same peer assistance team members continue to monitor
and support the dentist during the recovery process.[11] (This process should serve
as a model for the supportive peer review
mechanism, described previously as a
means of addressing poor quality dental
care.)

The profession has purposely created
these intra-organizational mechanisms for
identifying and referring afflicted colleagues so that such cases can be handled
within the professional association, thereby
preserving its self-regulatory privilege and
discharging its self-regulatory responsibility. Therefore, to blow the whistle on a
chemically dependent colleague publicly,
before first taking steps to address his or
her problem within the professional arena,
would be contrary to the essence of self-
regulation. Furthermore, those who use
external channels for reporting co-workers
are more likely to face organizational retaliation than those who pursue internal
channels.[16] (Interestingly, research suggests that an organization's threat to retal-
iate against those who "go public" results
in more, not less, external whistle blowing.[16] Perhaps the existence of internal
threats of retaliation suggest to responsible
professionals that internal channels of investigating alleged misconduct are unlikely
to operate ethically.) Nonetheless, having
brought the problem to the attention of
appropriate parties within the profession,
and finding that no action is being taken
or that no marked movement toward recovery is occurring, the dental staff member or colleague may be justified in making
a more public outcry. This might involve
informing patients as a protective warning
or contacting state licensing regulators for
proper redress.

In all cases of blowing the whistle on a
suspected impaired dentist, publicly or in-
traprofessionally, one must be guided by
clear conscience, an absence of malice in
motive, and accurate evidence justifying a
reasonable belief that a dependency problem exists. Such evidence therefore permits one to feel especially confident in
seeking assistance for a dentist whose dependency is currently and obviously im-
pairing his or her ability to provide quality
dental care. Suppose, however, that the
dentist's chemical dependency has not yet
caused any obvious impairment to his or
her ability to practice and that there is no
evidence of harm to others as a consequence of the affliction. How does one
justify intervening when there exists only
a perceived potential for harm? Consider
the following case.

CASE 2

Dr. Martin has practiced for nearly 20
years in a small midwest community. Ms.
Nathan, a recovering alcoholic and a divorced mother of two children, has worked
in his office as a dental assistant for the past
year and a half. It has been two years since
Ms. Nathan has come to terms with her
chemical dependency and received treatment. Through a program advocating employment for the rehabilitated chemically
dependent, Dr. Martin hired Ms. Nathan.
She is grateful for this work opportunity,
has earned Dr. Martin's trust and confidence
in her, and has received two salary increases.
Dr. Martin has indicated a future possibility
for her to become head assistant.

During the past 4 months, Ms. Nathan
had observed Dr. Martin during the day
routinely taking pills that she recognized as
a prescription tranquillizer. He also began
calling in, frequently at the last minute, to
break appointments, or would show up late
for morning appointments to which he arrived looking disheveled and appearing very
shaky. On several occasions, she had detected alcohol on his breath after long lunch
hours during which the patient was kept
waiting. He suffered from noticeable mood
swings. All these signs indicated to her that
Dr. Martin was probably struggling with
chemical dependency. Out of her personal
concern for his welfare and knowing the
hell of being in this disease state but being
unable to acknowledge it or overcome it
alone, she decided to speak to him confidentially.

Two months ago, after work, when Dr.
Martin was alone completing some patients'
charts, Ms. Nathan took advantage of the
moment. She approached the matter sincerely and openly described what she had
observed. She stressed that she did not wish

to interfere in his life, but that he was special to her because he had given her a fresh start and that she was concerned that his affliction would affect his practice and his health. She asked him to seek assistance and offered to put him in contact with a help group that would treat the matter confidentially.

Dr. Martin assured her that he had no problem and that he was just going through a difficult adjustment time. He was, in fact, going through a messy divorce and was in the midst of a child custody battle. Furthermore, he confided in her, a pending IRS investigation was increasing his feelings of stress. He thanked her for her obvious caring and promised not to come to the office in that condition again.

Less than a week later, Dr. Martin returned from his lunch break with glassy eyes and an odor of alcohol. His patient was already seated and waiting. As Dr. Martin proceeded into the operatory, Ms. Nathan felt that there was nothing she could do but follow him into the room to assist. When Dr. Martin completed a routine crown preparation procedure, Ms. Nathan was relieved that no mistakes had occurred from his noticeable tremors. That afternoon, she again called Dr. Martin aside and implored him to seek help. She pointed out that his chairside work was noticeably shaky and that even the patient had asked her if he was all right. She noted how embarrassed she felt having to cover for him. He snapped back that it was just a bad day, that everyone has bad days, and that she was overreacting. He suggested that her own past experience may be making her a little oversensitive to a nonexisting drinking problem and further reminded her that he had in fact given her a break, that he needed her utmost support as he worked through his outside troubles, and that her loyalty during these trying times would pay dividends to her and her family.

Four months have now passed, and Ms. Nathan notes that Dr. Martin's "lunch break highs" are continuing and his clinical performance seems increasingly hindered. Although she has not yet detected any resulting injury to a patient, she feels that it is time to do something. What are her options?

Ms. Nathan could approach Dr. Martin again, insisting that he get help this time, or she will have to inform the professional regulation agency of his impairment. Because she has done this twice already with little effect other than raising Dr. Martin's ire, it is unlikely that a third attempt would produce a successful outcome. Furthermore, her direct threat to expose him could result in his taking immediate retaliatory action against her (e.g., firing her), after which her accusations could be construed merely as those of a disgruntled employee.

Ms. Nathan could report Dr. Martin's substance abuse to the state board of professional regulation, which could initiate an investigation. Some type of disciplinary action, including the suspension or loss of his license to practice, could result if Dr. Martin were found to be practicing while his ability to practice was chemically impaired or if he were found to be "habitually drunk or dependent on habitual use of narcotics, barbiturates, amphetamines, hallucinogens, or similar drugs."[6] The investigation of the complaint would probably include the examination of prescription records, as well as the authorities' interviews of the accused dentist, his staff, his acquaintances, and perhaps his patients. Such an investigation would result in public exposure of his problem without really dealing with the dependency problem itself. Again, it is not unreasonable to anticipate his resentment and retaliation toward his previously trusted assistant, Ms. Nathan, as well as a deterioration of his health if he continues using alcohol and drugs in response to this additional pressure.

At this point, the situation remains in a largely preventive stage because there is no evidence that any patient has yet suffered more than inconvenience because of Dr. Martin's addictions. Therefore, taking such a drastic step as reporting Dr. Martin to the state board of professional regulation, although offering protection to the patient community, would be a no-win situation for Dr. Martin, Ms. Nathan, and other staff members and their families who depend on the income generated by Dr. Martin's practice.

At this stage, a more reasonable option for Ms. Nathan would be to anonymously contact a dental society intervention program and seek help for Dr. Martin. This action would seem to offer the best ethical balance among (1) her obligation to prevent harm to patients, Dr. Martin, his staff, and the profession (through an erosion of the public's trust); (2) her responsibility to remain employed and support her family; and (3) her desire to respect the autonomy of all those affected by Dr. Martin's chemical dependency—specifically, Dr. Martin and his patients.

Having been previously unsuccessful in motivating Dr. Martin to seek help, by now contacting a dental society intervention program, Ms. Nathan addresses the chemical dependency problem directly while still offering him maximal confidentiality and a chance for rehabilitation. Unlike state regulatory agencies, chemical dependency assistance programs take no punitive action against the dentist. By limiting the negative consequences for Dr. Martin as much as possible, while affording him the greatest opportunity for a positive outcome, Ms. Nathan also best protects her job and Dr. Martin's high regard for her. Although it is certainly not assured, "many times, the assistant who reported the abuse is later rewarded with a salary increase or promotion. It is not unusual for an employer and employee to become closer."[2]

If Ms. Nathan were not aware of a local peer assistance program, she could contact the ADA Council on Ethics, Bylaws and Judicial Affairs and, without identifying anyone, describe her situation and ask for guidance concerning the most ethically appropriate action. Ms. Nathan's situation as the concerned subordinate of the impaired practitioner has many parallels within the profession: for example, the dental student who observes the impairment or inappropriate practices of an instructor or the junior colleague who has concerns about a more senior or more prestigious member of the field. Turning to the ADA Council on Ethics, Bylaws and Judicial Affairs is an appropriate course of action for anyone seeking guidance about an impaired practitioner or someone whose professional practices appear substandard.

In reviewing possible courses of action for both Dr. Boley (Case 1) and Ms. Nathan, it should be clear that the "do nothing" alternative mentioned early in this chapter is unacceptable. In both cases, this chapter argues for third-party intervention, not for direct, personal intervention. Although there is no question regarding the acceptance of the third-party interven-

tion strategy as the prevailing practice in cases involving chemical dependency, there has not been the same level of professional acceptance for similar third-party approaches in cases of poor quality treatment. To bring the profession's responses to these two cases in line with each other, a greater effort should be made at the local level to ensure the availability of a well-publicized, nonpunitive third-party support system addressing cases of poor quality, similar to those support systems now in place for cases of chemical dependency. Although it is unlikely that the profession will be able to move quickly toward this objective, in light of the deficiencies of the personal intervention approach in identifying and monitoring the retraining of professionals providing poor care, we nevertheless advocate reporting poor-quality care to existing local peer review boards.

CONCLUSION

If they are to serve the public and deserve and maintain the public's trust and esteem, dentists must learn to be effective self-regulators. In the course of their dental school education and through continuing education programs and publications, dentists must learn to act autonomously, taking upon themselves the responsibility to promote and prevent harm to the dental health of patients. Educational, regulatory, and professional policies; structures; and mechanisms should seek to create an open and collegial environment in which dentists are expected to identify and seek help in correcting their mistakes and faults (e.g., a chemical dependency problem or a lack of preparation or skill), as well as those of their colleagues. A supportive and corrective professional response to mistake-making, rather than a punitive one, may encourage dentists to assume this self-regulatory responsibility.

Excellent-quality care is the primary goal of dentistry, and therefore poor-quality care is to be avoided. When, however, poor care has occurred or is likely to occur, dentists have a responsibility to correct or prevent it. In doing so, they promote good and prevent or correct harm, which are the goals of the ethical duties to act beneficently and nonmaleficently. By assuming this responsibility, by justifiably criticizing their own faulty work and that of their colleagues, and by informing patients of such faulty work when it occurs, dentists act as responsible, autonomous individuals and also promote the autonomy of their patients.

DISCUSSION QUESTIONS

1. Loyalty is a virtue invoked both in favor of and against blowing the whistle on colleagues' substandard practices. To whom might a dentist, who has knowledge of a colleague's misconduct, feel a duty of loyalty? Why? How should he or she weigh these conflicting loyalties? Why?

2. In his critique of the ADA Code, David Nash writes that "the practitioner not committed to lifelong learning and change in practice strategies has difficulty practicing ethically."[7] What is the relationship between competent practice and ethical practice in dentistry?

3. Evaluate the strengths and weaknesses of various responses to a colleague's poor quality patient care. If the colleague's substandard treatment resulted from his or her chemical dependency, would your response be different? Should it be?

4. If you choose to speak to one of your colleagues about his or her treatment error—for instance, a root tip left near the sinus following an extraction—and if he or she assures you that the error is an isolated one, that he or she will remedy the error free of charge to the patient, and that he or she will be more careful in the future, what will you then do? The error is the only one which has come to your attention.

   Next, suppose that you learn from other colleagues that this is not an isolated error that your colleague has made, but that it is one of several errors of a similar degree of seriousness. Does knowing this information lead you to a different course of action? If so, what and why? If not, why not?

   Now, suppose that your colleague explains why he or she believes the error was made; knowledge of another's reasons for mistake (or motives for action) often affects how one feels about the mistake (or bad outcome) and what one deems an appropriate response. Suppose that he or she explains that the error occurred because he or she had been up all night before performing the extraction with a colicky baby and was therefore tired, or instead that he or she had been out too late the night before with friends, had drunk a bit too much, and was therefore tired. Do these different explanations affect how you feel about the error or the course of action which you choose? Should they make a difference? How? Why?

5. What are your school's policies concerning chemically impaired dental students and faculty? What are the policies concerning poor quality patient care in the dental clinic of your school? How are patient grievances resolved? Do your clinic's structure, practices, and policies encourage students to blow the whistle on poor quality dental care? Do the grading practices of your dental school encourage students to be responsible professionals?

   If the dean of your dental school asked you to make recommendations concerning the curriculum and policies of your school so that they better reflected the school's commitment to training responsible professionals, what recommendations would you propose?

ACKNOWLEDGMENTS

The authors would like to acknowledge the contributions of Athena Beldecos, Re-

search Assistant, University of Pittsburgh;
and John Eisner, D.D.S., Ph.D., Associate
Professor, Department of Behavioral
Sciences, State University of New York,
Buffalo.

REFERENCES

1. Swazey, J.P., and Scher, S.R.: The whistleblower as a deviant professional: Professional norms and responses to fraud in clinical research. *In* Whistleblowing in Biomedical Research. President's Commission for the Study of Ethical Problems in Medicine and Biomedical and Behavioral Research, 1981.
2. Giangrego, E., and Oberg, S.W.: Chemical dependency: The road to recovery. J. Am. Dent. Assoc. *115*:26, 1987.
3. American Dental Association Principles of Ethics and Code of Professional Conduct. J. Am. Dent. Assoc. *120*:585, 1990.
4. Case adapted from Pollack, B., and Marinelli, R.: Ethical moral and legal dilemmas in dentistry: The process of informed decision making. J. Law Ethics Dent. *1*:28, 1988.
5. Waithe, M.: AIDS and dentistry: Conflicting rights and the public's health. *In* Biomedical Ethics Reviews: 1988. Edited by J.M. Humber and R.F. Almeder. Clifton, NJ, Humana Press, 1989, p. 142.
6. Moskowitz, J.D., and Farrell, J.D.: Professional disciplinary proceedings and the licensed dental practitioner. N.Y. State Dent. J. *50*:437, 1984.
7. Nash, D.A.: Ethics in dentistry: Review and critique of Principles of Ethics and Code of Professional Conduct. J. Am. Dent. Assoc. *109*:597, 1984.
8. Elliston, F., et al.: Whistleblowing Research: Methodological and Moral Issues. New York, Praeger Publications, 1985, p. 8.
9. Oberg, S.W.: Dependency. J. Am. Coll. Dent. *56*: 5, 9, 1989.
10. Council on Dental Practice: Chemical dependency and dental practice. J. Am. Dent. Assoc. *114*:513, 1987.
11. Peterson, R.L., and Avery, J.K.: The alcohol-impaired dentist: an educational challenge. J. Am. Dent. Assoc. *117*:743, 1988.
12. Atkinson, J.M., Millar, K., Kay, E.J., and Blinkhorn, A.S.: Stress in dental practice. Dent. Update. *18*:60, 1991.
13. Cannon, M.: Substance abuse is focus of Meharry conference. ASDA News *21*:4, 1991.
14. Van Dyk, W.: The disease called chemical dependency. J. Am. Dent. Assoc. *114*:568, 1987.
15. Deevy, P.E.: The moral status of loyalty: Whistleblowing. *In* Current Problems of Professional Ethics: An Interdisciplinary Approach. Edited by M. Barnes. Lincoln, NE, University of Nebraska Press, 1984, p. 46.
16. Near, J.P., and Miceli, M.P.: Retaliation against whistleblowers: Predictors and effects. J. Appl. Psychol. *71*:137, 1986.
17. Nash, D.A.: Ethics in dentistry: Review and critique of Principles of Ethics and Code of Professional Conduct. J. Am. Dent. Assoc. *109*:599, 1984.

SUGGESTED READING

Bok, S.: Whistleblowing and professional responsibilities. *In* Ethics Teaching in Higher Education. Edited by D. Callahan and S. Bok. New York, Plenum Press, 1980.
Heacock, M.V., and McGee, G.W.: Whistleblowing: An ethical issue in organization and human behavior. Business and Professional Ethics J. *6*: 35, 1986. (Criteria for determining when to blow the whistle and a survey of categories of whistle blowing)
Howard, W.W.: Integrity is part of the treatment plan. Dental Abstracts, August 1989, 384; reprinted from General Dentistry *37*:104, 1989. (A case of overtreatment, possible fraud)
Nash, D.A.: Ethics in dentistry: Review and critique of Principles of Ethics and Code of Professional Conduct. J. Am. Dent. Assoc. *109*:597, 1984.
Palat, M.: Legal aspects. *In* Guide to Dental Problems for Physicians and Surgeons. Edited by S.R. Thaller. Baltimore, Williams and Wilkins, 1988. (Suggestion of duties imposed by a standard of care)
Petersen, J.C., and Farrell, D.: Whistleblowing: Ethical and Legal Issues in Expressing Dissent: Dubuque, Iowa, Kendall Hunt Publishing, 1986. (Focused primarily on engineering, but relevant to all professions and a variety of employment settings)
Walters, K.D.: Your employees' right to blow the whistle. Harvard Bus. Rev. *53*:26, 161–162, 1975. (Suggestions of institutional mechanisms to obviate the need for external whistleblowing)

Chapter 8

Relationships with Dental Hygienists and Dental Assistants

Mary Alice Gaston
Marcia A. Gladwin

SUMMARY

A study of ethics in dentistry would be incomplete without a discussion of the ethical relationship between dentists and the support personnel within dental practices. This chapter examines the responsibilities that hygienists and assistants have toward their employer and their patients, and what they ought to do when these responsibilities appear to conflict. This discussion includes a historical review of dental assistants and dental hygienists to show the unique position of each within today's dental practice. We will also consider what it means that dental assistants and dental hygienists were originally young women recruited from the families of dentists and still continue to be primarily white women. This demographic profile sometimes creates problems related to personal moral values, and it influences how such problems are resolved within dental practices.

The chapter groups the professional relationships of dental hygienists and dental assistants into three general categories which by their very nature create ethical concerns: (1) relationships with the dentist-employer, (2) relationships with individual patients, and (3) relationships with the general public. A five-step problem-solving model is used in discussing a case study illustrating the ethical concerns present in the relationship between dental hygienists and their dentist-employers in a group specialty practice.

The chapter ends with a listing of additional questions and case studies useful for classroom discussion.

ETHICAL PROBLEMS IN DENTAL HYGIENE

A 1987 study of dental hygiene practice revealed that most dental hygienists encountered situations in practice they considered to be ethical problems, and they felt that they may not have been prepared to resolve them.[1] This chapter helps support staff to meet such challenges. It is important also for dentists to appreciate the moral dilemmas that their hygienists and assistants face, for those problems may affect the quality of care that dentists provide to patients. Being sensitive to the needs of support staff is also another way in which dentists fulfill their duties of beneficence and respect for persons. Because there are some morally relevant differences between the practices of dentistry and dental hygiene, we consider some of these differences by reviewing the history of dental hygiene and by examining the roles and responsibilities hygienists now have. We then analyze a moral problem facing hygienists and assistants, using a method similar to the one presented in

Chapter 3. This analysis may be applied to the cases we present at the end, or to any you face in your own practice.

HISTORICAL PERSPECTIVE

Like the medical profession, dentistry had very few women within its ranks until the middle of the 20th century. According to Motley, the first female dentist in the United States is thought to have been Emeline Rupert Jones, who was trained by her husband and began practicing in 1854 after his death. It was not until 1861 that the first woman graduated from a dental college.[2] Before the turn of this century, any assistant to a dentist was usually a newly graduated dentist or one in training. The practice of having a female "attendant" in the dental office became accepted practice only during the first decade of the 20th century. These early female assistants were usually the wives, daughters, or other relatives of the dentist. In addition to lending an air of respectability to the office, these early assistants carried out most of the menial tasks generally assigned to women of that period. The presence of the female dental assistant made it more acceptable for female patients to come to the dental office unattended. Gradually, the practice of engaging dental assistants became more widespread and later served as the basis for developing a category of employees who became known as dental hygienists.

The dentists who were the early leaders of the oral hygiene movement, which gained momentum around the middle of the 19th century, believed that women were not likely to be bored by repetitious tasks and were especially suited to perform preventive duties. Historical records do not indicate that any consideration was ever given to any group being trained in these new preventive procedures other than young women. Men were actually not allowed to become dental hygienists and were not accepted into early schools for dental hygienists.[3] Young women still appear to remain the most desirable candidates for careers in dental assisting and

dental hygiene; 99% of those practicing today are female.[4]

The growth and development of dental hygiene and dental assisting as disciplines within the practice of dentistry have been slow and have often been met with strong opposition. Initially, dentists trained dental assistants to perform the dental prophylaxis and allowed them to provide such care to their patients. The first formal training program for dental nurses, who were intended to be the counterpart of medical nurses, opened in 1910 at the Ohio College of Dental Surgery. This program remained in operation for only 4 years because of the bitter opposition from Ohio dentists.

The credit for coining the name "dental hygienist" is given to Dr. Alfred C. Fones, a Bridgeport, Connecticut, dentist who first adopted the theory and mastered the skills of dental prophylaxis. He taught his assistant and cousin, Irene Newman, to perform this procedure. Dr. Fones felt that the name of this new preventive dental specialist should express prevention rather than the treatment of disease, so he rejected the name "dental nurse," suggested earlier by an Ohio dentist, Dr. C. M. Wright. After Irene Newman's in-office training in 1906, Dr. Fones opened a school of dental hygiene in his carriage house in 1913 and graduated the first class in 1914. It is important to note that Dr. Fones publicly expressed his belief that dentists had a professional responsibility to serve the needs of the community. His primary goal in establishing this new auxiliary to dentistry was to promote oral health and educate school children of his city in the prevention of tooth decay. Therefore, many of the first graduates of The Fones School worked in the public school system providing oral prophylaxis and basic oral and general hygiene instruction.

Initially, local dentists opposed the work of these individuals who were referred to as "women operators in dental practice." Despite opposition, the movement grew, and dental hygienists were first licensed in Connecticut and Massachusetts in 1915 and in New York in 1916. Dr. Fones's carriage house dental hygiene school graduated three classes before other educational institutions such as Harvard and Tufts Universities, Forsyth Dental Infirmary for Children (Boston), Rochester Dental Dispensary (Rochester, NY), and Hunter College (New York City), began educational programs for dental hygienists.[2] Formal education of dental hygienists was a value instilled in the profession by its founder and serves as a source of conflict within dentistry today.

The problems encountered by dental hygienists and others delivering dental care are not unlike those experienced by nurses and allied health professionals who have similar working relationships and roles in providing health services with physicians. Problems often result from different interpretations of the proper roles and responsibilities of the various professionals involved in patient care. In the U. S. health care delivery system, physicians and dentists have traditionally been recognized as "rightful knowers" of knowledge in the health care arena.[5,6] For instance, even though a dental assistant is well trained and has observed dentists take many master impressions for fixed partial dentures, most states do not allow assistants to take a master impression because that procedure is reserved for the possessor of the highest level of knowledge. In other words, even though support professionals may be able to assess a situation and determine appropriate action, only the rightful knower has the sanction of society and individual states to make the final decision regarding appropriate care and to determine how that care is to be provided.

Individual dentists have always held opposing views as to whether these auxiliary professions should exist, how much education and training they should have, the duties they should be allowed to perform, where they should be allowed to practice, and the kind of dental supervision they require to ensure the safe treatment of the public. Even though many experimental projects have demonstrated the value of dental assistants and dental hygienists, many dentists still perceive any increase in education, lessening of dental supervision, or expansion of scope of practice as competition for the delivery of dental services.[7]

CURRENT PRACTICE: THE ROLES OF RACE AND GENDER

In 1990, the American Dental Association found that most dentists (90.1%) employed at least one nondentist staff person on a full- or part-time basis in their practice. Over half of the dentists (57.2%) employed at least one dental hygienist; most (92.2%) employed at least one chairside assistant and at least one secretary (85.4%). Of dentists employing dental hygienists and assistants, the average number of full-time or part-time dental hygienists employed per dentist was 1.3, and the average number of full-time or part-time dental assistants employed per dentist was 1.5.[8]

Approximately 80,000 dental hygienists and 187,000 dental assistants are currently employed in the United States. Ninety-nine percent of these are women, and 97.4% of the dental hygienists and 83.6% of the dental assistants are white.[9] Historically, both groups have been predominantly Caucasian females who are employed by Caucasian males. The majority (92.8%) of all private dental practitioners are white men.[10] We will refer to these statistics later in the chapter because they are relevant to the discussion of values and ethics in dentistry.

DENTAL HYGIENE TODAY: ROLES AND RESPONSIBILITIES

Dental hygienists must hold a current license to practice in the United States and Canada, and their practice is regulated by individual state and province dental practice acts. Currently, the minimum entry-level educational programs for dental hygienists are 2-year college or university programs. Many of these programs require at least 1 year of college before admission, which results in graduates actually having 3 years of education. In addition, some 2-year programs have at least 2 summer sessions, which also result in 3 years of education. Another type of educational setting is the 4-year program in which graduates are offered a baccalaureate degree. In addition to graduating from an accredited educational program, dental hygienists must pass a written national examination for dental hygiene licensure. Regional or state examinations are generally required which may be administered in a clinic practice and/or written format. In 1991, approximately 4000 dental hygienists completed educational programs, graduated and became licensed.[11]

Dental assistants can be trained in programs offered in community and junior colleges, trade schools, technical institutions, and in the armed forces. They can also be trained on the job by their employing dentist. Optional certification can be earned by passing an examination offered through the American Dental Assistants' Association. Approximately 4000 dental assistants graduate annually from accredited dental assisting programs.[11] A license to practice is not required, but a certificate may be required by some states to perform certain procedures. Many dental assistants have completed expanded-function auxiliary training programs and are prepared to assume more than the traditional chairside dental assisting duties. As with dental hygienists, the duties they may legally assume are also determined by individual state practice acts.[12]

More dental hygienists and dental assistants joined the work force during the 1970s than at any other time, when the demand for dental services exceeded the resources available. In response to this demand, the scope of training and practice for dental auxiliaries was expanded to include procedures that previously had been performed only by dentists. Tension was created between dentists and their auxiliaries during the 1980s when the demand for dental services declined and the number of dentists increased. This has led to challenges to state dental practice acts and general disagreement regarding roles in the dental care delivery system.[13]

The need to recruit and retain adequate numbers of support personnel in medical and dental practices has produced studies demonstrating that a practice environment that created positive personal relations and provided professional freedom to perform expanded duties tended to increase the degree of satisfaction felt by dental hygienists.[14,15] Practice management experts have even suggested using the job preview as a screening device to assess the moral values in a practice to determine if the likelihood exists that the employer and prospective staff will share the same goals and beliefs.[16]

THREE CATEGORIES OF RELATIONSHIPS AND SOME QUESTIONS THEY RAISE

Professional relationships of dental assistants and dental hygienists may be grouped into three general categories, with each category giving rise to moral concerns. These are (1) the relationship with the dentist-employer, (2) the relationship with individual patients, and (3) the relationship with the public. Problems in each relationship are likely to be generated by differences in social, cultural, economic, and moral values, and the relative priority given to those values. Dental assistants and dental hygienists may find themselves asking some of the following questions regarding their relationship with their employer, their responsibility to the patients in the practice, and their obligation to the public as healthcare providers. For purposes of abbreviation, we refer only to dental hygienists, although each category applies to dental assistants as well.

1. **The dentist-hygienist relationship.** Is the relationship with the employer collaborative and collegial or competitive? Is there a "dental team approach" and an attempt to nurture high ethical standards among all the office employees? Does the dentist make all the decisions affecting the practice, including those affecting the assistant and hygienist? Does the fact that most dentists are men and most assistants and hygienists women have any influence on the way office procedures and policies are established? If a dentist's management style is paternalistic and autocratic, is that style reinforced and even encouraged by the more passive behavior of the females in the practice? What role does gender play in these relationships? When moral

questions surface, which kind of relationship fosters effective problem solving? What are the rights and responsibilities of each member of the dental team, and how is each member accountable to the others?

2. **The hygienist-patient relationship.** Dental hygienists often consider the patients they treat as "theirs," because with respect to preventive dental care they are the major care provider. However, most state dental practice acts require dental hygienists to practice under direct, indirect, or general supervision of a dentist, which makes hygienists legally bound to act as an agent of the dentist. However, because the dental hygienist provides treatment during prophylaxis, is she not therefore accountable to the patient? Or is the dentist the only one accountable? (One might speak of being accountable not only in a *legal* sense, but in a *moral* sense as well.) Which dental team member should make the final decision regarding appropriate patient care? It is not unusual for the dental assistant also to provide individualized home care instruction to patients that is appropriate for their oral condition. If she is interrupted by a telephone call and forgets to fulfill this duty, who in the dental team is accountable to the patient? Information may be provided to patients by any dental team member, and such disclosure is one of the critical elements of informed consent. What role should hygienists play in obtaining informed consent?

3. **The relationship the hygienist has with the public.** The dentist and dental office employees may be asked to provide dental services to the needy and underprivileged as a community service. Do dental hygienists and assistants have responsibilities for providing service to the public outside of the private practice setting? If so, how much is required? Does the public have a right to receive quality dental health care at a cost they can afford? What is a fair or just distribution of dental health care? Further consideration of this relationship may be given when analyzing case number 6 at the end of this chapter.

We now turn to a case that raises many of these questions. We analyze the case by applying a five-step model, similar in content to the one presented in Chapter 3.

CASE ANALYSIS

Consider the following situation:

For the past several months, the dental hygienists in a busy periodontal specialty practice have been spending at least 10 minutes between patients taking steps to adhere to the strict infection control standards required by the Occupation Safety and Health Administration (OSHA). Patients are usually scheduled for regular dental hygiene maintenance care in 1-hour appointment periods, and despite the additional time required to carry out the necessary infection control procedures, no additional time between patients has been allotted. The dental hygienists are becoming more and more dissatisfied because they feel they do not have sufficient time to provide comprehensive patient care. Instead, they are forced to "cut corners" when providing services to each patient scheduled. In their opinion, the dentists have been less than supportive because the practice depends on the dental hygienists to generate a sizable percentage of practice revenue, and allowing 10 minutes between appointment periods would result in a daily loss of revenue equal to the fee assessed to two patients. The dental assistants in the office are unable to assist the dental hygienists because the assistants must also spend this additional time in keeping the dentists' operatories disinfected and instruments sterilized according to the same OSHA standards.

In attempting to resolve the impasse, the dental hygienists have organized the sterilization and disinfection procedures for greatest efficiency but have not been able to significantly reduce the time needed between patients to do a thorough job. The attempt made to fulfill their employer's wish has resulted in a lower level of patient care that does not meet the hygienist's professional standards. The level of stress generated by this situation has forced two of the dental hygienists to consider changing positions.

What should the hygienists do? There are several courses of action they *could* take. Which of these choices is the best from a moral point of view, and why? To answer these questions, we will do the following:

1. Describe the facts.
2. Identify the human factors involved.
3. Identify the values and ethical principles involved.
4. List alternative solutions and their justification.
5. Choose a course of action.

Facts in the Case

Infection control standards are not optional and every dental practice must adhere to them. The dental hygienists have tried unsuccessfully to shorten the time spent in this effort, and they cannot reasonably expect any assistance from the dental assistants, who have other responsibilities. The dental hygienists have become discontent, and have made a deliberate effort to resolve this problem with the dentists. Without resolution, the entire practice would be adversely affected.

In this practice the relationship between the dentists and office staff is hierarchical rather than collegial. The dentists own the practice, are responsible for controlling expenses, and must make sure that the revenue generated is sufficient to keep the practice financially profitable. Therefore, they assume the right to make most of the decisions. It is also apparent that both the dentists and the dental hygienists have similar knowledge and responsibility with respect to infection control and appropriate preventive patient care. The dental hygienists in this case would argue that they are, along with the dentists, rightful knowers by virtue of their education, licensure, and practice experience.[5] Some collaboration among individuals involved in this case is highly desirable and will be necessary to successfully resolve the impasse.

Human Factors Involved

When attempting to solve problems, especially moral ones, resulting from interactions between people, it is helpful to consider the situation from the unique perspective of each individual involved. Because human factors such as emotions, feelings, and perceptions that are present in this case have the potential to facilitate or inhibit problem resolution, it is important to identify and explore them as fully as possible before moving to the next step.

The dental hygienists feel a commitment to provide high-quality care to the patients in the practice and do not feel that the dentists have demonstrated the same level of commitment. The dental hygienists are probably powerless in this situation, because they have not been included in the scheduling decision but are expected to make it work. Their feelings of self-esteem and self-worth are lower than desirable, as expressed in their consideration of leaving the practice.

The dentists have the authority to set the schedule for those employed in the practice and have exercised that authority. The dentists feel pressure to keep everyone satisfied and still maintain a practice that is financially stable. They consider themselves to be the primary decision makers because they have the greatest financial investment in the practice. They have also acquired the highest knowledge level and have great accountability to the public.

However, the dentists have not demonstrated clearly to the dental hygienists a respect for their knowledge, skills, and ability to determine their own standards for excellent quality dental hygiene care. All indications are that the dentists believe they know what is best for their practice. This hierarchical relationship is probably a result of the historical social and economic position of women in dentistry discussed earlier in the chapter, and the dentists may be unaware that there is a problem.

The dental assistants in the practice are also affected by this problem because they have also had to spend additional time in preparing the dental operatory between patients. Because of the close working environment, they are presumably aware of the difficulties experienced by the dental hygienists and have felt the resulting tension between them and the dentists. Because they are employed by the dentists, they may feel little responsibility for making the situation better for the dental hygienists. They could view this situation as being of no concern to them.

The patients in this practice expect the office staff to maintain a level of environmental safety that protects everyone from harm such as contracting an infectious disease. Patients may not be receiving the best comprehensive dental care, even though steps are being taken to protect them. Long-time patients in the practice may be able to detect a difference in the length of time they now spend with the dental hygienists. It is possible, too, that they may notice subtle changes in the way they are treated as a result of this tension among the hygienists, assistants and dentists.

Values and Ethical Principles Involved

Identifying the values and ethical principles involved is the third step of the ethical analysis. From the dentists' perspective, one important value is respect for the law. The dentists have respect for the Dental Practice Act and value their privilege to practice dentistry. To keep their license in good standing, and to avoid fines or violations, they are obligated to abide by the OSHA standards. In addition, the dentists have a moral obligation to obey the law. At the same time, by following these standards they are well aware that they are doing good (fulfilling their duty of beneficence) and preventing future harm (fulfilling their duty of nonmaleficence) to their patients and staff. A related value is the trust that the dentists' patients place in them; promoting this trust is another way the dentists realize their general duty of beneficence. It is likely that the dentists also value their personal autonomy. This is reflected by their satisfaction and contentment in owning a dental practice, their financial stability, and their position as authority figures as owners of the practice. It is also the case that the dentists have a moral obligation to respect patient self-determination. Finally, the dentists value justice, because they hold themselves responsible in providing fair employment compensation to the office staff.

The dental hygienists value their relationships with the dentists as well as with their patients. They have correlative moral obligations to respect the dentists' authority, as well as to promote the welfare of patients and to protect patients from harm. The hygienists also believe it is important to be satisfied in their jobs, and may even believe that they have a moral obligation to be true to themselves. Like the dentists, the hygienists have a moral responsibility to respect the laws regulating dental and dental hygiene practice, as well as the dignity and autonomy of others.

The patients too, hold values in regard to receiving dental care. Patients value the freedom of selecting a dental office of their choice and the right to be respected by professionals, both examples of autonomy. In turn, the patient respects the professionals and the dental services that they provide. Although dental ethics focuses on the responsibilities of dentists and hygienists toward patients, it is also the case that patients have responsibilities toward those who provide health care to them, as Kahn and Hasegawa note in Chapter 4. For example, patients not only have a right to know what will be done to them, but they have an obligation to disclose all information that would be relevant to their oral health care.

ALTERNATIVE SOLUTIONS AND THEIR JUSTIFICATION

There are at least four courses of action that the hygienists *could* take. They could:

1. Leave the practice and find positions elsewhere;
2. Continue working for these dentists and simply do the best they can under the circumstances;
3. Attempt to persuade the dentists to be more relaxed with infection control requirements; or
4. Discuss the issue at a staff meeting and encourage the dentists to allow more flexibility in scheduling, so that the hygienists have enough time to provide high quality care while following the infection control protocol.

Which of these options is best from a moral point of view, and why? We will consider each in turn.

ALTERNATIVE ONE

In choosing the first alternative, the dental hygienists would be exercising their right to personal autonomy. To deny that the dental hygienists have the right to leave the practice would be to deny them due respect for personal independence and dignity. A decision to leave would also demonstrate their commitment to do no harm to patients, because the hygienists believe they are presently unable to provide an optimal level of care. However, in this case it is not clear that their leaving would avoid harming future patients, because subsequent dental hygienists would be placed in the same position and the quality of care could still be compromised.

One could argue that this is not an acceptable choice because the dental hygienists may be acting out of self-interest more than respect for duty to others, including the dental hygiene profession. The hygienists might be basing their decision to leave not on their obligation to avoid placing patients at risk, but rather on their desire to find a more personally satisfying job. From a moral point of view, one might conclude that the hygienists could justify leaving only if they could demonstrate that their actions were based primarily on their duty to protect patients from harm, rather than their desire to be less frustrated in their work. If they could not rule out self-interest as the primary concern, it would be difficult to say that they had good *moral* reasons to leave.[17]

Although the first alternative solution could possibly bring immediate relief for the frustrations of the dental hygienists, the underlying problem would not be resolved, patient care could be compromised, the financial status of the practice could be affected, and the resentment of the dental hygienists would remain unresolved. Discussion of this alternative leaves several other unanswered ethical questions that we will identify in considering the second alternative.

ALTERNATIVE TWO

In choosing to continue to work for these dentists and do the best they can under these circumstances, the dental hygienists would be placing the patients at risk of harm and might be jeopardizing the integrity of the profession. The assumption underlying professional privilege is that patients have the right to expect health professionals to act on each patient's behalf, and when making decisions concerning each patient's well-being, act as the patient would if the patient possessed the same level of knowledge and skill. Alternative two, like alternative one, would allow professionals to neglect their responsibility to do good and to do no harm. Although this choice might be *easier* for the hygienists to make, it is difficult to *justify* it from a moral point of view, because the hygienists would be failing to fulfill their primary ethical obligations.

If these dental hygienists chose this alternative, the credibility and standing of dental hygiene as a profession might be jeopardized because others might act in the same way. Also, the hygienists would have to disregard their right to self-determination. In addition, accepting this alternative would strengthen the role of the dentist as the primary decision maker in a traditional hierarchical relationship between dentists and the auxiliaries in their employ, and thereby reinforce paternalistic behavior. Many dental hygienists might choose this alternative because of the historical tendency to view themselves as having little power and being somewhat less than autonomous. However, this does not justify the choice *ethically*.

In choosing alternative two, the hygienists would fail to fulfill their duty to report unsafe procedures to appropriate agencies such as state dental boards, and the Occupation Safety and Health Administration. According to Barish and Barish, dental hygienists, like nurses, are capable of recognizing high quality care and are obligated to report inadequate and inappropriate patient care services to appropriate authorities.[18] The moral obligation to report violations of the law may be understood as an application of the duty of fidelity. When hygienists become licensed, they promise to abide by the law and the relevant rules and regulations. Because they are legally required to disclose OSHA violations to the proper authorities, alternative two would compromise their duty of fidelity.

It is useful to refer to the historical review of the development of dental auxiliaries provided previously in the chapter when considering this alternative. Although this alternative may have been somewhat acceptable to dental hygienists at the point in the development of the profession when they were relatives of their dentist-employer or socially and economically subservient to men in general, it is not acceptable in view of the changed role of women in today's society. Because personal autonomy and economic independence have become general values of women in today's society, and, because dental hygienists are almost exclusively women, it is unlikely that the dental hygienists in this practice could ever be satisfied after choosing alternative two.

In 1986, Rubenstein and May identified sources of stress during the training and practice of dental hygienists. They reported that attempting to do a thorough job in less than optimal time is a major source of stress. This kind of pressure is particularly harmful, because it is often constant and influenced by factors such as patients being on time and the dentist's schedule, both of which are beyond the dental hygienist's control. According to the report, another factor is the extent to which hygienists are participants in decisions related to patient care. They want to be given credit for the contribution they make to patient health, and when they are not, they find it extremely stressful.[19] Reports such as this indicate that alternative two would be psychologically unacceptable to most dental hygienists.

Finally, alternative two involves deception, because patients would falsely believe that the dental office is providing the highest standards of care. Truth-telling is a professional obligation and ensures support of the community, so failing to be truthful seriously undermines both the dental and dental hygiene professions. Because alternative two involves violating the moral duties of fidelity and truth-telling, most hygienists would find it an ethically unacceptable solution to the problem.

ALTERNATIVE THREE

Attempting to persuade the dentists to relax infection control requirements would, if successful, expedite the daily flow of patients in and out of the practice, but this choice presents a number of ethical problems that seem to rule it out as an alternative. Alternatives three and two are alike in that similar values and ethical principles are involved. The greatest concern with this alternative would be that any relaxation of infection control procedures has the potential to cause great harm to patients and office staff and would thus violate the principles of beneficence and nonmaleficence. Additionally, this alternative would violate the laws protecting the health and safety of employees. Perhaps most importantly, this choice would violate the rights of patients because dental hygienists are expected to act in the patient's best interest.

ALTERNATIVE FOUR

Through discussion with the staff, the dentists could work out a way to allow more flexibility in scheduling, so that the dental hygienists feel they have enough time to provide high-quality care while following the infection control protocol was the last alternative solution to solve this dilemma. Common-sense morality would lead us to conclude that this is the best alternative of the four. Beyond common-sense morality, however, selecting this alternative can be justified by appealing to generally accepted professional values and ethical principles. Open discussion between the members of the office staff respects the right of individual staff members to contribute to decisions that affect them. It would at the same time strengthen a more collegial and collaborative approach to resolving problems and would lessen the paternalistic tendencies expressed by the dentists.

Although competitive salaries and benefits may enhance the probability of retaining essential dental auxiliaries, less tangible values often have just as much impact. Studies of dental hygiene job and career satisfaction indicate that dental hygienists place high value on feelings such as inner harmony, happiness, self-respect, honesty, and responsibility. Achievement, independence, and altruism are also cited as values related to overall satisfaction with dental hygiene as a career.[15] Assuming that these research findings are valid, open discussion to solve this problem can only strengthen the commitment of these dental hygienists to this dental practice.

The dentists, by making the appropriate modifications, would be fulfilling their professional duties to provide a safe environment for patients and staff, and to place the interests of patients above their own. This alternative would also be the most acceptable because many, rather than few, people would benefit by this choice of alternatives.

This alternative still leaves some important questions unanswered. Even though alternative four could possibly resolve ethical concerns, the dentists might still feel pressure to make certain that the practice remained profitable enough to ensure the economic well-being of everyone in the practice. As stated previously, allowing more time between patients would lessen the income generated by the dental hygienists. Would it be fair to pass that cost on to the patients in the form of a fee increase? Would it be fair to ask employees to share in the loss of income by agreeing to work with no annual raise or perhaps a smaller bonus or none at all? How long would staff be content with such an arrangement? Should the dentists absorb the cost and just accept a reduced personal income? A fuller ethical analysis of this case would do well to address these questions.

SUMMARY

This chapter has provided a description of dental hygienists and, to a lesser extent, dental assistants. It has briefly reviewed the history and roles and responsibilities of each. The chapter has illustrated the connection between the origin and early development of dental assisting and hygiene with respect to their relationship to dentists and some of the ethical concerns within current dental practice. The chapter also identified and discussed one of three general areas in which individual dental professionals are forced to make value judgments and ethical decisions. Sources of conflicts that might result when individuals encounter situations, react to them, and make decisions using personal interpretations of standards of ethical behavior were identified. An analysis of a case illustrated how ethical principles might be applied to the resolution of an ethical problem. Further discussions of ethical issues in dental hygiene might consider the accountability of hygienists to their patients and the nature and scope of the hygienist's obligation to promote the public health. Cases on these and other issues are provided for this purpose.

DISCUSSION QUESTIONS

1. Recalling the material on the nature of dental ethics from the first section of the book, which of the questions listed in the section, "Three Categories of Relationships and Some Questions They Raise," are truly ethical ones? Why?
2. What should a hygienist or assistant do when he or she has good reasons to believe that a member of the team is compromising patient care because of a chemical dependency or other impairment? Refer to chapter 7 in your answer.
3. Activities central to the profession of dental hygiene, such as accreditation of educational programs and national testing of graduates, are conducted by agencies established and staffed by the American Dental Association. Additionally, dental hygiene practice is regulated by individual state dental practice acts. Although these ADA agencies and state dental boards include some dental hygiene representation, the majority of the members are dentists. What involvement should the dental profession have in the education, testing, and licensing of dental hygienists, or the

regulation of hygiene practice? Is there a moral justification for one profession exercising such a strong influence over another?

4. The dental workplace requires close personal interaction. Because most dentists are men and most hygienists and assistants are women, what are the rights and responsibilities of each member of the team regarding sexual harassment? What ethical principles apply? What should dentists do to promote professional and respectful treatment of support staff?

5. Many state dental practice acts permit dental hygienists to practice only under the supervision of a dentist. Are these supervision requirements morally justified, in view of the education and licensure requirements for dental hygienists? What harms, if any, might result from making supervision laws less restrictive? What benefits? Do they outweigh the potential harms?

ADDITIONAL CASE STUDIES

CASE 1

You are a dental hygienist who is presently unemployed and have been looking for a job for 2 months. Employment is necessary because you are single and must support yourself. You hear, through a friend, that Dr. Jones might be considering terminating Ms. Smith, a dental hygienist whom she has employed for the last 10 years. You arrange an interview with Dr. Jones, and, during the discussion, you learn that Ms. Smith has been providing high-quality care for patients in the practice. You also learn that Dr. Jones is experiencing some financial problems and must cut her expenses. Because Ms. Smith has been with Dr. Jones for so long, her salary and benefits are considerably higher than she would feel it necessary to pay a new employee such as you. Should you, or would you, take the position if it is offered? Are there any ethical principles illustrated by this case? If yes, what are they? Using the problem-solving model, work through to a satisfactory resolution of this problem.

CASE 2

Susan, a new patient, is a 16-year-old single young woman who is seeing you for dental hygiene care for the first time. In your practice, radiographs are taken of every new patient as a part of the diagnostic data gathering. As a safety precaution, before taking radiographs of all women of childbearing age, you always ask them whether or not they are pregnant. Susan, aware that her mother is in the waiting room, very quietly tells you that she is pregnant. She also says that her parents are unaware of her condition, and sincerely asks you not to tell her mother or the dentist. How do you treat this confidential information? Should you take the radiographs? What questions will arise if you do not? What do you owe this patient? What, if anything, do you owe this minor's mother? Would you, or should you, involve your dentist-employer in this matter?

CASE 3

You are employed in a large group practice with four dental hygienists, some part-time and some full-time. Patients are scheduled for preventive care and are assigned to a dental hygienist at random. For some time now, patients have confided in you their displeasure with the treatment received when seen by one particular dental hygienist in the practice. Patients commonly complain that the hygienist rushes them in and out, and that the patients' mouths are sore for several days after each appointment with her. Some of the patients say that if they keep getting assigned to this particular hygienist, they will probably find a new dentist, to avoid this bad experience. Now that you have been made aware of this situation, what responsibilities do you have in this case? What are some possible ways of handling the situation? What do you owe the patients, the employing dentist, the other dental hygienist, and the profession of dental hygiene?

CASE 4

You are a female dental hygienist who has been employed in the same dental office for 5 years. You have enjoyed your work and have felt fairly compensated. The practice has grown and there is a need to employ another dental hygienist. The person who is hired is a male dental hygienist who has been out of school for one year. Within the next few months, you discover that he forgets to take medical histories on new patients and review those that exist for established patients. Many times, you have discovered localized substantial subgingival deposits on patients with 2- and 3-month recalls. You also notice that he habitually arrives to work late, making the patients wait 15 to 20 minutes before being seated. Up to this point, you have decided to say nothing to him or the dentist.

Then one day, because of carelessness on the part of the bookkeeper, you find out that this new dental hygienist is receiving a salary higher than yours. You are shocked and feel that your years of experience and particularly your loyalty to this practice should result in your earning a significantly higher salary than a new graduate.

There are a number of options in this case. What would be the appropriate action for you to take? What would you do first? What will be the result of these possible alternative actions? Are any ethical principles present in this case? If so, what are they?

CASE 5

In your practice, you are paid a percentage of the fees you charge for each service provided to your patients. In addition to the percentage, you are also given an incentive bonus for each patient you see each day in excess of 8 patients or 12 if some of the patients are children. With this method of compensation, it is possible for you to earn a substantial salary. As a matter of fact, it is possible to increase your earnings simply by working faster and getting patients in and out of your operatory as quickly as possible.

You decide to buy a new car because you can earn the amount of the car payment just by making sure that you see one additional patient each day and by making a few more full-mouth x-ray series each week. You can also increase your income by placing dental sealants for a broader selection of patients, including those whose need you would term as "marginal." Occasionally you can cut an appointment session short so that you can see an extra patient because you can always make sure to provide more thorough treatment on the next appointment. Dental x rays pose a minimal health hazard, and dental sealants are always more helpful than not. What, if any, are the ethical conflicts present in this case?

CASE 6

A dental hygienist manages a preventive dental program with the public health department in a large metropolitan area. The program is supported primarily through state Medicaid funding. Dental assistants and dental hygienists conduct dental screening, dental health education, fluoride rinse, and dental sealant programs within the public schools and community health clinics. The population served does not have adequate financial resources or insurance to receive preventive care through any other method.

Although dental hygienists and assistants can provide preventive services, patients who have restorative or other treatment needs must be referred to local dentists. State Medicaid reimbursement for such care is lower than the fees that local dentists normally charge other patients. This presents a problem for the dental hygienist program manager who must make the referrals, because many dentists refuse to treat these patients because it is so unprofitable. Dentists who accept these patients actually donate services equal to the income lost.

The department has three unfilled dental hygienist positions that the manager has been unable to fill because the salary she can offer is less than the salaries offered dental hygienists in private dental practice. Because she has not been able to recruit dental hygienists, she has had to hire two dental assistants to carry out the dental health education programs. Dental assistants are capable of performing this task and are happy to work for the salary offered.

After reading Chapters 2 and 9, which discuss the concept of justice, use the five-step process for solving ethical problems and analyze this case to determine a just solution.

CASE 7

Jane Smith, a pregnant woman in her mid-20s, informs her hygienist that she is HIV-positive and asks that her private disclosure go no further than the hygienist's treatment room. Specifically, Jane requests that nothing be written on her dental record which reveals her HIV seropositive status, fearing that such information will stigmatize her, and cause people to treat her and her baby as dying patients. Over the last few years, Jane has not required any operative dentistry and therefore feels it unnecessary to inform the dentist of her HIV status. Jane trusts that the hygienist will respect her request. She assures the hygienist that if circumstances arise that she feels are pertinent to her well-being and the well-being of the dentist, she will reveal the diagnosis herself. What should the hygienist do? (Case provided by B. Bizup Hawkins)

REFERENCES

1. Gaston, M.A., Brown, D.M., and Waring, M.B.: Survey of Ethical Issues in Dental Hygiene. J. Dent. Hyg. *64:*216, 1990.
2. Motley, W.: History of The American Dental Hygienists' Association, 1923–1982. Chicago, American Dental Hygienists' Association, 1983.
3. Watterson, J.: Wilma Motley: ADHA Historian, An Interview. Dental Hyg. *57:*25, 1983.
4. Employment of Dental Practice Personnel: The 1990 Survey of Dental Practice. Chicago, American Dental Association, 1990.
5. Davis, B.G.: Specialized Accreditation: The Relationship Between Attitudes Toward Outcome Oriented Standards and the Professionalization of Medical Technology. A Dissertation to the Faculty of the Graduate School, Memphis State University, 1985, p. 52.
6. Rehr, H., and Bosch, S.J.: A professional search into values and ethics in health care delivery. *In* Ethical Dilemmas in Health Care. Edited by H. Rehr. New York, PRODIST, a division of Neale Watson Academic Publ., 1978.
7. Dunning, J.M.: Principles of Dental Public Health. 3rd Ed. Cambridge, Harvard University Press, 1980.
8. Employment of Dental Practice Personnel: The 1990 Survey of Dental Practice. Chicago, American Dental Association, 1990.
9. Employment and Earnings. Bureau of Labor Statistics, U.S. Department of Labor, Washington, DC, January 1990.
10. General Characteristics of Dentists: The 1990 Survey of Dental Practice. Chicago, American Dental Association, 1990.
11. Annual Report Allied Dental Education 1990/91. Chicago, American Dental Association, 1991.
12. Torres, H., Ehrlich, A.: Modern Dental Assisting. 3rd Ed. Philadelphia, W.B. Saunders. 1985.
13. Rosen, J.: The political evolution of the American Dental Hygienists' Association. Dental Hyg. *58:* 402, 1984.
14. Loiacono, C.: Manager's guide to reducing dental hygiene turnover. J. Dent. Hyg. *63:*328, 1989.
15. Body, K.L.: Dental hygiene job and career satisfaction, a review of the literature. J. Dent. Hyg. *62:*170, 1988.
16. Cianflone, D., and Riccelli, A.E.: Ethical considerations for dental hygienists in private practice settings. J. Dent. Hyg. *65:*277, 1991.
17. Kant, I.: Some examples of major ethical theories. *In* Moral Problems in Medicine. Edited by Gorovitz, et al., Englewood Cliffs, New Jersey, 1976.
18. Barish, N.H., and Barish, A.M.: The ethical dilemma of the dental hygienist. J. Am. Coll. Dent. *39:*169, 1972.
19. Rubenstein, L.K., and May, T.M.: Stress in the training and practice of dental hygiene. Dent. Hyg. *60:*166, 1986.

ADDITIONAL READINGS

Books

Beauchamp, T.L.: Principles of Biomedical Ethics. Third Edition. New York, Oxford University Press, 1989.
Cianflone, D., and Riccelli, A.E.: Ethical considerations for dental hygienists in private practice settings. J. Dent. Hyg. *65:*277, 1991.
Clouser, K.D.: Teaching Bioethics: Strategies, Problems, and Resources. Hastings-on-Hudson, New York, Institute of Society, Ethics, and the Life Sciences, 1980.
Enos, D.D., and Sultan, P.: The Sociology of Health Care: Social, Economic, and Political Perspectives. New York, Praeger Publishers, 1977.
Francoeur, R.T.: Biomedical Ethics: A Guide To Decision Making. John Wiley & Sons, 1983.
Hardin, J.F.: Supportive periodontal therapy: Long-term maintenance of the treated case. *In* Clark's Clinical Dentistry. Edited by J.F. Hardin. Philadelphia, J.B. Lippincott Co., 1990.
Kupperman, J.J.: The Foundations of Morality. London, George Allen & Unwin, 1983.
May, W.F.: Notes On The Ethics of Doctors and Lawyers. Bloomington, Indiana, Indiana University Foundation, 1977.
O'Rourke, K.D., and Brodeur, D.: Medical Ethics: Common Ground for Understanding. St. Louis, The Catholic Health Association of the United States, 1986.
Pavalko, R.M.: Sociological Perspectives on Occupations. Itasca, Illinois, F.E. Peacock Publishers, 1972.
Roberts, M.: Responsibility and Practical Freedom. Cambridge, Cambridge University Press, 1965.
Shannon, T.A., and DiGiacomo, J.J.: An Introduction to Bioethics. New York, Paulist Press, 1979.
Shelp, E.E.: Justice and Health Care. Dordrecht, Holland, D. Reidel Publishing Co., 1981.
Vaux, K.: Powers That Make Us Human. Urbana and Chicago, University of Illinois Press, 1985.

Journals

Journal of Public Health Dentistry: Vol. 50, No. 2, Special Issue, 1990.
Journal of Dental Education: Vol. 49, No. 4, 1985.
Journal of the American Dental Association: Vol. 120, May, 1990.
American Dental Hygienists' Association Policy Manual. 1991.

Chapter 9

Race, Gender and Class: What Can the Profession Do to Promote Justice?

Teresa A. Dolan
Linda C. Niessen
Mary B. Mahowald

SUMMARY

Despite the recent increase in enrollment of women and minorities in dental school, the dental work force continues to be stratified by race, gender, and socioeconomic class. Women outnumber men in the dental profession, yet they continue to cluster in the lower paying and less prestigious occupations. Likewise, the percentage of women African-, Hispanic-, Asian- and Native-American dentists in the United States is not reflective of the general population. Equal opportunity and affirmative action legislation has expanded opportunities in the health professions to women and minorities. But this desirable outcome has not ended the gender and racial imbalance in the dental work force.

The purpose of this chapter is to examine the effects of the variables of race, gender, and class on the profession, its members, and those it serves. We review the data on the changing ethnic and gender composition of the dental profession and the ethical concerns that these changes introduce.

Current evidence suggests that women are practicing differently from men. Although they practice only slightly fewer hours per week than their male colleagues, they earn significantly less income from the practice of dentistry. Women dentists are less likely than men dentists to be practice owners. Preliminary data suggest that women are more likely to see a greater percentage of patients who are of minority groups, have handicapping conditions, have low income, and receive public assistance for dental care. Mean dental procedure fees show little difference by gender. Unfortunately, there has been little research on the practice patterns of minority dentists. The overwhelming majority of dentists, regardless of race or gender, resides in counties not classified as high poverty areas. However, except for Asian-Americans, minority practitioners are more likely than white dentists to reside in such areas.

Data reveal inequities in the dental profession, including a gender and race wage gap among dentists, gender and socioeconomic differences between dentists and hygienists, and socioeconomic differences between dental providers and the patients they serve. The key ethical question that such disparities raise is one of distributive justice. Different theories of justice and concepts of equality provide different criteria for resolving conflicts. Whether any of these constitutes an adequate theoretical construct is disputed. Nonetheless, most concepts of justice provide grounds for assessing racism, sexism, and classism as wrong.

Accordingly, we propose a modest strategy for dealing with conflicts, namely, to consider all of the factors that are pertinent to the goal of dentistry, which necessarily involves the health of patients. In general, race, gender, and class are not pertinent to the goal of dentistry because dental health is not essentially related to these factors. The moral challenge for professionals is to ascertain and implement ways of correcting the injustice that arises when such factors are treated as pertinent.

We illustrate this ethical strategy by considering two cases in which differences in race, gender and class arise. One involves hiring within a dental practice, the other involves admission into dental school. Our conclusion poses questions intended to facilitate further discussion.

EMPIRICAL CONCERNS

The past twenty years have witnessed an enormous expansion in both the size of the health workforce and the number of new job titles and specialties. . . . In spite of these changes, the hierarchical organization of the health sector has remained intact. The workforce continues to be stratified by class and race. Superimposed on both strata is a structure which segregates jobs by sex. Female health workers outnumber men by three to one yet they continue to be clustered in occupations which are lower paying, less prestigious and less autonomous than those which are predominantly male.[1]

Women and Asian-, African-, Hispanic- and Native-Americans are sorely underrepresented in the dental profession in the United States. The participation of women and minorities as dentists in any significant numbers is a recent phenomenon. Until the 1950s, African-American dentists were denied admission to most educational institutions and professional societies.[2] Discrimination against African-Americans in dentistry mirrors discrimination against them in society generally. Slavery was legally permitted until 1865, African-Americans were not recognized as citizens until 1868, and the right to equal access to education did not legally include African-Americans until the 1954 United States

Supreme Court decision *Brown v. Board of Education*.[3] Yet African-Americans have a long history in American dentistry, most being products of the apprenticeship system. One such apprentice, Robert Tanner Freeman, resigned from his apprenticeship to enroll in the first class of Harvard University's School of Dental Medicine, and was one of the first six students to receive a dental degree from that institution in 1869. Departments of dentistry organized at Howard University, Washington, D.C., in 1881, and at Meharry Medical College, Nashville, Tennessee in 1886 educated nearly all African-American dentists in the United States until the 1960s.[2-3] Today, fewer than three percent of dentists in the United States are African-American, even though they comprise twelve percent of the nation's population.

Emeline Roberts, the first woman dentist in the United States, learned her profession through an apprenticeship with her husband, Dr. Daniel Albion Jones.[4] She became her husband's partner in 1859 in Danielson, Connecticut, and practiced for 60 years after his death.[5] Lucy Beaman Hobbs graduated from the Ohio College of Dental Surgery in 1866, becoming the first woman in the U.S. to receive a dental degree. However, her admission to dental school and her acceptance as the first female delegate to the American Dental Association convention in 1865 were opposed by her male colleagues.[2] In 1920, when apprenticeship was still a means to pursue dental training, 3% of the dentists were women. By 1960, when a formal dental school education was the norm, women represented less than 1% of dentists in the workforce, and remained so until the late 1970s, when their numbers in dental school increased dramatically.[4]

Many factors contributed to the lack of women and minority dentists before the 1970s. The failure of many dental schools to accept women, African-Americans, and other minorities is only one factor. Other considerations are the lack of financial aid for students, deficient guidance and counselling at the high school and college level, inadequate recruitment measures by the dental schools, and expanded employment opportunities for women and minority students in fields other than dentistry.[6]

The purpose of this chapter is to examine the effects of the variables of race, gender, and class on the profession, its members, and those it serves. We review the empirical data on the changing ethnic and gender composition of the dental profession and the ethical concerns that these changes introduce. Next we offer two cases to illustrate the issues raised by race, gender, and class and present an ethical analysis of each case. Finally, the chapter poses additional questions for the student to reflect upon to gain insight regarding ethical aspects of the profession.

Women and Minorities as Dentists

Trends in dentistry mirror those in society as a whole, with a growing number of women and minorities applying to and enrolling in dental school since 1970.[7–9] However, dentistry remains a predominantly white male profession. As illustrated in Figures 9–1 and 9–2, 94.2% of dentists are men, and 92.2% are white. The data for dental faculty members are similar; over 80% are men, and over 85% are white.

Although the number of African-American dentists has increased in the past 20 years, only 2.6% of dentists are African-American. A recent report estimated that in the United States there is only 1 African-American dentist for every 7297 African-Americans in the population, as compared to 1 dentist for every 1571 people in the general population.[10] Likewise, other minority groups including Asian-, Hispanic-, and Native-Americans are underrepresented or not reflective of the US population. For example, only 2% of dentists in the United States are Hispanic-American, even though Hispanics comprise about 9% of the U.S. population.[11]

Equal opportunity and affirmative action legislation has expanded opportunities in the health professions to women and minorities. But this desirable outcome has not ended the gender- and race-based imbalance in the health work force. The literature suggests that, although women and minorities are able to gain entry into these professions, they are notably underrepresented in high-level positions, leadership roles, and settings critical to resource allocation and priority deter-

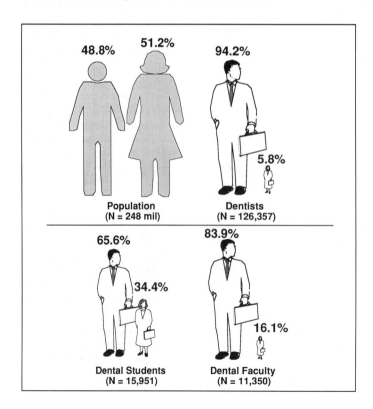

Fig. 9–1. Gender composition of the United States population, total predoctoral dental school enrollment, dental faculty, and dentists. Sources:
1. United States Population: 1990 Census Data, Department of Commerce, Bureau of Census.
2. Dentists: Includes active private practitioners in the United States in 1987. Distribution of Dentists in the United States by Region and State, 1987. American Dental Association, Bureau of Economic and Behavioral Research.
3. Dental students: Annual Report on Dental Education 1990/91. The American Dental Association, Council on Dental Education, Division of Education, Department of Educational Surveys.
4. Dr. Eric Solomon, American Association of Dental Schools, personal communication. Includes administrators as well as faculty from the basic, clinical, and behavioral sciences.

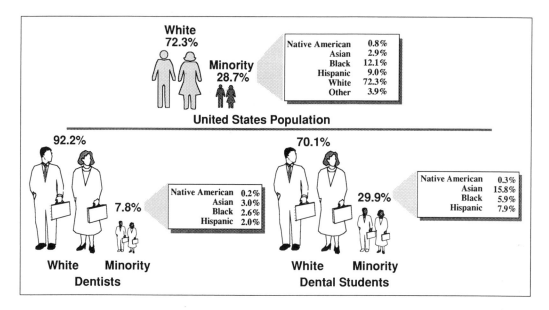

Fig. 9–2. Minority composition of the United States population, predoctoral dental school students, and dentists.
Sources:
1. United States Population: 1990 Census Data, Department of Commerce, Bureau of Census.
2. Dentists: Personal communication, the American Dental Association, Bureau of Economic and Behavioral Research.
3. Dental students: Personal communication, Dr. Eric Solomon, The American Association of Dental Schools.

mination.[1] For example, the American Dental Association has been in existence since 1859, yet Dr. Geraldine Morrow was the first woman elected to the ADA Board of Trustees in 1984, and became the first woman president in 1991. Likewise, in dental education, very few women and minorities hold administrative titles, including department chairman, program director, or dean.[12,13]

The future of the dental profession is in its students. Trends over the past three decades suggest that predoctoral dental school enrollment is slowly becoming more diverse in terms of its gender and minority composition (Fig. 9–3). In 1970, only 1.4% of dental students were female, and about 5% were nonwhite. Although total enrollment in dental schools in the United States peaked in 1980 and has since been grad-

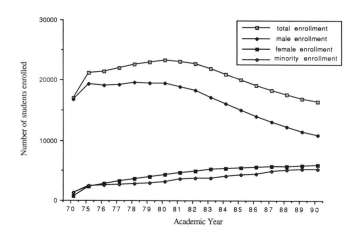

Fig. 9–3. Enrollment in United States dental schools by gender and minority status, 1970 to 1990.
Sources:
1. Trend Analysis, The Annual Report on Dental Education 1984/85, Supplement 11. The American Dental Association, Council on Dental Education.
2. Trend Analysis, The Annual Report on Dental Education 1990/91, Supplement 2. The American Dental Association, Council on Dental Education.

ually declining, the number of women and minority students has consistently grown. For the 1990–91 academic year, women comprised 34.4% of the total dental school enrollment.[8] Minority groups are still underrepresented in the dental student body, despite increased participation in recent decades. In fact, because of declining dental school enrollment since the mid-1970s, the proportional representation of African-American first-year students in schools of dentistry has actually declined slightly, whereas the proportional representation of Hispanic-Americans in the first-year dental classes has doubled since 1975. Increases in first-year enrollments of minority students were insufficient to bring the active supply of minority dentists to population parity.[10]

Current Trends in Dental Practice

PRACTICE LOCATION

A study of dentists and other health providers suggests that practitioners from each of the racial/ethnic minority groups was much more likely than white practitioners to cluster in certain geographic areas, according to the race of the practitioner and, to some extent, the profession.[10] For example, significant percentages of African-American practitioners reside in the East North Central and South Atlantic areas, whereas Hispanic practitioners reside in large percentages in the South Atlantic, West South Central, and Pacific Divisions of the United States. Asian dentists reside overwhelmingly in the Pacific Division. Native American practitioners reside in large part in the South Atlantic, West South Central and Pacific Divisions. In general, the location of minority practitioners is highly associated with the presence of a substantial proportion of that population group in the area. There are exceptions, of course, with the most notable disparity among African-Americans in the East and West South Central Divisions, where the proportion of African-American dentists is about half of the proportion of the African-American population.[14]

The overwhelming majority of dentists, regardless of race or gender, reside in counties not classified as high poverty areas. However, except for Asians, minority practitioners are more likely than white practitioners to reside in such areas.[14] Health professionals from all racial groups were disproportionately located in heavily populated areas in 1980. This is partially explained by the fact that nearly 40% of the population of African-, Hispanic-, and Asian-Americans resided in communities with a million or more inhabitants. In a study of recent dental graduates, women tended to be in larger practices, in areas of higher per capita income, and in areas with a greater number of dentists per 10,000 population.[15]

PRACTICE OWNERSHIP

Recent national studies of gender trends in dental practice patterns suggest important differences in personal characteristics, practice ownership status, and income from the practice of dentistry.[15-17] Unfortunately, fewer data are available regarding these issues for minority dentists.

Most dentists are owners or share in the ownership of their practices, but a greater proportion of male dentists than female dentists are practice owners (Fig. 9-4). Men are more likely to be solo private practitioners. Among owner dentists, staff sizes are larger for male than for female dentists. A larger proportion of male dentists employ hygienists compared with female practitioners.[15] Because male dentists on the average are older than women dentists, some differences may be accounted for by age.

Male dentists are more likely to begin their practice activities as practice owners.[17] In a recent survey by the American Dental Association, about 89% of the men said that they were currently practice owners, as compared to 68% of the female respondents. Among dentists under age 45, about 50% of the women and 70% of the men respondents started as owners in the practice. As expected, the highest proportion of dentists in nonownership positions occur among recent graduates. However, at all categories of years since graduation, the percentage of women in nonownership positions exceeded the corresponding proportion of men.[17]

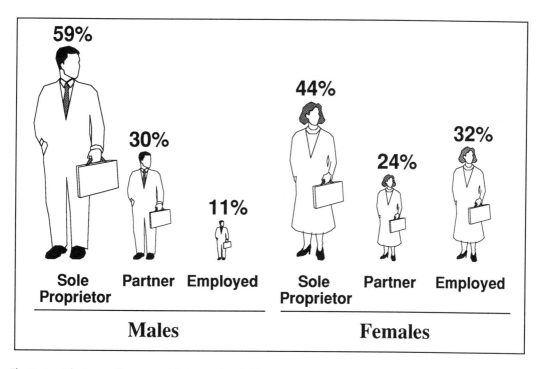

Fig. 9–4. Private practice ownership by gender, 1988.
Source: A comparative study of male and female dental practice patterns. Bureau of Economic and Behavioral Research, Council on Dental Practice, American Dental Association. May 1989. (Includes only dentists under age 45.)

These findings are consistent with other reports in the medical and dental literature, which concur that women are more likely to practice as employees in group practices, health maintenance organizations, governmental agencies, and private institutions.[18–19] Historically, women physicians have had a propensity to cluster in salaried employment and in organization work settings, in contrast to the highly autonomous, self-employed practice mode of their male peers. Surveys of medical and dental students indicate that male and female students expect to practice in different settings. Male students expect to establish independent or group practices; female students expect salaried positions.[20–21] Thus, differences in practice arrangements between male and female students are likely to persist.

DENTAL PRACTICE PATTERNS

Numerous studies have compared the professional work effort and other dental practice patterns of male and female dentists and physicians. The stereotype of female professionals having weak and unstable commitments to the work role was perhaps reinforced by early studies of women dentists.[22–24] However, recent studies suggest far greater professional work effort and productivity of women dentists than earlier reports.[15–17]

Recent data suggest similarities in time spent in practice activities by male and female dentists.[15–17] Women, on the average, work slightly fewer weeks per year, and slightly fewer hours per week. Work effort is associated with ownership status in the practice. Data suggest similar work effort for men and women when they are sole owners of their dental practices with a difference of only 2.1 hours worked. However, for employed men and women, there is a 7-hour difference in favor of the men. Single, divorced, and separated men and women worked about the same number of hours per week. Married women, however, worked 5.8 hours less per week than their married male counterparts. In addition, women spend slightly more time with each patient, with the net finding that women tend to see fewer patients per year, on average, than their male colleagues.[17] Wilson, Branch, and Niessen reported that women were more likely to see a greater percentage of patients who were of minority groups, had handicapping conditions, low income, and received public assistance for dental care.[16] Mean dental procedure fees show little difference by gender.[17]

These findings represent a very preliminary examination of trends in dental practice patterns of women and minority dentists. Additional research is needed to fully understand any similarities or differences in practice trends by dentists, particularly as the number of women and minorities increases over time.

GENDER WAGE GAP

Two recent national surveys of dentists suggest a significant gender wage gap.[15,17] In the study of recent dental school graduates, women dentists earned 75.4% of the pretax income of their male counterparts from the private practice, administration, or teaching of dentistry, with a mean annual difference of almost $10,000 (Fig. 9–5).[15] Men consistently earned greater income from the private practice of dentistry, regardless of ownership status. The smallest difference ($6740) was found for sole proprietors, and the largest difference ($17,984) for dentists who were partners or shareholders in their dental practices. Married women earned significantly less income than married men ($33,095 versus $45,748). There was no significant difference in income for single, divorced, or separated men and women. An important similarity is that male and female dentists employed by federal or state government or the armed services earned equitable incomes. This can probably be attributed to Equal Opportunity and Affirmative Action legislation.

IMPLICATIONS OF INEQUITY

Cultural diversity is a bellwether issue for the future of American business as well as the professions. The question of whether women or members of minority groups can become dentists is no longer an issue. The more relevant question is how the practice of dentistry will be altered as a result of their participation. Will they

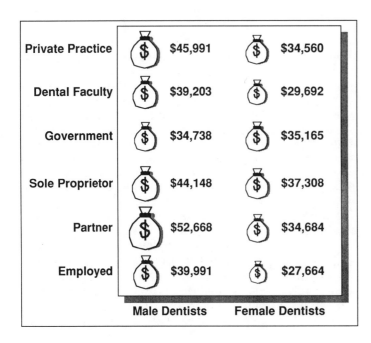

	Male Dentists	Female Dentists
Private Practice	$45,991	$34,560
Dental Faculty	$39,203	$29,692
Government	$34,738	$35,165
Sole Proprietor	$44,148	$37,308
Partner	$52,668	$34,684
Employed	$39,991	$27,664

Fig. 9–5. Mean annual income by gender and primary dental occupation and practice ownership status for recent dental school graduates.
Source: Dolan T.A., and Lewis, C.E.: Gender trends in the career patterns of recent dental graduates. J. Dent. Educ. 11:639, 1987, Table 2.

be granted the same rights, privileges, and responsibilities as other dentists?

Current evidence suggests that women are practicing differently than men. Women are redefining their practice options to accommodate their needs, most notably the biological need of integrating a professional career with parenting responsibilities. In fact, although there are more two-parent families than ever before, women still bear the burden of child care.

Women and minority dentists also serve as role models to members of the community at large as well as to prospective and current dental students.[25] Dr. David Nash recently observed that despite the absence of female role models, women students have done remarkably well in dental school.[26]

The gender and race wage gap is another inequity that must be resolved. The fact that women and minority groups are generally paid less than white men puts some white men at a disadvantage with regard to obtaining employment. If one prospective employee would work for $0.58 and the other would work for $1.00, the former is more likely to be hired. Thus the majority gender and race also have a stake in equality of salary for women and minority dentists.[28]

Other inequities in dentistry include gender and socioeconomic (class) differences that occur within dental practice between dentists, who are still predominantly men, and dental hygienists, who are still predominantly women (see Chap. 8). Racial and class differences also occur between dentists and hygienists as a group and the patients whom they serve. Patients in general are much more likely than professionals to come from minority groups. In both sets of relationships, not only an income differential but also a difference in prestige and power separates the groups. Across the entire range of health professions, women and minorities are more numerous at the less rewarded levels of the professions, and more numerous as patients.[28] The power discrepancies that result sometimes lead to sexual harassment and other forms of discriminatory behavior. Even when these practices are inadvertent, they place obstacles in the path of women and minorities.

ETHICAL CONCERNS

The key ethical principle at stake in situations involving discrimination based on race, gender, and class is justice. Justice may be viewed as a mediating principle between the principles of beneficence and respect for autonomy that have become "canonical" in contemporary biomedical ethics. Although some authors distinguish between nonmaleficence (avoiding harm) and beneficence (doing good), we here collapse the former meaning into that of the latter (see, for example, Chap. 2). Doing good thus includes avoidance of harm. Justice demands equitable distribution of harms and goods, including the good of respect for autonomy. It is *distributive* justice rather than other forms (such as procedural justice) that performs a mediating function when conflicts arise between the preferences of those involved, or between burdens and benefits to those affected.

Beauchamp and Childress list the following candidates for different concepts of distributive justice:

1. To each person an equal share.
2. To each person according to need.
3. To each person according to effort.
4. To each person according to contribution.
5. To each person according to merit.
6. To each person according to free-market enterprise.[29]

The first concept is the most difficult to defend if equal shares mean the same shares. Literally equal shares (same shares) of resources are neither needed nor desired by all persons. A dentist who lives in a city where the cost of living is high, for example, may require a higher income to meet expenses than one who lives in a rural area. On the other hand, if equal shares are assumed to take account of differences among individuals and groups, then they are equally pertinent shares, and different criteria for pertinence are embodied in the other concepts of justice. In the United States, for example, need is sometimes the basis for distribution of goods that are crucial to subsistence, such as food and some forms of health care. Jobs and promotions are usually awarded on the basis of merit, and the higher income of some is supported on grounds of the free-market system, which is based on equal competition. The higher status of some professionals may be justified because of their greater social contribution, and effort is often seen as deserving of reward on moral grounds as well.

Admittedly, different concepts of distributive justice are not always theoretically or practically compatible. In fact, some are essentially related to economic theories that are diametrically opposed such as capitalism and socialism. Ethical theories associated with different concepts of justice include utilitarianism, libertarianism, and egalitarianism. Each of these theories has its strengths as well as weaknesses, and none has been universally, or even generally, accepted as adequate for the resolution of ethical conflicts. Accordingly, we propose a modest strategy for dealing with conflicts involving distributive justice, that is, to consider all of the pertinent factors. Pertinent to what? Pertinent, in the field of dentistry, to the goals of dentistry, which necessarily involve the health of patients. On this account, it is not just or fair to treat all individuals or groups in exactly the same way, as long as the individuals or groups differ in pertinent ways. Putting this positively, justice demands taking account of pertinent differences and disregarding differences that are not pertinent.

In general, race, gender, and class are not pertinent to the practice of dentistry because dental health is not essentially related to these factors. Nonetheless, the data cited in this paper suggest that such factors have influenced decisions made in dentistry, as well as in other areas. Strictly speaking, these situations do not constitute ethical dilemmas because dilemmas as such present intellectual rather than practical challenges. Any of the preceding concepts of justice provides clear grounds for assessing racism, sexism, and classism as wrong. Nonetheless, there is often a gap between what individuals know to be right and what they choose to do. A tension may arise because of what Campbell and Rogers consider "moral weakness." In such situations, "moral responsibility points in one

direction and personal inclinations in another" (see Chap. 2). When recognizing the injustice of discrimination, therefore, professionals face the practical challenge of ascertaining and implementing ways of correcting the injustice.

Class is pertinent to achievement of the goals of dentistry only if it impedes fulfillment of those goals either qualitatively or quantitatively. (The same is also true of race and gender.) A free enterprise system allows for disparities in income within dentistry, and between dentists and others. Limitations to free enterprise are generally introduced by government in order to avoid deprivation of basic dental care in those who cannot pay for it. To the extent that dentistry is construed as a profession rather than a business, the free enterprise rationale is inadequate. Milton Friedman writes that "there is one and only one social responsibility of business—to use its resources and engage in activities designed to increase its profits."[30] In contrast, one of the distinguishing marks of a profession is its human service orientation.[31–33] Economic inequities are not entirely overcome by this orientation, but they are reduced. A radical overhaul of the privatized system of dental care would be necessary to eliminate such inequities in their entirety.

Although biomedical ethical principles are useful in addressing ethical dilemmas in dentistry, the interpretation and application of these principles is dependent on the nuances of specific cases. To illustrate the way in which principles can mesh with particulars (and vice versa), consider the following cases.

CASE 1. DR. VAN DIVER HIRES AN ASSOCIATE

Dr. Robert van Diver has been in private practice in the San Francisco metropolitan area since 1978. His practice has grown steadily throughout the years, and he feels that he has more patients than he could possibly treat. He has always been the only dentist in the practice, but he employs a dental hygienist and six dental assistants and office staff to help him with his busy daily schedule. Dr. van Diver considered "taking in" an associate several times over the years, but came to realize that he felt comfortable "being the only man in the office." Recently he has become more professionally active with both his state and national dental association. With these new professional commitments, he thinks it might be time to hire someone to help maintain the practice productivity and income, while he attends professional meetings. He'd also enjoy having more time to spend with his wife and family, and to improve his tennis game.

Dr. van Diver recently attended a local dental society meeting, where two colleagues were discussing their new associates. They suggested that, with the glut of new dental graduates and the shortage of dental hygienists, it costs almost as much to hire a hygienist as it does to hire a new dentist. And the dentist can work more independently and profitably! Dr. van Diver did not like the idea of "exploiting a fellow dentist," but after all, "business is business," and he did need some help in the practice. Later that week, he put an advertisement in the local newspaper, seeking a dentist associate 3 days per week.

Six dentists, all recent graduates who had California Dental licenses, inquired about the position. The applicants included one African-American woman, one white woman, one Hispanic-American man, one Asian-American man, and two white men. Dr. van Diver interviewed all the dentists and their references, and found them all to be quite personable and competent. Dr. van Diver's wife, who was the office manager, also interviewed the candidates. After the interviews, her first comment to Dr. van Diver was that the patients would never accept an African-American woman as a dentist. All of the men wanted too much money and seemed "too independent." Dr. van Diver was also worried that the men would work the other 2 or 3 days/week in nearby practices. He was afraid that, if they opened their own practice, that they would take patients from his practice. After much deliberation, Dr. van Diver hired the white woman dentist because she seemed most willing to "do hygiene" when she wasn't booked with restorative patients, and was willing to accept the lowest salary. In fact, he found he could pay her less than he paid his dental hygienist. The African-American woman was willing to do the same, but Dr. van Diver was concerned that his wife, staff, and patients would not accept her as readily as they did the new white female associate.

Ethical Analysis

Apparently, concerns about beneficence toward patients are not problematic in this case, because all of the applicants for the position are "personable and competent." What is problematic, however, is whether Dr. van Diver is obligated to respect the alleged preference of his patients for having someone other than an African-American woman as their dentist. In light of what has been said previously, this is an unjust preference because it is not pertinent to the goals of dentistry. Although the ethical obligation to respect autonomy extends to others besides patients, it does not extend to respect for decisions that reflect prejudice.

Respect for autonomy of prospective employers does call for disclosure to them of criteria for hiring that are not obviously relevant to the applicant, but may be relevant to the employer. In this case, Dr. van Diver made several assumptions about the differences between male and female applicants, apparently without such disclosure. He assumed, for example, that the male candidates would work elsewhere as well, and that the female candidates would not. In fact, of course, either or both assumptions might be false, or neither might be true. Dr. van Diver might have communicated this concern to all of the applicants and inquired about their intention in that regard. It would then be their responsibility to respect his autonomy by their own disclosure.

Dr. van Diver's decision to hire the white woman may be viewed as "affirmative action," but it is apparently based mainly on his own interests and those of his practice rather than those of others in society. Affirmative action is generally defined as a preference among equally qualified candidates for a member of a group that has been discriminated against in the past. It is intended to reduce social inequities based on gender, race, and class differences. Unfortunately, Dr. van Diver rejected the opportunity he had to practice affirmative action toward African-Americans as well as women. His decision could be supported by a concept of justice consistent with free enterprise, but not by a concept of justice based on greater social need, merit, contribution, or effort. In fact, he missed (we believe) a golden opportunity to overcome or reduce racial stereotypes or prejudices among his staff. Hiring an equally qualified African-American would at least have contributed toward that end.

CASE 2. ANITA RODRIGUEZ APPLIES TO DENTAL SCHOOL

Anita Rodriguez is a senior student at the University of Michigan majoring in zoology. She is the daughter of Jose and Ana Rodriguez, who immigrated from Cuba to the United States in the 1950s. The Rodriguez family had been quite wealthy and were well educated in their native Cuba. They fled Cuba to avoid political persecution, leaving behind most of their wealth and possessions. They initially relocated in South Florida, but because of the prejudice they experienced, as well as difficulty in obtaining employment, the family moved to New Jersey, where they joined relatives who had immigrated earlier.

Jose Rodriguez found a job as janitor for the local county school system. Ana Rodriguez worked at a small embroidery factory while raising her two young daughters, Anita and Rosa. Although Anita's parents were disappointed that they could not find higher-paying jobs, they were grateful that they could live modestly on their two incomes. As the daughters grew up, the parents stressed the importance of education to them. They were bright and attentive students.

Anita Rodriguez benefitted from state and federal assistance, and was able to attend the University of Michigan under a special minority recruitment program. She was reluctant to leave her family in New Jersey, but welcomed the opportunity to attend this academic institution. Anita worked hard, but had trouble adjusting to the new environment. She particularly missed the strong family support she received while living at home. By her senior year, she had a cumulative average of 2.9 (on a scale of 0 to 4, 4 being the highest score).

During the previous 2 years, Anita had worked part-time at a local dentist's office, assisting with the front desk and patient billing. As she learned more about dentistry, she thought this profession would suit her well, particularly because she enjoyed working with people and was industrious and entrepreneurial. She knew that she had some trouble with her science courses and organic chemistry, but felt that she would be able to manage the difficult course work in dental school. In the spring of her junior year, she took the dental admissions examination, and later applied to seven dental schools.

Initially, Anita was not accepted for admission by any of the dental schools. However, late in the fall, one university notified her that it had received a federal grant to recruit minority students into a special Minority Dental School Program. She was invited to participate. At first Anita was thrilled, but later she felt concerned that she was offered admission because of her minority status. She could not decide whether to accept a position in the program.

Ethical Analysis

This is another case that seems to involve affirmative action. Note, however, that affirmative action (as defined in the preceding analysis) does not mean "reverse discrimination" or "preferential hiring," either of which suggests that individuals have been deprived of opportunities for which they are better qualified than others. Presumably, the admissions officers who first rejected the application of Anita Rodriguez did not consider the broader context in which her qualifications might be equal to or better than those of other candidates. Equal qualification is a complex concept, and neither human judgments nor test results are adequate indicators in this regard. Dental school admissions officers are generally interested only in past performance as a means of assessing future performance. Past performance, in fact, involves multiple factors that are not measured and often go unmentioned on applications. In this case, for example, the stressors of the applicant's life were probably greater than those of most of her peers. That she achieved as much as she did suggested strengths beyond her grades. When admissions officers later recognized this, she would be offered admission not because of her minority status, but because they recognized ability that had been obstructed and that might well surpass that of her peers if the obstructions were removed.

The preceding rationale obviously supports a decision to accept Anita's admission into dental school. But need, effort, contribution, and merit may also be cited as relevant to the decision. From the dental school's standpoint, there are added benefits if Anita accepts its offer. The school will then be able to take advantage of the federal grant, utilization of which may benefit other students as well. Other students also stand to be enriched by the diversity that recruitment of minorities contributes to their own education and socialization. Because minorities form so great a part of the patient population that dental students will one day serve, their presence within the ranks of professionals-in-training is no small contribution to the development of their peers.

It is not surprising that Anita Rodriguez is hesitant to accept the admissions offer. Women and members of minorities tend to be more used to missed opportunities over which they have little or no control than are their white male counterparts. Socioeconomic disadvantages and the demands of pregnancy and child care contribute to the incidence of missed opportunities among these groups. Moreover, because they have become inured to a system that defines the worth of individuals on the basis of criteria developed without regard for such complexities, it seldom occurs to them that their actual qualifications may never have been adequately assessed.

These cases illustrate generic problems involving gender, race, and class differences. Whether they occur among individuals or groups, the crucial ethical principle for addressing them is justice or fairness. Although different concepts and theories of justice may yield different resolutions of specific questions, it seems clear that some interpretation of this principle should be applied. We have proposed that a literal concept of justice as sameness is morally inadequate because of the human diversity that gender, race, and class introduce, a diversity that enriches society as a whole. A literal concept is also inadequate because it fails to respect the uniqueness of individuals and groups. The social and economic disparities based on race, gender, and class documented in the first part of this chapter are not differences that ought to be tolerated in a just society. Such disparities are unjust because they are not based on pertinent differences. Pertinent differences may be based on need, contribution, merit, effort, or procedural consistency. The free enterprise system, despite its limitations, defines a procedural model of justice.

Developing a specific theory of justice is obviously beyond the scope of this chapter. What we have attempted is to sketch an empirical picture revealing injustice with regard to race, gender, and class, and to propose some concepts that may be simultaneously applicable to situations in which a just solution is sought. In the questions that follow, you are asked to think further about how that might be done.

DISCUSSION QUESTIONS

1. Revisit the case of Dr. van Diver. Did he have a moral obligation to choose a woman or minority candidate for the position? Why, or why not?

2. Dr. van Diver's search for an associate was based on the notion that "business is business." Compare or contrast the defining characteristics of businesses as profit-making enterprises, with professions as oriented towards human service. What ethical rationale supports either concept? In what ways are they, or are they not, compatible in the practice of dentistry?

3. Dr. van Diver's decision to hire the white woman as his associate was based in part on her willingness to accept a lower salary than her male counterparts, and her willingness to "do hygiene" as well. How does this reflect a concept of justice as free enterprise? What does this suggest regarding justice between genders?

4. Dr. van Diver was unwilling to hire the African-American woman despite her willingness to accept a lower salary and "do hygiene." What does this suggest regarding justice between races?

5. Revisit the case of Anita Rodriquez. What moral considerations might lead her to reject the offer of admission into dental school? What moral considerations might lead her to accept the offer?

6. If you were the dean of admissions at the dental school, what moral arguments would you offer for accepting or rejecting Anita Rodriguez as an applicant?

7. Consider your own race, gender, and class. In what ways, if any, are these traits pertinent to moral decisions that you make as a person and as a professional?

ACKNOWLEDGMENT

The authors would like to thank Wallace L. Mealiea, Ph.D., for his graphics assistance.

REFERENCES

1. Butter, I., Carpenter, E., Kay, B., and Simmons, R.: Sex and Status: Hierarchies in the Health Workforce. Public Health Policy Series, American Public Health Association, March 1985.

2. Ring, M.E.: Dentistry: An Illustrated History. New York, Harry N. Abrams, Inc., 1985.

3. Haynes, H. An Historical Perspective of Blacks in American Dentistry. The Dental School Quarterly V:5, 1989.

4. Niessen, L.C., Kleinman, D.V., and Wilson, A.A.: Practice Patterns of Women Dentists. JADA 113: 883, 1986.

5. Commencement Exercises. Dent. Reg. 20:145, 1866.

6. Kidd, F. Profile of the Negro in American Dentistry. Washington, D.C., Howard University Press, 1979.

7. Council on Dental Education, Division of Educational Measurement. Annual Report on Dental Education 1990–91. Chicago, IL: American Dental Association.

8. Council on Dental Education, Division of Educational Measurement. Annual Report on Dental Education 1985–86. Chicago, IL: American Dental Association.

9. Inglehart, J.K.: Datawatch: Trends in health personnel. Health Affairs 5:128, 1986.

10. U.S. Department of Health and Human Services, Bureau of Health Professions. Estimates and Projections of Black and Hispanic Personnel in Selected Health Professions 1980–2000. DHHS Publication No. (HRA)-82-10, Washington, D.C., Government Printing Office, September, 1982.

11. Baez, R.: Hispanics in Dentistry. The Dental School Quarterly. V:1, 1989.

12. Neidle, E.: President's Address. J. Dent. Educ. 50:380, July, 1986.

13. Solomon, E.S., Gray, C.F., and Whiton, J.C.: Promotion and appointment to administrative positions of dental school faculty by gender. J. Dent. Educ. 54:530, 1990.

14. U.S. Department of Health and Human Services, Bureau of Health Professions. Location Patterns of Minority and Other Health Professionals. ODAM Report No. 4-85, Washington, D.C., Government Printing Office, 1985.

15. Dolan, T.A., and Lewis, C.E.: Gender trends in the career patterns of recent dental graduates. J. Dent. Educ. 11:639, 1987.

16. Wilson, A.A., Branch, L.G., and Niessen, L.C.: Practice patterns of males and female dentists. J. Am. Dent. Assoc. 116:173, 1988.

17. Bureau of Economic and Behavioral Research, Council on Dental Practice, American Dental Association. A comparative study of male and female dental practice patterns, May, 1989.

18. Cohen, E.D., and Korper, S.P.: Women in medicine: A survey of professional activities, career interruptions, and conflict resolutions. Trends in Career Patterns. Conn. Med. 40:195, 1976.

19. Mitchell, J.B.: Why do women physicians work fewer hours than men physicians? Inquiry 21: 361, 1984.

20. Kutner, N.G., Brogan, D.R.: A comparison of the practice orientations of women and men students at two medical schools. J. Am. Med. Wom. Assoc. 35:80, 1980.

21. Solomon, E., and Pait, C.: Women dental students exhibit different career and income expectations. J. Dent. Educ. 44:619, 1980.

22. Linn, E.L.: Professional activities of women dentists. J. Am. Dent. Assoc. 81:1383, 1970.

23. Rosner, J.F.: Career patterns of female and male dentists. J. Dent. Pract. Adm. 1:89, 1984.

24. Tillman, R.S., and Horowitz, S.L.: Practice patterns of recent female dental graduates. J. Am. Dent. Assoc. 107:32, 1983.

25. Price, S.S.: A profile of women dentists. J. Am. Dent. Assoc. 120:403, 1990.

26. Nash, D.A.: The feminist mystique in dental education: A feminist's challenge. J. Am. Coll. Dent. 58:33, 1991.

27. Niessen, L.C.: Women dentists: From here to the 21st Century. J. Am. Coll. Dent. 58:37, 1991.

28. Mahowald, M.B.: Sex-role stereotypes in medicine. Hypatia 2:21, 1987.

29. Beauchamp, T.L., and Childress, J.F.: Principles of Biomedical Ethics. 3rd ed. New York, Oxford University Press, 1989.

30. Friedman, M.: Capitalism and Freedom. Chicago, University of Chicago Press, 1982.

31. Bales, M.: Professional Ethics. Belmont, CA, Wadsworth Publishing Co., 1981.

32. Flexner, A.: Is social work a profession? National Conference of Social Work 2, 1915;

33. Goldman, A.H.: The Moral Foundations of Professional Ethics. Totowa, NJ, Rowman and Littlefield, 1980.

Chapter 10

Advertising

Linda S. Scheirton
Thomas H. Boerschinger*

SUMMARY

For many decades, advertising was considered unethical behavior for professional dentists. Announcements of name and address were allowed, but genuine advertisements that intended to promote an individual's practice were not sanctioned. However, under pressure from various Supreme Court decisions and Federal Trade Commission policies, since 1979 the dental associations and state boards no longer prohibit dental advertising if such advertising in not false or misleading.

In this chapter, it is argued that the moral status of advertising by dentists cannot be established independently from the ethical perspective one holds regarding the appropriate ethical model for the occupation of dentistry. Two main models are distinguished: (1) the professional model, in which the trust between the public and dentists as a group is considered the most important value; and (2) the commercial model, in which the free and unrestricted trade relationships between the individual dentists and their clients are considered the most important value. In the professional model, any practice that could harm this relationship of trust is considered unethical. Because advertisements intend to make patients believe that there is a qualitative difference between the advertising dentist and his or her colleagues, and because, therefore, patients may lose their trust in the dental profession as a whole, advertisements are not allowed in a professional model. On the other hand, in a commercial model, it is thought that patients are best served when dentists can advertise because this leads to competition, price decreases, innovations, and a larger array of available services. It is shown that either model allows for simple announcements of name, address, opening hours and specialty, whereas neither model will sanction false or clearly misleading advertisements. But consensus between the two models is less likely with regards to other advertisements, such as persuasive or price-promoting advertisements.

It is maintained that a minimum demand for an ethically acceptable stance towards the issue of advertising is consistency. However, many contemporary dental ethics codes and practice acts reflect an undesirable mixture between two incompatible models: professionalism and commercialism.

* To the extent that Mr. Boerschinger has contributed to this chapter, the views expressed are his own, and should not be attributed to the policies or views of the American Dental Association.

ADVERTISING IN DENTISTRY

Advertising in dentistry is a reality. Because the United States Federal Trade Commission (FTC) determined in 1979 that dentists should be allowed to advertise and the American Dental Association (ADA) consequently changed its code of ethics to read that advertising would no longer be considered unethical, as much as $250,000 annually for group and multidiscipline practices are being spent on advertisements, according to one author.[1]

Discussions about the morality of advertising by dentists now focus mostly on limits to advertisement, the appropriate style, and the media of choice, but not on advertisement as such. Yet the ruling of a powerful government agency, and even a change in a code of ethics do not settle an ethical dilemma. Advertising once was considered prototypical behavior of nonprofessionals, of businessmen, for-profit companies, of crooks and quacks. And although advertisements containing impertinent self-aggrandizement and bold lies about miraculous treatments have become very rare, advertising remains a morally troublesome practice. Dental advertising is at the crossroads of two very different philosophies about what the occupation of dentistry is or should be.

The traditional view opposes advertising which it deems demeaning to the profession and a potential harm to the public's well-being. The marketing of health care, it is maintained, cannot be equated with the marketing of other services in business. On the other hand, the more prevalent contemporary view holds that dentistry is commercially oriented and that increased advertising is an encouraging sign of legitimate competition.[2]

In this chapter, the moral status of dental advertising is examined. Because dental advertising was an ardently debated dilemma long before 1979, when dental advertising was liberalized, a short excursion into the history of dentistry is undertaken, from the date at which the first known advertisement was published to the situation in this decade. The current moral status of dental advertising, as reflected by different dental practice acts and judicial decrees, is examined in detail. The descriptive division of the chapter is followed by a careful ethical analysis of dental advertising. Various ethical arguments in favor and against advertisement by dentists will be evaluated. However, the arguments are not weighed on an imaginary scale because choosing the kind of scale would imply a subjective and thus questionable judgement about the morality of dental advertising. Rather, the various arguments in favor and against will be shown to reflect different opinions about the appropriate moral model for the occupation of dentistry. Two main interpretations can be distinguished, each of which, when abiding the principle of consistency, implies a very different image of the dental occupation. Yet, the current debates on advertising and professionalism usually reflect a mixed and very inconsistent philosophy. However, because reality will most likely remain unchanged despite a plea for consistency, the chapter closes with an examination of a number of different advertisements from both ethical perspectives.

SOME HISTORICAL FACTS

The Early Days (1735–1866)

It is often thought that advertising by dentists is a recent phenomenon.[3] In fact, dental advertisements, despite previous prohibitions, are as old as American dentistry itself. There is a distinct ethos of the first American dentists and the ethical standards of professional dentistry in those days. In his "An Introduction to the History of Dentistry in America," Weinberger has compiled a marvelous collection of early advertisements. Advertisements can be encountered as early as the 18th century. The oldest known newspaper advertisement of a "tooth drawer" dates back to 1735.[4] In the late 18th and early 19th century, advertisements seemed to have become customary and considered in "good professional form."[4] Not unlike modern advertisements, early advertisements had a double function. First, they were intended to provide "neutral" information, in modern terms: to stimulate informed consent. In a society that lacked fast modern communications, yet was spread over a vast country land, it was a way of informing potential clients about the availability of dental care and to distinguish oneself from quacks. Operators John Watts and Samuel Rutter from the Company of Barber-Surgeons felt it necessary to stress in their 1744 advertisement that they "apply themselves wholly to the said business,"[4] much unlike James Daniel who, in 1766, in one advertisement announced his qualities as "Operator of Teeth, Wig-Maker and Hair-Dresser."[7] If we are to believe Benjamin James' 1814 publication "Treatise on the Management of the Teeth," itinerant dentists were impostors, who called themselves dentists, yet practiced deceitful tricks and then disappeared.[4]

Advertisements were part of the great campaign that dentists of the 19th century waged against quackery and hucksterism.[5] The only problem with this strategy was that quacks advertised as well. The Publics Most Humble Servant Philodontalkikos announced in a page-long advertisement in the Virginia Gazette of February 18, 1768, that he had returned from a visit to Constantinople where he learned from the great dentist Mustapah Ben Achmet, enabling him to draw teeth without the least imaginable pain or inconvenience.[4]

Whether it was such aggrandizement and bluffing that drew dentists themselves to "misuse" advertisements is not clear. But 18th century advertisements, much like modern advertisements, clearly served a second purpose—to promote profitable business.[6] For example, as many as three different 1744 almanacs contain the same advertisement by operators John Watts and Samuel Rutter from the Company of Barber-Surgeons, claiming: "Artificial Teeth set in so firm, as to eat with them, and so exact, as not to be distinguished from Natural."[4] And upon returning to Philadelphia in 1771, Poree announces in the local Gazette that "the great encouragement he has met with in New-York, determines him to fix himself in America, and proposes in future to divide the year between that city and Philadelphia, if he meets with the same approbation."[4]

In the 1800s, according to Dummett, "unsubstantiated claims to scientific verifications cultivated a melange of false, misleading, and useless information foisted onto an unsuspecting public. To this improbity was added the itemization of costs and services, discount coupons, work guarantees, and special gimmicks to lure patients."[7] Consequently, toward the end of the 19th century, the overt soliciting of patients and dramatic claims of painless treatment and cures had brought the profession of dentistry into serious disrepute. To stimulate the growth and strength of the newly formed dental profession (the American Dental Association (ADA) had been formed in 1859), a campaign was mounted to identify quackery and to control the conduct of practitioners by setting national standards. Advertisement was no longer part of the strategy. On the contrary, it had reached such exaggerated and flamboyant levels that it had become a disreputable practice. And in 1866, the ADA moved to ban advertisements.

The Gentleman's Era (1866–1979)

The ADA determined that any advertisements, exceeding a business card or sign with name, title and address, were to be considered unprofessional.[8] This first formal ban was not the result of a fear of competition, but the recognition that the public was being misled and the image of the profession damaged by exaggerated claims of individual superiority.[9] To improve the profession's image, it was needed to attract more "gentlemen," and because it was not considered a gentleman's style to advertise, advertisements were prohibited.[8] The language was clear, but the ADA lacked the necessary power to enforce its verdict. Anxiety over possible loss of newly gained members withheld the Association from attaching stringent requirements to its membership. The ADA confined itself to exerting moral pressure.[10]

In the following years, some local associations issued similar decrees. For example, in 1894, California's first Dental Code of Ethics contained a paragraph dealing with advertisements:

> Sec. 6.—It is unprofessional to resort to public advertisements, cards, handbills, posters, or signs, calling attention to peculiar styles of work, lowness of prices, special modes of operating, or to claim superiority over neighboring practitioners, to publish reports of cases or certificates in public prints, to go from house to house to solicit or perform operations, to circulate or recommend nostrums, or to perform any other similar acts.[10]

In the 1935 Supreme Court decision of *Semler v. Oregon Board of Dental Examiners* the ADA's stance against advertising to ensure the quality of the profession and to protect the public against fraud was legally established.[11] But the revised version of the California Dental Code of Ethics, issued in the very same year, already reflected a much more liberal stance toward advertising, making it unethical to deceive or mislead the public, advertise free dental treatment and examinations, and guarantee painless dental treatment.[10] In spite of such local shifts toward liberalization, a few decades later the 1962 ADA's *Principles of Ethics* still prohibited explicitly any advertisement:

> The dentist has the obligation of advancing a reputation for fidelity, judgement, and skill solely through professional services to patients and to society. The use of advertising in any form to solicit patients is inconsistent with this obligation.[12]

The prohibition was clear, but the language used no longer reflected the emphatic opposition against advertisement that characterized the codes in the second half of the 1800s. In October, 1978, the ADA again went one step further toward freedom of advertising in that it retained the prohibition on providing false, misleading, deceptive or fraudulent representations, but permitted a dentist to advertise "the availability of his services and the fees that he charges for routine procedures."[13] The 1978 revisions in the ADA position may very well have been a capitulation to a superior force, rather than an authentic change of mind. For in the years prior to that revision, the United States Supreme Court had issued two decrees that announced the inevitable end to the nonadvertising position of the professions. *Goldfarb v. Virginia State Bar* (1975) held that there was no "professional" exemption to the antitrust laws, and that the antitrust laws applied to the "learned" professions with the same force and effect that is applied to the rest of industry and commerce.[14] *Bates v. State Bar of Arizona* (1977) held that the First Amendment protection of free speech included advertisements of professionals. The Court found that lawyer advertisement of specific fees for uncomplicated legal services in particular, was commercial free speech and protected from government interference by the First Amendment of the U.S. Constitution. Moreover, the court lauded commercial free speech as an integral part of commerce which informs the public of the availability, nature, and prices of products and services, and thus performs an indispensable role in the allocation of resources in a free enterprise system.[15] Foreseeing the consequences of these decrees, the ADA started moving toward liberalization of advertisement. In 1977, the ADA placed a moratorium on the initiation of disciplinary actions against members "who only advertise in the public press the availability of their services and fees which they would charge for routine dental procedures." Furthermore, it ruled not to deny membership solely on the basis of legally permitted advertising.[16]

However, this movement apparently was not fast enough in the eyes of the Federal Trade Commission, which had been watching the competitive enclave of professions. The ink was hardly dry on the *Bates* opinion before the FTC took the opportunity to strike at ethical code restrictions on advertising by filing formal complaints against the advertising restrictions of the American Medical Association (AMA) and the American Dental Association.

The FTC complaints against the ADA and AMA were basically antitrust actions. The complaints alleged that the associations, and their physician and dentist members, were seeking to restrain the trade by limiting the commercial information available to the consumer. Section 5 of the FTC Act prohibits unfair methods of competition in commerce and unfair or deceptive acts or practices in commerce. Because the associations, unlike sovereign states, were subject to the antitrust laws, any combination that did in fact restrain trade was vulnerable. In March 1979, the ADA decided to enter a consent decree, which settled the issue out of court, yet did not constitute an admission of the ADA that it had violated any laws, but provided that advertising was to be allowed and the ADA code of ethics would be revised accordingly. The era of gentlemanliness had ended.

The Supreme Court's absorption of professional advertising into the protective folds of the First Amendment under the doctrine of commercial free speech placed severe limitations of the ability of the states to regulate dental advertising under their dental practice acts. Previously, the state dental practice acts had largely reflected the views of the dental profession which severely limited the ability of the dentist to advertise. The Supreme Court's decision in the *Bates* case, pre-empted the restrictive states laws. After the *Bates* decision, the states were effectively limited to prohibiting advertising that was false or misleading in a material respect or proving that advertising which was not false or misleading contravened a legitimate public interest which gave the states a right to regulate. The limited rights of the states to prohibit even nonmisleading advertising when a legitimate public interest existed was seen to arise from states' inherent police power to protect the health and welfare of the public. Professional associations, such as the American Dental Association, American Medical Association, and American Bar Association, obviously do not have this inherent police power. Nor are they subject to the First Amendment because theirs is a voluntary membership and members voluntarily agree by joining to waive their First Amendment rights. However, the combination of the *Goldfarb* and *Bates* case decisions did subject advertising regulation by professional association ethical codes to the antitrust laws.

Any doubts about the applicability of *Goldfarb* and *Bates* to the professions were laid to rest by the Supreme Court's decision in *National Society of Professional Engineers v. U.S.* (1975).[17] The Department of Justice sued this professional association, alleging that its ethical code prohibiting the submission of competitive bids on prospective projects constituted price fixing. Although the case dealt with outright price control rather than advertising, the message was clear. The professions had to bring their activities which affected commerce into compliance with the antitrust laws. Thus the Court struck down the ban on price

bidding, finding that it prevented:

> . . . all customers from making price comparisons in the initial selection of an engineer, and imposes the Society's views on the costs and benefits of competition on the entire marketplace. It is this restraint that must be justified. . . , and (the engineer's) attempt to do so on the basis of the potential threat that competition poses to the public safety and the ethics of the profession is nothing less than a frontal assault on the basic policy of (the antitrust laws). (The antitrust law) reflects a legislative judgment that ultimately competition will produce not only lower prices, but also better goods and services.

Under the views of these court decisions, the ethical codes of professional associations will be limited for the foreseeable future to regulating advertising that is determined to be false and misleading in a material respect.

Developments Since 1979

The consent order provided that the ADA would regulate advertising only to the extent that it was "false or misleading in any material respect." Pursuant to this order, the ADA repealed its existing ethical code and all advisory opinions thereunder and issued a new revised code that was subject to the following provision:

> Advertising, solicitation of patients or business, or other promotional activities by dentists or dental care delivery organizations shall not be considered unethical or improper, except for those promotional activities which are false or misleading in any material respect.

The courts, federal and state regulatory agencies, and professional associations soon learned that it is one thing to permit regulation of advertising which is "false or misleading" and quite another to determine what this phrase means.

The first Supreme Court decision to address this issue was *In Re RMJ* (1982).[18] In this case, a lawyer appealed a reprimand from the state disciplinary agency for the attorney licensing authority. This would be equivalent to a censure or reprimand issued by a dental board in the case of a dentist. The lawyer had advertised, describing his areas of practice, in a manner that deviated from language prescribed by the state bar association, e.g., "personal injury" and "real estate" instead of "tort law" and "property law." His advertisement also said that he was licensed to practice in Missouri and Illinois and, in large capital letters, "ADMITTED TO PRACTICE BEFORE THE UNITED STATES SUPREME COURT." The Supreme Court reversed the reprimand and restated the commercial free speech doctrine as follows:

> When the particular content or method of advertising suggests that it is inherently misleading or when experience has proved that in fact such advertising is subject to abuse, the States may impose appropriate restrictions. Misleading advertising may be prohibited entirely. But the States may not place an absolute prohibition on certain types of potentially misleading information, e.g. a listing of areas of practice, if that information also may be presented in a way that is not deceptive. . . .

In short, the Court found terms such as "real estate law" and "personal injury" not to be misleading and not so inherently harmful to the public that the state could entirely prohibit their use.

The Court was troubled by the lawyer's reference to being admitted to practice before its own Supreme Court bar because this is a fairly meaningless piece of information; this privilege is granted almost automatically to any duly licensed lawyer who applies. However, the state agency had not used this as a basis for the reprimand issued and so the Supreme Court passed over this issue with the following comment:

> The emphasis of this relatively uninformative fact is at least bad taste. Indeed, such a statement would be misleading to the general public unfamiliar with the requirements of admission to the Bar of this Court. Yet there is no finding to this effect. . . .

In a subsequent application of the commercial free speech doctrine to the professions, the Supreme Court ruled that, when states were concerned about an advertisement being misleading, they should act in a manner that met their concerns but give the greatest possible deference to the First Amendment. To accomplish this, the Court suggested that requiring additional information in the advertisement or requiring disclaimers was preferable to prohibiting the advertisement altogether.[17] A federal appellate court applied this concept to a dental board's attempt to prohibit a general dentist from advertising "orthodontics" (*Parker v. Kentucky Board of Dentistry*, 818 F. 2d 504 [6th Cir. 1987]). The Kentucky Dental Practice Act prohibited general dentists from holding themselves out as specialists and also from "inserting the name of the specialty, or using other phrases customarily used by qualified specialists that would imply to the public that he is so qualified. . . ." (818 Ibid., F. 2d at 506). The federal appellate court reasoned that if a state permitted a dentist to perform orthodontic procedures, there is nothing inherently misleading in a dentist who chooses to do so saying that he or she does "orthodontics." The court went on to state:

> To the contrary, by suppressing such speech, the public will possibly be misled into believing that only orthodontists can perform orthodontic procedures. Since this information is truthful and related to a lawful activity, it is entitled to the First Amendment protection. . . . A disclaimer . . . would adequately address the State's concern (about the public being misled with respect to whether the dentist they choose is a specialist). (Ibid., 818 F. 2d at 510.)

Some states such as Illinois,[20] Missouri,[21] and Pennsylvania,[22] require general dentists who announce services in specialty areas or specific areas that might be interpreted by the public to be specialty areas to accompany such advertisements with a disclosure that the services are being offered by a general dentist.

CURRENT SITUATION

State Practice Acts in the 50 States

Each state has a dental practice act that defines how the practice of dentistry shall be conducted in that jurisdiction and who shall be entitled to practice dentistry. All of the practice acts, in one form or another, address the subject of advertising, usually under the heading of unprofessional conduct. Some states merely prohibit, under the direction given by the recent Supreme Court cases, advertising that is false or misleading in a material respect. Others are quite detailed and set forth particular modes or types of advertisements that are prohibited.

Such statutes are of vital concern to dentists because the dental board, or the dental board in conjunction with a separate enforcement agency, has the authority to revoke and suspend licenses, place dentists on probation, and issue fines and letters of censure for violations of the dental practice act. Therefore, before a dentist becomes involved with advertising, the appropriate dental practice act of the jurisdiction must be consulted because the very right of the dentist to continue the practice of dentistry is at stake.

The states that go further than generally prohibiting false and misleading advertising, do so under the concept that the specific prohibitions enumerated are false or misleading or that the state has an overriding public interest in controlling some types of advertisements. For example:

The regulations of the Texas Dental Board deem advertisements that would "appeal to an individual's anxiety in an excessive or unfair way," or "create unjustified expectations concerning the potential result of any dental treatment" to be false or misleading.[23]

The Rules for the Administration of the Dental Practice Act of Illinois, issued by the Illinois Department of Professional Regulation, deem advertisements that contain "testimonials ... pertaining to the quality of dental care" to be misleading.[24]

Many states also have requirements that, if broadcast media are used, copies of the commercials that are broadcast must be retained for a certain period. This permits the authorities to check the advertisements in the event there is a subsequent complaint that an advertisement was misleading.

The Role of Professional Associations

The disciplinary authority of professional associations relates solely to the ability of the association to control retention of membership. In dentistry, Chapter XII, Principles of Ethics and Code of Professional Conduct and Judicial Procedure, of the American Dental Association's *Bylaws*, sets forth the procedures for the discipline of members. Section 20 provides that a member may be subject to discipline for "(1) having been found guilty of a felony, (2) having been found guilty of violating the dental practice act of a state, District of Columbia, territory, dependency or country, or (3) violating the *Bylaws, Principles of Ethics and Code of Professional Conduct*, the codes of ethics of the constituent or component societies."

Chapter XII goes on to outline the procedure for disciplinary procedures. Generally, the charges are brought at the local or state dental society level with an appeal to the Council on Ethics, Bylaws and Judicial Affairs of the ADA. The minimum penalty which may be imposed is censure. The other two possible penalties are suspension of or expulsion from membership. Membership may also be put on a probationary status as a result of a disciplinary proceeding. Probation is usually applied in conjunction with supervision or expulsion.

Of course, with respect to advertising, any discipline imposed by a dental society as a result of a member's advertising would be subject to review outside of the procedures of organized dentistry by the government antitrust enforcement agencies. At the federal level, these are the Federal Trade Commission and the Antitrust Division of the U.S. Department of Justice. States' Attorneys General offices also have antitrust enforcement branches. Any of these government enforcement agencies can seek to restrain the dental society's activities by filing an action, either civil or criminal, in a court of law alleging a violation of the antitrust laws. Individual dentists also have the right to initiate civil actions in court if they believe their rights are being infringed upon.

Although the threat of lawsuits from

these many sources cannot be discounted, dental societies have been given a fair amount of insulation from antitrust lawsuits by the courts. The courts have recognized that professional associations fulfill an important role in society by issuing and enforcing ethical codes. An example of this is the federal appellate court opinion that affirmed the FTC finding that the AMA violated the antitrust laws by issuing ethical canons that prohibited all physician advertising. Although finding for the FTC, the court nevertheless made an important modification in the final FTC order issued against the AMA. This modification, which is applicable to all professional health associations, including dentistry, provides that such associations may enforce *reasonable* ethical guidelines governing the conduct of its members with respect to advertisements, when the professional association has a *reasonable belief* that such advertisements would be false or misleading.[25]

ETHICAL ANALYSIS

Arguments in Favor of Advertising

The arguments in favor of advertising can be classified in three related but separate categories: (1) advertising disseminates information to nonutilizing or underutilizing asymptomatic people about the need to regularly seek dental services; (2) advertising provides the public with information that may assist them in choosing a dentist; (3) advertising stimulates competition among dentists, which in turn has a great number of beneficial consequences both for the dentists and the public.

The first category of arguments—providing information to nonutilizers—does not really justify genuine advertising as that word is used in everyday language. The kind of advertising referred to would more appropriately be called "dental health education" because no commercial intentions whatsoever are involved. The purpose of such educational advertisements is to persuade asymptomatic people to regularly visit *any* dental office for a preventive examination. Getting more people to seek and receive the care they

need generally is considered an ethically acceptable practice, even if advertising techniques are employed.[26] In most countries advertising by individual dentists is still prohibited, but the local, regional, and national dental organizations may arrange "institutional" educational advertisements. Many American dental organizations engage in similar campaigns. For example, in 1979, the ADA House of Delegates approved the expenditure of up to two million dollars for a nationwide campaign aimed at motivating more Americans to seek regular dental care.[27] According to an Academy of General Dentistry's Institutional Advertising Test Market Project, successful dental health education can increase the nationwide sum of dental visits by as much as 14%.[28] In 1983, the ADA House of Delegates provided seed money for an additional public education campaign, which included the development of television commercials and print advertisements, which mainly emphasized the benefits of regular visits to the dentist in preventing periodontal disease. In 1984, the ADA House of Delegates failed to adopt the dues raise necessary to fund the purchase of television time and print space to carry out this campaign. Although a slight majority of the House of Delegates voted in favor of this campaign, the proposal was unable to garner the two-thirds majority necessary for the dues raise. The commercials and print advertisements were subsequently made available, and utilized by constituent dental societies in campaigns funded locally.[29] Consequently, an increased demand for dental care may increase the income of an individual dentist as well. But that increase is not the primary goal of the advertisement, it is merely a welcome side effect.

The second category contains advertisements that usually are not purely educational, but not plainly commercial either. Patients in need of dental care must be able to quickly locate a dentist. Not only are advertisements such as those placed in the telephone directory Yellow Pages mentioning the dentist's name and address seldom questioned (even in the heyday of the anti-advertisement movement at the end of the 19th century), but one may even argue that such "announcements" are a moral obligation of any dentist. Physicians and dentists alike are expected to be easily accessible in emergencies, and announcement in the telephone directory serves that purpose well. Although prohibited from private advertisements for commercial purposes, dentists could be obligated to have their names added to an inventory in the Yellow Pages, listing address, hours, specialty and other relevant information in a similar, standardized manner. Because nearly half of the U.S. population moves every 5 years, "announcement" advertisements help many people find dental services once they have relocated to a new community. Furthermore, it can be argued that patients have a right to choose a health care provider of their liking, which can be eased by allowing dentists to announce their opening hours, specialty, and other practical information. Additionally, to make informed choices, patients may want information about office location, nature of services, and the qualifications of the dentist. Although advertising does not provide a complete foundation on which to select a dentist, at least some relevant information needed for an informed decision is provided. It seems difficult, if not impossible, to justify withholding such basic information from patients. Information allows the patient with perceived oral health needs to find a dentist who is equipped to treat those specific needs.

Obviously, most, if not all, of the advertising dentists in this second category are not merely interested in the benefit of the patients; they hope also to foster their own practice and not dentistry in general, let alone their colleague's practice. Empirical research has shown that advertisements (contrary to health education campaigns) do not attract the underutilizer into the dental care system.[30] It persuades newcomers in the area to visit the advertising dentist's office (rather than some other dentist's office or no office at all); it may remind people to visit a dentist (or their own dentist, which would actually improve the non-advertising dentist's practice instead of the advertising dentist's practice); and it causes a (temporary) shift in patients from a nonadvertising to an advertising dentist. In all these situations, the advertisements are not likely to materially improve the dental health of the population. Rather, any improvement in health is incidental to the improvement in the business of the advertising dentist. Consequently, the line between altruistic beneficence and self-centered commercialism is a very fine one, as subsequent examples will show.

The third category of arguments pertains to genuine advertisements. Such advertisements are part of competition strategies directly aimed at improving the economical "health" of the advertising dentist. The interrelationship between socioeconomic conditions and advertising becomes clear when we look at impoverished third-world countries. In many of these countries, there are so few dentists that there simply is no need to attract patients by means of advertising. In Western Europe, on the other hand, there is an oversupply of dentists; and although individual advertising is generally still prohibited, some countries (such as Great Britain and New Zealand) are moving toward a liberalization of advertising.[31-33]

According to advertising advocates such as the FTC, advertisements not only benefit the dentists, but the public as well. Advertising can prevent price-fixing, it can stimulate the use of new innovative systems, and it can force dentists to continuously improve their practice.[34] Although no empirical studies demonstrate the effect of advertising on the price of professional dental services, there is revealing evidence with regard to products. When suppliers advertise price information, retail prices often are considerably lower than they would be without advertisement.[35,36] However, suppliers of products generally do not have as much influence over their purchasers as professional health care providers have over their patients. This influence is readily susceptible to misuse by the doctor recommending additional and unnecessary procedures. Even if the fee for most services is slightly reduced by advertising, if the advertisements are paid for by the doctors pushing more services, the savings from lower fees are illusory. It would be interesting to see what research on the advertising of health care services would show with respect to the overall expenditures by society and by individuals for health care.

Arguments against Advertising

The most commonly voiced arguments against advertising fall into two categories: (1) those denying the positive effects suggested by advocates, such as price decreases and quality increases, and (2) those contending that advertisements harm the professional nature of dentistry.

Those opposing advertising by dentists have argued that, in reality, advertising simply does not work, or at any rate is not worth the money. The increase of patients caused by advertisements is minimal and negligible. Others have claimed that advertisement actually defeats its purpose, that is, it increases instead of decreases patient fees. Havard has pointed out that this is a foreseeable consequence in countries with socialized health care systems, such as the British National Health Service, as the costs of advertising will form a integral part of the practice expenses pool.[33] But also, in a free-market system, the patient may have to pay the price. "Inevitably, as more and more dentists advertise, the ante is raised. Spurious referral services and guarantees intensify the contest, advertisements become larger and more strident, the costs of the advertising increase, and inevitably, so do fees."[9] What is even more, not only may the advertising of fees increase patient fees, because it is the patient who in the end pays for the advertisement; price advertising paradoxically may also drive prices up if consumers take fees to be a measure of quality and consequently perceive higher priced professionals as better.[3]

More important than the arguments that simply deny the benefits of advertising suggested by advocates are those arguments against advertisement that belong to the second category. It is argued that eye-catching advertisements, like billboards and neon signs, are not in accordance with the standards of professional and collegial practice. Advertisements undermine the confidential relationship between dentist and patient, because patients begin to distrust the authority of dentists when appeal for services is created more by imagery than by substance.[37] In fact, advertisements are usually aimed at manipulating behavior rather than fostering informed choices by patients. Creating needs is incompatible with a model of health *care,* in which the dentist solves the patients' problems rather than creating them. Jonsen brings to mind the doctor who is rejoicing: "We are really lucky in this hospital, we've got a lot of nosocomial infection here. That means more business."[38] Equally baffling would be a dentist who is delighted about his or her patient's need of a root canal.

Profession or Commerce

Before an evaluation of the ethical strength of the arguments presented against or in favor of advertising by dentists, it must first be decided what counts as morally good dental practice. This question, however, is not discussed in the literature on advertising, either by those in favor or by those against. The explanation for this failure lies in the fact that both groups take for granted a different moral model for the occupation of dentistry, that is, a commercial model versus a professional model. Which of these models is morally superior is quite a different question than the one pertaining to the moral status of advertising; the former transcends the latter, and the latter cannot be answered decisively without the former being answered first.

That is not to say that only the question pertaining to the moral model of dentistry is a serious ethical question, and that the past prohibition of advertisement was merely a matter of etiquette[39] or even a psychological barrier to be overcome.[40] It is true that the "sentiments" of dentists toward advertising have quite rapidly changed since the ADA decided in 1979 that advertising would no longer be considered unethical. A review of the literature reveals that, before 1979, dentists had strong negative attitudes toward dental advertising.[41–44] On the other hand, one more recent study suggests a less negative and increasingly positive attitude towards advertising.*[45] This shift suggests that the issue of advertising is merely one of taste, rather than values. But that would be too hasty a conclusion. A closer examination of the empirical data reveals that advocates of advertising are likely to favor a more commercially than professionally oriented occupational model of dentistry. Often, those opposed to advertising are older, settled dentists, whereas those in favor tend to be younger dentists with less than 10 years experience and needing to develop their practice, or dental students.[46–51] The moral stance of the dentists towards advertising reflects his or her choice of occupational model. Thus, the issue of advertising is not merely a matter of taste, but part of the overreaching ethical dilemma of the most appropriate model for the occupation of dentistry as a whole.

Solving that dilemma, however, is not within the realm of this endeavor (see, however, Chaps. 1 and 4). Instead, this chapter shows how the professional and commercial models imply very different answers to the question of the moral status of advertising by dentists.

Elsewhere in this book (see Chap. 4), three models, rather than two, are distinguished: the commercial, guild, and interactive models. The first of these corresponds with our commercial model; the second corresponds with our so-called "professional model." The interactive model is an attempt to unite the former two more extreme models while at the same time adding certain notions for which neither of those two models can adequately account. Since those special notions are of minor relevance to the issue of advertising, while on the other hand the differences between the first two more extreme models are of paramount importance, we have decided to limit this chapter to the commercial and professional (guild) models.

Furthermore, we have chosen to adjust slightly the vocabulary used in other chapters. Instead of using the generic term "models of professionalism" for all model variations, we use the term "occupation models." If it is argued that the commercial

model implies a classic business approach such that the commonly assumed moral differences between dentistry and, for example, selling automobiles fade away, and if dentistry nonetheless is characterized as a commercial *profession,* this implies one of two confusing things: either selling automobiles is a profession as well, or there are commercial professions (such as dentistry) and commercial non-professions (such as selling automobiles). The former seems not to be in accordance with everyday language, while the latter raises the question of what feature accounts for the difference. After all, the commercial model was introduced as a classic business approach. By employing the more neutral term "occupation," we are able to reserve the term "profession" for those occupations which traditionally and intuitively are thought to be distinct from classic commercial occupations.

In this chapter, when the two different models of dentistry are discussed, the terms "commercial" and "professional" function only as a label.[1] Obviously, in doing so, we are referring to the common use of the terms: generally it is understood that a profession is an occupation that is concerned more with the ethical nuances of the craft, business, or trade.[52] But in employing the labels, we do not want to accept from the outset all the connotations and vagueness implied in these terms. For example, the professional model does not necessarily imply that the dentist's interests are of less importance than those of the patient. Many a dentist, physician, or lawyer has made more money from his or her altruistic services than the local butcher, the housekeeper, or the ice-cream vendor from his or her private for-profit business. Similarly, the commercial model does not necessarily imply that the provider stands to benefit more than any other party. In the *Bates* decision, the United States Supreme Court assumed that, in a free-market economy, lawyer advertising may well benefit the administration of justice, because it is the traditional mechanism for a supplier to inform a potential purchaser of the availability of the product or services and terms of exchange.[15] Consequently, the question emerges, what differentiates a profession from other occupations, no-

---

* Some recent empirical studies, however, deny that dentist attitudes towards advertising have become more positive.[46,47]

tably business? Traditional criteria such as specialized knowledge no longer apply because computer specialists and biochemists have highly specialized knowledge, probably more specialized than that of dentists. Self-regulation through a body of behavioral rules, a so-called "code of ethics," is an equally weak criterion. First of all, any occupation, whether commercial or professional, has to function within the boundaries of the law of the nation (such as, for example, the antitrust laws); self-regulation, therefore, is always regulation within the limits of and guided by external, imposed regulation. More importantly, such limited self-regulation through codes of ethics has become a customary habit of almost all occupations: architects, bankers, journalists, moving companies, car dealers, even lobbyists have drafted such codes.

It seems that the only distinctive criterion is the particular tripartite relationship between occupational organization, provider, and client. In a commercial model, the client deals with the provider and not directly with the latter's occupational organization. For important deals, a client does not trust just any businessperson, simply because he or she represents a certain trade; the client shops around until he or she finds the businessperson who provides the product of his or her liking and who offers a good price. For less important purchases, the client may be willing to pay less for less quality. Clients accept differences in the quality of the products and services; clients want those differences. When a client is satisfied, he or she praises that particular businessperson, not the whole trade; when he or she is dissatisfied, he or she complains or even sues that particular businessperson, not the whole trade.

In a professional model, on the other hand, the client (or patient) first of all deals with the occupational organization, the profession, not with the individual provider. A patient suffering from a severe toothache should be able to trust any dentist, simply because he or she is a representative of the occupation of dentistry. There should be no need to first check with a friend at work, the neighbor around the block, or Consumer Reports, whether Dr. X can be trusted as a dentist. The trust concerns primarily the profession of dentistry, not the individual provider; and the profession, consequently, is responsible for the quality of the provided services by each of its members.

The essential difference between the commercial model and the professional model is not the degree of altruism, of placing the benefit of the patient or client under or over the provider's. Misleading clients, enriching oneself by abusing the needs and weaknesses of clients, or breaking a promise to a client is never justifiable, either in a professional relationship or in a commercial relationship. What differs is the method to promote client benefit, which in turn is based on a dissimilar interpretation of the nature of "product" exchanged in the relationship between dentists and patients.

In the commercial model, more specifically, a free-market commercial model, it is assumed that dental care is essentially the same as any other kind of product offered by one person and, if so desired, acquired by another. In this relationship, ideally, the client is the steering force because it is his or her desires, wishes, and preferences that cause certain products to be offered in the first place, and lead him or her to decide whether to buy the product offered. Therefore, in the commercial model, it is thought that the client's benefit is realized best by allowing competition among providers and a variety of choices for clients. The price that the client pays for this competition and variety is the increased chance to deal with an unscrupulous crook and the need to look around for a good deal.

In a professional model, it is thought that the product offered is not a commodity, but aid and relief. The person in need of aid and relief does not have time to shop around for an appropriate "product;" he or she must be able to find it quickly. In the professional model, therefore, the client is guaranteed a standard level of quality so that he or she can trust every single representative of the profession. Thus, if someone develops an acute dental ailment while traveling in an unfamiliar part of the country, it would be unnecessary to shop for a dentist because every dentist in the area should be practicing the standard level of quality care. In the professional model, to sustain general trustworthiness of dentists the patient cannot be offered a variety of dental practice styles to choose from because every dentist has to practice in the manner dictated by the profession.

Obviously, both theoretical models in reality can be corrupted. In a commercial model, major companies can acquire a hard-to-break monopoly and consequently too much power. In a professional model, the occupational organization, i.e., the profession may fail to maintain a basic quality level among all of its members. In both instances, the fundamental principle itself is undermined: in the first, that of freedom of choice; in the second, that of trust.

The 1866 ADA prohibition on advertising reflects the professional model: professionals should not try to improve their personal image by suggesting they provide better service than their professional colleagues. Advertisements undermine the trust in other members of the profession. As Havard has summarized, "Self promotional advertising is inconsistent with the philosophy of a caring profession. It leads to the introduction of a *caveat emptor* (let the buyer be aware) into the relationship."[33]

On the other hand, the FTC's position reflects the commercial model. It holds that competition is a method to promote low-cost dentistry and better services. Advertising is an important strategy to promote competition and therefore may not be prohibited by the ADA.[11,53] Restraints on advertisement can be justified, according to the FTC, but "only if they promote competition, rather than merely other social goals."[54] This statement clearly reflects the assumption, which is simply taken for granted by the FTC, that competition is the single most important value and that all other social goals are "merely" secondary. Prohibiting false and misleading advertisements does not limit competition because it forces dentists to provide accurate information to consumers, which, in turn, may promote competition.[83] Similar assumptions concerning the legitimacy of advertising are made by other authors. Schiedermayer, in his lecture at the 1987

Annual Meeting of American College of Dentists, maintained that truthful, verifiable advertisements do not harm professionalism (the patient always has the option of suing if the dentist does not fulfill his or her promises), and such advertisements are part of "*legitimate* competition."[55]

The decision in favor of or against advertisement depends on the occupational model of dentistry chosen. It may even be the case that no decisive arguments can be found to justify the choice between one of these two models. Those favoring a commercial model have claimed that patients want advertisements. And indeed, empirical studies have verified this contention.[47,48,56] However, dentists opposing a commercial model may counterargue that this empirical fact does not prove the moral surplus of a commercial model. On the contrary, it merely underscores the need to protect patients against their lack of insight in the complexity of the treatment process. Competition among dentists may do the patients more harm than good.[47]

Similarly, those favoring a professional model have tried to argue that advertising increases instead of decreases patient fees. But even if this prediction is true (which will be hard to prove empirically because the decrease in fees resulting from increased competition may even out the increase caused by advertisements and, conversely, dentists could choose to augment decreases in fees by recommending additional procedures or treatment), this contention is not a valid argument against the commercial model. It merely shows that the patient has to pay for the information offered. But in a commercial model, it is legitimate to assume that patients are apparently willing to pay for this price increase because they have always kept the freedom to seek the services of non-advertising dentists. One observer has advised professionally oriented dentists to collectively insert into the Yellow Pages an announcement reading: "Seek the services of a non-advertising dentist."[9] If patients nonetheless do not visit non-advertising dentists and advertisements become more frequent, bigger, and more glaring, that indicates that patients, in spite of increased fees, apparently prefer this expansion of the commercial model over the professional model in which advertisements are discouraged.

Next, the ethical status of various examples of advertisements is examined from the perspective of both the commercial model and the professional model of dentistry. Some forms of advertising are found reproachable from both perspectives because the commercial model does not grant carte blanche for any advertisements. False and deceiving advertisements are not acceptable in the framework of a professional model, but are not acceptable in a commercial model either. On the other hand, both the commercial and the professional model may allow certain neutral informative advertisements, because as Havard's statement aptly indicates, advertisements are incompatible with a professional model only when they are self-promotional.[33] An advertisement that does not suggest a greater trustworthiness may very well be acceptable within a professional model of dentistry.

Examples of Various Advertisements

ANNOUNCEMENT OR ADVERTISEMENT

The simplest form of an advertisement is what is often called a threshold or tombstone advertisement: a name and address, opening hours, and possibly a specialty announcement. Obviously, by placing such an advertisement in the telephone directory, a dentist increases the chances that a patient will visit him rather than a non-advertising dentist. The appealing nature of this advertisement lies in the fact that this dentist makes himself easier to be found. Note that there is no suggestion that Dr. Doe is a superior dentist. As argued earlier, such an advertisement is not a genuine, that is, commercially oriented, advertisement, but a mere announcement.

Announcements, as shown in Figure 10–1, are generally accepted by the public and by a majority of dentists as well.[47] Dispute about the morality of tombstone advertisements arise when the advertisement intends to do more than just announce the dentist's existence. A bold or larger letter

```
┌─────────────────────────────────────────┐
│            JOHN A. DOE, D.D.S.           │
│                                          │
│          Announces availability of       │
│                                          │
│    EVENING AND SATURDAY APPOINTMENTS     │
│                                          │
│      in addition to regular appointments for │
│                                          │
│          GENERAL DENTAL CARE             │
│                                          │
│  123 Main Street              Tel. 555-1212 │
│  Anytown, USA                for appointment │
└─────────────────────────────────────────┘
```

Fig. 10–1. Announcement advertisement. With permission from Shapiro, I.A., and Majewski, R.F.: Attitudes of dental students and faculty toward advertising. J. Am. Dent. Assoc. *105:*468, 1982.

type, a little logo, or a portrait photograph intends to catch the attention of the reader and to keep him or her from scanning the other dentists' announcements in the Yellow Pages. Those advocating a professional model of dentistry may oppose big and flashy advertisements as unprofessional because such advertisements do not present information in a reasonably dignified and restrained manner that contributes to the esteem of the profession.

Similarly, adding information beyond name, address, and hours may meet with disapproval. The name under which a dentist conducts his or her practice may be a factor in the selection process of the patient, but the use of a trade name or an assumed name can be misleading. Some states prohibit the use of "trade names" such as "Southmost Dental Center" as their practice name. Other states allow trade names as long as the dentist(s) also include their individual names.

Furthermore, mentioning a specialty implies a qualitative difference between oneself and other dentists, because a specialty implies that one has specialized knowledge and skills, that is, knowledge and skills other colleagues may not have. For that very reason, in 1866, the year in which the ADA deemed advertisements to be unprofessional, some people argued that mentioning a specialty on a business card constituted disguised advertising.[8] Recently, those favoring a professional model have become less opposed to specialty advertising because such information may assist patients to find the dentist who can best solve their specific problems. However, to prevent the public from being misled into believing that the dentist has met the educational requirements for a certified specialty, he or she must advertise his or her field of practice in such a way that the public is not misled. From the perspective of the professional model, announcing oneself as a dental specialist is allowed only when the dentist has successfully completed a post-doctorate course approved by the Commission on Dental Accreditation of the American Dental Association in a specialty recognized by the board. The special areas approved by the ADA for specialty announcement and limitation of practice are dental public health, endodontics, oral pathology, oral and maxillofacial surgery, orthodontics, pediatric dentistry, periodontics, and prosthodontics. For example, it is misleading for a dentist to advertise that he or she is a specialist or limits his or her practice to the diagnosis and treatment of temporomandibular joint disorders, facial pain therapy, or implantology because these are not Board-recognized specialties.

In a commercial model, these restrictions on specialty advertising are often considered an unacceptable limitation of legitimate business. In concert with the Supreme Court rulings on commercial free speech and restraint of trade, ADA's *Principles of Ethics and Code of Professional Conduct* recognizes the right of general dentists to announce services in which they take a particular interest, whether or not these services are in a specialty area, so long as this is done in a manner that does not express or imply the status of a specialist. The ADA Code indicates that this should be done by a specific statement that the advertiser is a general dentist. The ADA Code also prohibits general dentists from using the phrase "practice limited to" on the premise that, in dentistry, this phrase has become a synonym for specialization. The ADA Code does not prohibit the use of specialty terms, such as, orthodontics, prosthodontics, or endodontics. Nor does it require any disclaimers. It has been interpreted as prohibiting a general dentist from using the term orthodontist, prosthodontist or endodontist.[57]

JOHN A. DOE, D.D.S.
GENERAL DENTIST

Examination $5
  Extractions $20
    Cleaning and X-Rays $20
      Fillings $10 per surface

Other fees explained upon request

123 Main Street   Anytown, USA
Tel. 555-1212   for appointment

Fig. 10–2. Fee-listing advertisement. With permission from Shapiro, I.A., and Majewski, R.F.: Attitudes of dental students and faculty toward advertising. J. Am. Dent. Assoc. *105:*468, 1982.

FEE LISTING AND PRICE PROMOTION

A common topic of dispute involves the advertisement of fees. Because the Bates decision of 1977 held that the advertising of fee information for services provided could not be prohibited by a licensing authority,[15] fee listing has become common practice. But such listings can easily become misleading, when, for example, the dentists fails to indicate to the public the length of time for which that fee shall be in effect. Figure 10–2 shows a simple, easily verifiable and clear price listing. Figure 10–3, on the other hand, is an example of a very suggestive yet multi-interpretable and thus misleading price promotion.

Empirical studies have shown that, indeed, price promotion advertisements are rejected by both consumers and dentists. But neutral price listing does not draw

CUSTOM FITTED
DENTURES—$99 and up!

All other dental services at
INFLATION FIGHTING FEES!

Credit cards and time payments

Call now! **JOHN A. DOE, D.D.S.**—555-1212
123 Main Street   Anytown, USA

10% DISCOUNT WITH THIS AD!

Fig. 10–3. Price promotion advertisement. With permission from Shapiro, I.A., and Majewski, R.F.: Attitudes of dental students and faculty toward advertising. J. Am. Dent. Assoc. *105:*468, 1982.

general disapproval. Although one study showed some 87% of consumers approved of such a message, 84% of dentists disapproved.[47]

Various state dental practice acts require services to be advertised with a stated fee to include all components of providing that service without additional charges added or without additional unstated restrictions. Likewise, when an office charges a range of fees for a dental service, any advertisement of the fee for that service should disclose the range and include a listing of all the factors that cause the fee to vary. For example, advertising of denture prices often fails to include whether or not the dentures are preformed/prefabricated or custom-made, and whether the advertised price includes both upper and lower dentures. Special discount offers should include the nondiscounted or full price and the final discounted price, and it should be clear whether the dentist provides the same quality and components of service and material that he or she provides at the normal, nondiscounted fee for that same service. Some state dental practice acts require that any fee advertisement should be exact, without the use of comparative phrases such as "from," "between," "as low as," "and up," or "lowest prices," or claims of implied "bargains." On the other hand, a former Director of the FTC Bureau of Consumer Protection opined that language such as "lowest cost" or "as low as" were useful because they commanded consumer attention![58]

PERSUASIVE TECHNIQUES

Although in Figure 10–3 the advertisement appeals to the desire of every person to get the best bargain in town, other dental advertisements intentionally appeal to the particular anxieties and fears and people in need of dental care. Promises of "painless dentistry," "pain-free dentistry," or "gentle dentistry" play with people's past experiences and commonplace myths. Such promises can be deemed immoral simply because they are misleading; they create unjustifiable expectations that a dentist cannot achieve.

However, it is much more difficult to argue against advertisements that play with the current worldwide phobia for AIDS. Some dentists have advertised that they take special infection control precautions against AIDS. Again, this is misleading because every dentist is required by law to take the necessary precautions prescribed by the Centers for Disease Control (CDC) and the Occupational Safety and Health Administration (OSHA). Any so-called extra precautions are not necessary and do not significantly increase the effectiveness of infection control in a dental office. Both advocates of a professional and a commercial model consequently ought to renounce such advertisements. However, consensus is less likely to occur on the issue of advertising the HIV status of the dentist.

Dentists have the right to communicate to their patients that they have been tested and are HIV-negative if this information is accompanied by an explanation that places this fact in the proper perspective within the overall subject of infection control in the dental office. This can be best done in a conversation directly with the patient. However, some dentists have started advertising their own negative HIV status. As of 1992, available tests have a lag time of up to 6 months before the virus might be detected. Thus, even if a dentist were tested every six months, it would be possible for the dentist to be HIV-positive any time during a period of up to 1 year before the test would reveal this. There is some contention that the virus is most virulent and easily spread when it is in the very early stages. Some patients, being fully informed by the advertisement of all the scientific implications surrounding testing, may take much less solace from the advertised HIV test results than the advertiser intends. Yet, in spite of such scientific explanation, many other patients may attach undue significance to the advertisement and become afraid to visit a dentist who does not announce his HIV status. Consequently, in professional model advertising HIV status is unacceptable since it is likely to harm the trust between dentists and the public. On the other hand, in a commercial model, HIV status advertisements that include all relevant scientific information are not misleading in any material respect and therefore cannot be prohibited. The issue of HIV status constitutes an apparent example of an area where the commercial and professional models are divergent.

A similar disagreement is likely to occur about advertisements that play with people's desire to look attractive. The text of Figure 10–4 is not misleading in any material respect. The advertisement merely inquires whether a person is afraid to smile, or embarrassed to show his or her teeth. No guarantees of a better job, a happier life, or a Miss America title are made; just some help is offered to improve a part of one's image. A former Director of a Regional FTC Office argued that such statements pertaining to patient appearances may be difficult to verify objectively, but are not inherently deceptive. "Prohibition of nondeceptive subjective claims may reduce the effectiveness of advertising in lowered frequency, increasing costs for consumers."[59] In a commercial model, salespersons and dentists alike do not have the moral obligation to warn a client that he or she is not really in need of the product he is about to purchase.[33] On the contrary, suggesting needs is a common advertisement strategy, and health care advertisements are no exception.[60] If one adopts the commercial model, it seems inconsistent and unfair to allow the advertisement of special interests, price listings, and even HIV status, but not an appeal to all-too-common vanity.

FALSE AND MISLEADING ADVERTISEMENTS

In the Pennsylvania Gazette of 1799, a certain Dr. Hamilton boldly claimed that

---

ARE YOU AFRAID TO SMILE?

Are you embarrassed to show your teeth? Let me help you rebuild an important part of your image . . .

"YOUR SMILE"

JOHN A. DOE, D.D.S.

123 Main Street   Anytown, USA

Tel. 555-1212 now . . . for your future!

Fig. 10–4. Persuasive advertisement. With permission from Shapiro, I.A., and Majewski, R.F.: Attitudes of dental students and faculty toward advertising. J. Am. Dent. Assoc. 105:468, 1982.

Painless treatment GUARANTEED through our use of sweet air !!

JOHN A. DOE, D.D.S.

"The Dentist with a Heart"

MODERN STATE OF THE ART MATERIALS

CALL NOW AT 1-800-555-1212

Anytown Civic Award	Main Office at
Anytown High School Booster	123 Main Street
Finalist, Mr. Anytown Contest	Anytown, USA

Fig. 10–5. Misleading advertisement

"he cleans and removes tartar from the teeth so effectually, as to restore them to *native* whiteness, without the *least* injury to the enamel."[61] Guaranteeing any dental procedure with such terms as "satisfaction guaranteed," "under no obligation," "indestructible," or a claim that a manifestly incurable disease can be permanently cured, was and still is misleading, because it makes a promise that seldom if ever can be kept (Fig. 10–5). There is general agreement that false and misleading advertising is immoral. After all, any lie or deception is immoral. Thus, statements that misconstrue the nature of dental procedures, or do not tell patients all that they need to know about them, are unacceptable. (For more on the subject of disclosure, see Chapters 5 and 6.) Advertising nitrous oxide as twilight sleep borders on recommending it for recreational use. No anesthetic or medication is completely without side effects; obviously, it would be inappropriate to use such drugs for the pleasure of the patient rather than therapeutically. However, the dentist who advertises sweet air and twilight sleep is in a poor position to resist patient demands for such services on the grounds that they are inappropriate in the case of the patient making the request. The same applies to dentists advertising that they do not use or place amalgam restorations. How far can such advertisements go before they create public apprehension that has no basis in scientific research with respect to the presence of mercury in amalgam restorations? Again, the basic question is which advertisements are false and misleading. It is often difficult to determine where to draw the line (Fig. 10–5.).

Disagreement arises when it comes to advertisements that can be misread, but are not necessarily deceptive. The statements in these advertisements can be either literally correct or, if not correct, at least very difficult to disprove. Advertisements mentioning superior equipment such as the "latest modern equipment," "modern offices," "quality dentistry," "scientifically equipped," "modern methods and devices," or the use of such terms as "high level performance," "fast results," and "progressive," may be read to imply that the advertising office is "up to speed" with the rest of the profession. But they are more likely to intend and infer professional superiority over neighboring practitioners. These messages convey the message that one dentist is more trustworthy than another. After all, nobody advertises that his or her office is not modern or that nonquality dentistry is delivered. Yet such extravagant claims, aggrandizement of abilities or self-laudatory statements that are calculated to attract patients, are seldom objectively false. A similar effect may be obtained by the use of celebrities or celebrity endorsements, statements of benefits from dental services received, expressions of the appreciation for dental services, and character references. Although such testimonials clearly *imply* superiority and exceptional trustworthiness, they may not be objectively accurate.

Consequently, although those advocating a professional model of dentistry will renounce such self-promotional advertisements, those advocating a commercial model may have considerably less objections. In the 1989 letter quoted previously from a former Director of a Regional FTC Office, it was actually suggested that "consumers may benefit from the kind of comparative statements that the Board's regulations prohibit. Some consumers may want to know, for example, which dentist believes he or she is the 'kindest' or 'most sympathetic.' Such statements clearly are puffery, yet may provide useful information to consumers on the elements of a practice that a dentist considers most important."[59]

However, even the FTC might be changing. It recently commented with respect to a proposed FTC consent order against the Connecticut Chiropractic Association, which would have prohibited the Association from barring its members from making claims in advertisements that they possess "unusual expertise." The ADA comment expressed concern that this proposed consent order would prevent the Chiropractic Association from barring unsubstantiated false and deceptive claims. In responding to the ADA concerns, by letter of November 19, 1991, the FTC pointed out that the language of the order, as provided by the decision in *American Medical Association v. FTC* case, provided that the Association could prohibit advertisements it "reasonably believes to be false or deceptive. . . ." The letter from the FTC concluded "unsubstantiated representations are among those that the Commission considers to be deceptive under Section 5 or the Federal Trade Commission Act"[62] Therefore, it may be that future rulings on professional advertising from both the dental boards and professional associations may come to hold that false impressions generated by unsubstantiated statements in advertisements constitute deceptive advertising.

CONCLUSIONS AND SUGGESTIONS

We have seen that the morality of advertising depends to a large degree on the occupational model dentistry adopted. Certain advertisements are immoral regardless of the model one chooses, whereas others are acceptable in both models. Ethical dilemmas arise in regard to the category of advertisements that are neither flagrantly deceptive nor purely neutral. Unfortunately, this category is the biggest. Lacking decisive arguments to choose between the two occupational models, it is pertinent to, at any rate, be consistent in one's stance towards advertising. One cannot have one's cake and eat it too: when adopting a professional model, one has to accept that most forms of advertisements are simply unacceptable. When one adopts a professional model while at the same time allowing self-promotional advertising, a necessary condition of moral life, that is, consistency, is undermined. Without consistency, morality is downgraded to subjective, arbitrary preferences.

Unfortunately, many regulations currently reflect a very inconsistent stance toward advertising. Some practice acts, for example, do allow dentists to offer and advertise special low fees, but not free services. It is argued that free dental examinations or x rays are an inducement to secure dental patronage, yet that is the very purpose of all competition and advertising. Some dental practice acts state that dentists may advertise or offer free examination or free dental services, but it shall be unlawful, however, for any dentist to charge a fee to any new patient for any dental service provided at the time that such free examination or free dental services are provided. Again, the authors of such guidelines opened the door to a commercial approach in dentistry, yet at the same time tried to save as much professionalism as possible.

Many contemporary dental codes of ethics and practice acts still list traditional professional duties such as: (1) the dentist's primary professional obligation shall be service to the public, and (2) dentists are expected to maintain and elevate the esteem of the profession. Yet the very same regulations and guidelines allow dentists to employ a typically commercial method to solicit patients, namely to advertise name and address, hours, specialty, prices, discounts, even HIV status—anything that is not false or misleading in any material respect.

In defense of the authors of these codes and practice acts, one may argue that the officers, members, and staff of those professional organizations and boards never agreed wholeheartedly with the FTC regulations in the first place. The FTC regulations against prohibiting advertisement have frustrated the professions' (e.g., law, dentistry, medicine) attempts to maintain a professional model. This is not because of the fact *that* the FTC imposed regulations, thereby limiting the area of self-regulation, for any occupation, including professions, is bound by the nation's laws. The professions' attempts were frustrated by *what* the FTC mandated, that is,

unrestricted freedom of advertisement for their members. One may, therefore, argue that the professions, to save a little bit of professionalism, had to "sit on the fence, run with the hare, and hunt with the hounds," that is, evade the very choice between the two models while attempting to secure some traditional professional values and complying at the same time as much as possible with FTC regulations. The question remains whether such a political strategy can be successfully realized and guarantee high moral practice standards in the long run.

DISCUSSION QUESTIONS

1. An ethical standard common among advertising businesses is not to promote one's own business by presenting incorrect information about competitors. However, it is considered acceptable to refer to a competitor's product of lesser quality when this difference in quality is verifiable. Do you think it is acceptable for dentists in advertisements to compare themselves with colleagues when the facts mentioned about those colleagues are verifiably true (e.g., fewer years of practice experience, lacking specialization, reprimanded by professional organization, or positive HIV status of colleague).

2. Advertising is a common method in business to attract clients, but not the only one. Another such strategy is to reward old customers for bringing in new ones. If dentists are granted the right to promote their own practice by means of advertising, do you think they should also be allowed to do so by rewarding old patients for bringing in new ones?

3. When a dentist advertises HIV negative test results, what is the statement to the public?
   a. HIV testing is an important aspect of infection control in a dental office.
   b. There is no risk to the patient because the dentist is HIV-negative.

c. There is a risk if the dentist has not been tested.

d. There is a risk of HIV infection in visiting dentists.

4. What are the strongest moral arguments *against* advertising one's HIV status to patients? What are the strongest moral arguments that might *support* it? Which are more persuasive, in your opinion?

5. An office advertised mercury testing and analysis. Is this a signal for soliciting patients to have sound amalgam restoration redone? Is it a trick code for alleging that dental offices that are continuing to place amalgam restorations are harming the public by placing "toxic" substances into the body? Suppose another office advertised merely that it does not use amalgam restorations. Are your answers to these two questions the same?

REFERENCES

1. Berning, R.K.: Marketing dentistry . . . without breaking the law. Dent. Pract. *3:*22,23,25,27, 1982.
2. Margo, C.E.: Selling surgery. N. Engl. J. Med. *314:*1575, 1986.
3. Sanchez, P.M.: The case for/against the effectiveness of dental services advertising: Implications and recommendations. J. Dent. Pract. Adm. *5:*25, 1988.
4. Weinberger, B.W.: An Introduction to the History of Dentistry. St. Louis, The C.V. Mosby Company, 1948.
5. Ward, H.N.: Professional medical advertising. J. Kansas Med. Soc. *80:*436–444, 1979.
6. Guerini, V.: A History of Dentistry From the Most Ancient Times Until the End of the Eighteenth Century. New York, Milford House, Inc., 1969, p. 245.
7. Dummett, C.O.: Bioethics and history: Neglected essentials of modern dentistry. Compend. Contin. Educ. Dent. *7:*232, 1986.
8. McCluggage, R.W.: A History of the American Dental Association: A Century of Health Service. Chicago, American Dental Association, 1959, p. 190.
9. Steinholtz, L.H.: Advertising and the deprofessionalization of dentistry. N.Y. State Dent. J. *52:*10, 1986.
10. Poupard, J.: Advertising: A challenge for the 1980s. CDA Journal *9:*53, 1981.
11. Friedman, P.K.: Implications of advertising in dentistry. J. Dent. Pract. Adm. *1:*21, 1984.
12. American Dental Association: ADA Principles of Ethics and Code of Professional Conduct. Chicago, January 1962.
13. American Dental Association: ADA Principles of Ethics and Code of Professional Conduct. Chicago, October, 1978.
14. *Goldfarb v. Virginia State Bar*, 421 U.S. 773, 1977.
15. *Bates v. State Bar of Arizona*, 433 US 350, 53L.Ed. 2d 810, 97 S. Ct. 2691, 1977.
16. Anonymous: People and events. J. Am. Dent. Soc. *97:*1065, 1978.
17. National Society of Professional Engineers versus U.S., 421 u.s. 773, 1975.
18. In Re RMJ, 455 U. S. 191, 1982.
19. *Zauderer v. Office of Disciplinary Council of Supreme Court of Ohio*, 471 U.S. 626, 1985.
20. Illinois Revised Statutes, Ch. III, Section 2311(b), Rules of the Illinois Department of Professional Regulation, Title 68 §1220.421(f) (g).
21. *Parmley v. Missouri Dental Board*, 719 S.W. 2d 745 (S.C. Mo.), 1986.
22. Pennsylvania State Board of Dentistry, Rules and Regulations §33.31.
23. Texas Statutes, Article 4548f. Section 1 (C) (3) (4).
24. Illinois Dental Board Regulations, Part 1220.421(b) (4).
25. *American Medical Association v. FTC*, 638 F2d. 443 (2d. Cir. 1980), aff'd by an equally divided court, 455 U.S. 676 (1982), reh. den. 456 U.S. 969, 1982.
26. Griffin, A.M.: The controversial effects of advertising in dentistry. Dent Hyg. *59:*540, 1985.
27. Jennings, W.: Dental organizations advertising good care: A summary. J. Michigan Dent. Assoc. *63:*801, 1981.
28. Millenson, L.J.: Increasing demand for dental care: AGD advertising pays off. J. Acad. Gen. Dent. *30:*206, 1982.
29. Anderson, P.E., Senior Editor: ADA House of Delegates Votes Down Funding for National Advertising Program. *Dental Economics 74:*35, 1984.
30. Friedman, P.K., Jong, A.W., DeSouza, M.B., et al.: An investigation of the effect of advertising on dental consumers. J. Dent. Pract. Adm. *5:*166, 1988.
31. Horst, G. ter: Advertising in dentistry. Int. Dent. J. *37:*137, 1987.
32. Collinge, J.: Competition, law, and the dental profession. N. Z. Dent. J. *85:*59, 1989.
33. Havard, J.D.J.: Advertising by doctors and the public interest. Br. Med. J. *298:*903, 1989.
34. Stock, F.: Professional advertising. Am. J. Publ. Health *68:*1207, 1978.
35. Benham, L.: The effect of advertising on the price of eyeglasses. J. Law Econ. *15:*337, 1972.
36. Cady, J.F.: Drugs on the market. Lexington, MA, Lexington Books, 1975.
37. Jacobs, A.: The commercialization of dentistry (Editorial). Int. J. Orthodont. *20:*5, 1982.
38. Jonsen, A.R.: Ethics remains at the heart of medicine: Physicians and entrepreneurship. West. J. Med. *144:*480, 1986.
39. Jong, A.W.: Dental advertising. Dentistry *87:*9, 25, 1987.
40. Cunningham, M.A., and Logan, H.L.: Dentist's

attitudes toward dental marketing tactics and yellow page advertisements. *4:*30, 1987.

41. American College of Dentists. Sections oppose advertising. J. Am. Coll. Dent. *46:*150, 1979.

42. Meskin, L.H.: Advertising of dental services: A consumer and dentist attitude survey. J. Am. Coll. Dent. *45:*247, 1978.

43. Swerdlow, R.A., and Staples, W.A.: The views of Iowa dentists on professional advertising. Iowa Dent J. *64:*22, 1978.

44. Darling, J.R., and Blussom, R.S.: A comparative analysis of the attitudes of dentists toward the advertising of their fees and services. J. Dent. Educ. *41:*59, 1977.

45. Darling, J.R., and Bergiel, B.J.: A longitudinal analysis of dentists' attitudes toward advertising their fees and services. J. Dent. Educ. *46:*703, 1982.

46. Shapiro, I.A., and Majewski, R.F.: Attitudes of dental students and faculty toward advertising. J. Am. Dent. Assoc. *105:*468, 1982.

47. Majewski, R.F., and Shapiro, I.A.: Attitudes of dentists and consumers toward advertising. J. Am. Dent. Assoc. *108:*345, 1988.

48. Shapiro, I.A., and Majewski, R.F.: Should dentists advertise? . . . Contrasting attitudes of dentists and consumers in a community. J. Advertising Res. *23:*33, 1983.

49. Anderson, P.E.: More non-advertising dentists in higher income brackets. Dent. Econ. *74:*42, 1984.

50. Anderson, P.E.: 1984 survey shows advertising dentists making income gains. Dent. Econ. *75:*89, 1985.

51. Anderson, P.E.: 1985 survey shows more advertising dentists in higher income brackets. Dent. Econ. *76:*81, 1986.

52. Schultze, Q.J.: Professionalism in advertising the origin of ethical codes. J. Communication *31:*64, 1981.

53. Johnson, E.P.: An FTC view on codes of ethics: The legal limits for the 80's. J. Am. Coll. Dent. *50:*10, 1983.

54. Federal Trade Commission: FTC Opinion in *FTC v. AMA* case, *94 F.T.D. at 1009.*

55. Schiedermayer, D.L.: The process of deprofessionalization. J. Am. Coll. Dent. *55:*10, 1988 (p. 15; emphasis added).

56. Rakhvalsky, A.: Dental Advertising: A patient attitude survey. N.Y. State Dent. J. *56:*47, 1990.

57. American Dental Association: ADA Principles of Ethics and Code of Professional Conduct, Section 5-C, Announcement of Specialization and Limitation of Practice, and 5-D, General Practitioner Announcement of Services. Chicago, January 1991.

58. Crawford, C.T.: March 1985 Letter of Director of the Bureau of Consumer Protection to the Executive Secretary of the New Jersey State Board of Dentistry.

59. Kindt, M.D.: April 24, 1989 letter from Director of the FTC Cleveland Regional Office, to the Pennsylvania Independent Regulatory Review Commission.

60. Schick, I.C., Schick, T.A.: In the market for ethics: Marketing begins with values. Health Progress *70:*72, 1989.

61. Weinberger, B.W.: An Introduction to the History of Dentistry. St. Louis, The C.V. Mosby Company, 1948, p. 28 (emphasis added).

62. Federal Trade Commission: Letter to ADA of November 19, 1991 (in response to ADA comment regarding FTC consent order against the Connecticut Chiropractic Association, which would have prohibited the Association from barring its members from making claims in advertisements that they possess unusual expertise.) Proposed consent agreement published at 56 Fed.Reg. 23586 (v.56 #99), May 22, 1991.

Chapter 11

Dental Research

Eric M. Meslin
Patricia A. Main

SUMMARY

This chapter examines several issues in dental research. Unlike the clinical care of patients, about which codes of ethics provide helpful commentary, the relationship between the dental researcher and the subject is infrequently addressed. The purpose of this chapter is to explain how ethics is related to clinical dental research. We intend to do this by first outlining the way in which normative principles and theories of ethics provide a framework for assessing bioethical issues in general, and research issues in particular. We review the way in which ethical principles of respect for persons, beneficence, nonmaleficence and justice provide a foundation for assessing research studies. Second, we outline some of the ethical issues that arise in dental research. Here we will use the research protocol—the researcher's plan for conducting an experiment—as a paradigm for explaining these issues in chronological order. These issues are the justification for conducting the particular study, research design, identifying and recruiting research subjects, assessing harms and benefits, obtaining informed consent, and protecting privacy and confidentiality.

Third, we describe three broad approaches for ensuring that dental research is conducted ethically. First we examine the existing international codes of ethics for research and discuss several of their common features. Second, we describe the two national approaches for ensuring ethical research—regulation and professional guidelines. Third, we explain how the institutional research ethics committee, known in the U.S. as the Institutional Review Board (IRB), functions as a gatekeeper for research conducted within its institution.

Finally, we comment on several issues that affect the climate for ethical investigations in dentistry. These include issues of sponsorship, fraud, and misconduct, reporting data, and the dental curriculum. Two appendices are included, the first providing a brief guide to protocol review (with references to others), and second, the ADA *Guidelines for the Use of Human Subjects* (1978).

DENTAL RESEARCH ETHICS

Like all health professionals, dentists and dental hygienists encounter ethical issues in their practice. Many of the chapters in this textbook outline these issues and provide cases and analyses of the relationship between dentists and their patients, referring, when necessary, to professional codes and legal requirements regarding the behavior that is expected of dentists, and the rights of patients. In this chapter, we consider a particular aspect of the relationship between dentist and patient, one in which the principal goal is not therapeutic, but rather to gain new knowledge that will benefit future patients.

Understanding this distinction between "research" and "therapy" is a prerequisite to any analysis of the ethical issues that arise in dental research. Indeed, physicians and researchers have sometimes blurred the distinction.[1] Dental practice (or therapy) is an activity that is carried out with the intention of benefitting a particular patient. When we refer to "research," we are following the definition recently adopted in the U.S. legislation governing human subjects research:

> "*Research* means a systematic investigation, including research development, testing and evaluation, designed to develop or contribute to generalizable knowledge."[2]

This general definition holds for dental research which covers a broad spectrum of investigation, from studies that are designed to assess patient attitudes about dental care[3] to those involving the evaluation of new dental surgical procedures.[4] Describing an activity as research carries with it several implications, many of which we discuss as follows: it changes the relationship between health professional and patient, it demands a higher and more exacting standard for informed consent, and it introduces the requirement that the intervention be subjected to scientific and ethical peer review. We use the term "research" in this way to distinguish it from "therapy," and more particularly to avoid the conceptual debate about defining research as "therapeutic" or "non-therapeutic," terms that we and others consider unsatisfactory.[5]

The purpose of this chapter is to explain how ethics is related to dental research. We intend to do this by first outlining the way normative principles and theories of ethics provide a framework for assessing bioethical issues in general, and research issues in particular. Secondly, we outline some of the ethical issues that arise in dental research. Here we use the research protocol—the researcher's plan for conducting an experiment—as a paradigm for explaining these issues in chronological order. Thirdly, we describe the mechanisms for assuring that dental research is conducted ethically, by examining the existing codes and regulations intended to guide behavior, and at the review process

conducted by institutional review boards. Finally, we comment on several issues that create a climate for ethical investigations in dentistry.

ETHICS AND CLINICAL RESEARCH

Ethical consideration of human subjects research can be linked to several factors, including the historical precedent set by reports of unethical research and the public concern this created. These reports, coupled with a growing public interest in the conduct of medical experimentation, led to an articulation of ethical principles meant to guide research.

Reasons for Ethical Concern in Research

Discussion of the ethics of human experimentation has a rich legacy, punctuated by several important cases of unethical research. The experiments conducted on nonconsenting and vulnerable persons in Nazi concentration camps during World War II are the most horrific examples of the potential for abuse in scientific medicine. It is known that dentists took part in the selection of prisoners for medical extermination.[6] Rothman has recently argued that the critical time in U.S. history may well have been the period between 1966 and 1978, when reports of unethical research finally led to the implementation of a regulatory framework for the oversight of research involving human subjects.[7] The year 1966 is selected for two reasons: it was the year when the U.S. Public Health Service issued the first federal policy statement requiring "peer review" of funded research,[8] and it was the year that Beecher's article appeared in the *New England Journal of Medicine* detailing 22 cases of unethical research reported in prestigious medical journals.[9] Among the cases reported were studies in which known effective treatment was withheld, studies involving significant risk, and studies involving nonconsenting children or infants unrelated to any disease or condition. The year 1978 is selected because it was the year when the U.S. National Commission for the Protection of Human Subjects for Biomedical Research (The National Commission) published the guidelines and ethical principles for the conduct of research that have come to be known as *The Belmont Report*. This period is also important from the international perspective. In 1967, Pappworth documented many cases of unethical research in Britain, much as Beecher had done.[10]

Ethical concern was heightened as a result of this history for two reasons. First, these cases of unethical research are affronts to our sense of morality. Morality consists of our shared beliefs and values about right and wrong, about conduct and behavior toward others, and about decisions and judgments we make. Philosophers have explained this psychological disposition in several ways. Mill grounded his theory of utilitarianism upon the belief that all persons have a basic desire for unity and harmony with their fellow human beings.[11] Gert has recently argued that human beings share a common view regarding all harms such as disease, injury, and death: we universally view them as evils to be avoided.[12] Even though individuals (or societies) differ as to *what* constitutes an evil or harm, basic among such aversions are the loss of functional abilities, loss of freedom, and pain. It is not surprising, therefore, that the Hippocratic maxim, *primum non nocere* (first, or at least, do no harm) has survived for 2500 years and been regarded as the first principle of medical ethics.[13]

The second explanation for our moral concern with these cases may be attributed to our beliefs about the nature of medical relationships, particularly the relationship between a physician and patient and between a researcher and subject. The cases illustrate a violation of the trust relationship which lies at the root of the therapeutic relationship. Society has come to expect, apart from and in addition to the usual duties that reasonable people owe each other, responsibilities, obligations, and duties that are role-specific—that physicians and investigators have and other citizens do not. Violations of those duties engender additional moral concern on our part. Reports of unethical research, particularly in the wake of public concern about the responsibilities of the government to protect and promote individual rights,[14] has provided the impetus for action. Interestingly, this action took two forms. The first was a careful, publicly supported effort to define the ethical principles that were to guide research, which we address next. The second was the establishment of a sophisticated regulatory framework in the U.S. (and an equally sophisticated non-legislative framework elsewhere in North America and Europe) for assuring the ethical conduct of human research, which we address in Section III.

Ethical Theory and Principles

Motivated partly by reports of unethical research, the U.S. Congress passed the National Research Act (1974), creating the National Commission with a mandate to:

> ... identify the basic ethical principles that should underlie the conduct of biomedical and behavioral research and to develop guidelines which should be followed to assure that research is conducted in accordance with these principles.[15]

In its *Belmont Report*, the Commission recommended that three principles or "general prescriptive judgments" be used in the review of research protocols: respect for persons, beneficence, and justice.[16] Not only were these principles formally adopted by the Commission, they (or principles very much like them) have emerged as fundamental in reports of other deliberative bodies in medical research. They have been used to provide the specific criteria used to appraise the ethical appropriateness of research protocols. We discuss the criteria in more detail in the following paragraphs. First, we explain the content of these principles. (See also Chap. 2.)

RESPECT FOR PERSONS

Respecting persons has two manifestations in moral philosophy. The first refers to the respect owed to patients as persons, specifically with regard to their legal and moral rights as individuals. This interpretation follows from deontology and utilitarianism, two dominant ethical theories in western philosophy. Deontological ethicists, following the work of Immanuel Kant, regard respect for persons as an obligation owed to all rational moral agents. Kant stated the principle formally as: "So act as to treat humanity, whether in thine own person or in that of any other, in every case as an end withal, never as a means only." Philosophers have debated the nuances of this maxim (e.g., does the qualifier "merely" imply that persons can be treated as a means to another's end, so long as they are not treated exclusively in this way?), but the central point remains clear: one has an obligation as a rational moral agent to respect the unconditional worth that persons have to determine their own destiny.[17] Utilitarians, particularly in the liberal tradition, are concerned with respecting individuals—but focus on personal autonomy of action and thought. Whereas Kant's theory focuses on the obligation to treat persons with respect, utilitarian theory such as Mill's focuses on the obligation to respect individual choice, and particularly on the justifiable limits to exercising choice. This has been more carefully described by Beauchamp and Childress as respect for autonomy.[18] The implications of grounding the principle of respect for persons on either utilitarian or deontological theory is somewhat more relevant for moral philosophy than for the review of research protocols. Capron argues that respecting personal rights according to either theory

> ... implies that those in charge of a research project must provide prospective subjects with information that will enable them to decide whether it is acceptable to choose whether or not to participate according to their own values and goals and must then permit the subjects to choose whether or not to participate.[19]

The second application of the principle of respect for persons assumes that individuals who are not able to participate fully in decision making are, nevertheless, entitled to the same degree of respect as those who are fully autonomous. The National Commission described this as an obligation to "protect those with diminished autonomy." Individuals may be less autonomous than fully competent adults

for many reasons, including age (e.g., very young children), degree of mental capacity (e.g., individuals with developmental handicap or a dementia), or medical status (e.g., patients unconscious from a disease or accident). These persons may be vulnerable to certain risks (the most obvious of which in research are the risks from the research itself) to which they cannot voluntarily agree to expose themselves and from which they cannot protect themselves.

Anticipating the decisions an incompetent family member would make about medical treatment is problematic; anticipating these decisions for research is even more challenging for families, especially when the patient's wishes regarding research are not known. This creates the potential for coercion if parents believe that they have no legitimate choice to obtain a possible therapy but to enroll a child in research. Not only might this be regarded as a denial of existing benefits to patients (an issue better explained using the principles of beneficence and nonmaleficence explained subsequently), but a limitation on individual choice. The requirements to obtain the informed consent of research participants and to ensure that confidential or sensitive information is protected are directly associated with the principle of *respect for persons.*

BENEFICENCE

We have suggested how protecting the welfare of incompetent persons was an example of the principle of respect for persons. A second, separate requirement in protocol review is to balance the potential harms and benefits of research. We can see how this might work by considering vulnerable persons. The obligation to respect their rights is supported not by treating them as autonomous agents, but rather by protecting them from harm. This obligation often falls on parents (for children) and on grown children (for older parents) because family members are expected to understand the decisions their relative would have made had they had decision-making capacity, and in the absence of such knowledge, to make decisions in the best interest of the patient. This requirement evolves from the principles of beneficence and nonmaleficence. Beneficence refers to the positive obligation to maximize possible benefits from an action, and is decidedly consequentialist. The positive obligation to promote individual well-being presumes there are certain values and outcomes that are good. Health is such a value. In research, fulfilling this positive obligation is mediated by the fact that the principal intention of clinical research is to produce knowledge that is both valid and valuable. The benefits from current research studies accrue to future patients.

But the National Commission saw beneficence expressing two complementary and general rules "(1) do no harm and (2) maximize possible benefit and minimize possible harms." The principal focus of beneficence, therefore, becomes the avoidance or reduction of harm to research subjects, understood as nonmaleficence. This is consistent with Frankena's analysis of beneficence, which includes the following obligations:

One ought not to inflict evil or harm
One ought to prevent evil or harm
One ought to remove evil
One ought to promote good.[20]

Others, particularly Beauchamp and Childress,[18] regard beneficence and nonmaleficence as separate ethical principles. It is not a trivial matter of philosophic concern whether one's principal obligation is first to "do no harm" or first to "benefit the patient": because all research causes some degree of inconvenience, a strict interpretation of nonmaleficence might prohibit research entirely. In some instances, beneficence has also been taken to include the obligation to do or promote research for the benefit of the community tempered by one's obligations to benefit those to whom one has a commitment (e.g., one's employer or family). Beneficence can also require that research maximize good and minimize harm. Thus, as Branson has argued, at issue in biomedical research is the need to weigh the potential benefit against potential harm.[21]

JUSTICE

Justice is perhaps the most complex of the several ethical principles relevant to research. In general, the concept of justice refers to giving to each person his or her due. Injustice, therefore, refers to the denial of that to which someone is entitled.[18] This concept has been defined more carefully by describing types of justice: *compensatory* justice provides payment for loss of benefits; *retributive* justice provides punishment for transgressions of the law. The principal focus for ethical assessment of research, however, is *distributive* justice, the formal, *comparative* version of which is that equals must be treated equally and unequals treated unequally. One is treated equally or unequally only in regard to morally relevant criteria:

> More fully stated in its negative form, the principle says that no person should be treated unequally, despite all differences with other persons, until it has been shown that there is a difference between them relative to the treatment at stake.[18]

Beauchamp and Childress point to the lack of substance in this formal principle: "who is equal and who unequal? what respects are relevant for purposes of comparing which individuals and which range of cases?" One can distribute burdens and benefits according to strict equality (everyone getting an equal share) or, according to need, effort, potential social contribution, merit, or free-market exchange.[18] In research, these criteria begin to have moral weight when applied to potential participants in research. Who is entitled to participate in research? Who should benefit from research? Who should bear the burdens (especially, the risks of harm) from research? Different answers to these questions will emerge depending on the theory that informs the distributive justice principle. An *egalitarian* theory of justice might support the requirement that all dental patients participate in research, because all may potentially benefit from the knowledge gained. In contrast, a *utilitarian* theory might support the requirement that only research that is likely to produce the most useful knowledge at the least cost (moral, financial) should be conducted. One can envision this theory supporting research into better methods of preventing dental disease and caries for many thousands of individuals rather than studies that would ameliorate conditions in only a few (e.g., a rare oral condition such as necrotizing sialometaplasia).

With this background, we now turn to the ethical issues that arise in dental research, as they emerge in the lifespan of a research protocol.

ETHICAL ISSUES IN DENTAL RESEARCH

One of the characteristics of research that distinguishes it from clinical therapy is that research typically has as its principal goal the generation of knowledge or data, whereas therapy has as its principal goal the treatment of a specific patient.[5] This difference does admit some blurring. For example, individuals who participate in research may benefit from this participation, and data about medical treatments for patients may be valuable for other patients. A further distinction (which also admits some blurring) is the adherence in research to a formal protocol. Although it is true that, in dental practice, the dentist examines the patient, refers to the patient's history, reviews additional diagnostic procedures and completes a treatment plan, in research, the protocol is a more rigorous instrument. Ordinarily, a research protocol that involves the use of human subjects includes: the reasons for proposing to conduct a particular study, an explanation of the study's design, the methods for identifying potential research participants, a listing of the possible harms and benefits to the participants involved (and the methods to be used for minimizing risk), and the process of obtaining the informed consent of the participants. In this way, it is more comprehensive than a clinical treatment plan. At each point in the development and conduct of research, ethical issues arise.

Justification

The first consideration in any ethical assessment of a dental research protocol is the justification for conducting the study in the first place. Because research is an activity that is not principally intended to benefit particular patients, providing a justification that is ethically and scientifically defensible is a necessary prerequisite for enrolling human beings in any study. Several authors have noted the surprisingly little attention paid to discussions of justification. Beauchamp and Walters have observed that:

> . . . [t]his silence at the most general level of justification is particularly striking when one considers that the traditional ethic of medicine has been exclusively a patient-benefit ethic. The motto *primum non nocere* [first, do no harm] has been interpreted to mean "do nothing that is not intended for the direct benefit of the patient." We must ask, then, whether good reasons can be given to deviating in any way from therapy.[22]

Capron elaborates this point by explaining why justification is necessary:

> In an era as dependent upon science and technology as ours, it may seem unnecessary to examine the justifications for research with human subjects, since such research is an indispensable link between theory or initial observation, and the application of scientific findings and technology developments to benefit people and society at large. But in ethical terms, such scrutiny is needed because the question is not whether to have all possible research or none at all, but rather how much research to have at what cost, when "cost" includes possible harm to values other than the advancement of knowledge.[19]

We would add that one of the "costs" is the loss of opportunity to use these resources elsewhere. This becomes increasingly a component of justice when, as now, research resources are diminishing or scant. These comments suggest that research must first be justified as a general enterprise before any justification can be offered for a specific study. Two arguments provided by philosophers summarize the types of justification for research in general. Using the language of ethical principles, the first appeals to beneficence and the second to respect for persons. One of the early examples of the beneficence-based argument is defined by the French physiologist Claude Bernard, who suggested that the goal of medical research was "the pursuit of scientific solutions to the problem of conserving health and curing disease." This laudable goal, claimed

Bernard, was limited by the following rule:

> So among the experiments that may be tried on man, those that can only harm are forbidden, those that are innocent are permissible, and those that may do good are obligatory.[23]

A more contemporary version of Bernard's argument is defended by Leon Eisenberg, who claims that there is a social imperative to do research.[24] The social imperative to which Eisenberg refers can be explained using the principles of beneficence and non-maleficence. Research on human subjects is justified because it has the potential to eliminate harmful products or procedures from the therapeutic arsenal. By conducting "controlled clinical trials," science will be able to determine whether what is traditional does harm rather than good. Eisenberg's justification is similar to Bernard's in that both are based on the premise that research is permissible (perhaps even obligatory) when it can produce beneficial results or prevent harms.

In contrast, Hans Jonas is often quoted for his eloquent defense of a more cautious approach to research, particularly the pace that research ought to take when it involves human beings:

> Let us not forget that progress is an optional goal, not an unconditional commitment, and its tempo in particular, compulsive as it may become, has nothing sacred about it. Let us also remember that a slower progress in the conquest of disease would not threaten society, grievous as it is to those who have to deplore that their particular disease be not yet conquered, but that society would indeed be threatened by the erosion of those moral values whose loss, possibly caused by too ruthless a pursuit of scientific progress would make its most dazzling triumphs not worth having.[25]

This argument, although cautious of the pace of progress, does not discount research altogether. Research is a justifiable, and indeed a laudable, social goal, but not at any cost. This too can be understood using the language of ethical principles: Jonas defends the position that research is justified only to the extent that the individuals involved are treated with respect.

Research that fails to respect patients as persons cannot be justified because it fails to consider the rights of research subjects, regardless of the degree of benefit to others or the amount of knowledge to be gained. Similarly, as Thomas Malone has recently observed, the general moral imperative to do research will be increasingly influenced by its stakeholders:

> There is now the prospect—actually under way—that big science biomedical research will follow in the footsteps of the military, the nuclear, and the space establishments to become part of a medical industrial complex in which the researchers, the health care providers and the manufacturers who supply them will be closely linked. There is merit in such an arrangement . . . However, there are also obvious dangers . . .[26]

Thus far, we have reviewed the justification for research in general. What justification is necessary for a particular study to proceed? The following questions may provide a guide[27]: should this research be done at this time? Answers to this question would require that a researcher be convinced that the use of human subjects is essential, and be based on previous research using animal or other models. Is the research as a whole ethically acceptable? Answers to this question would require that researchers recognize the importance of research to a particular community, for reasons apart from the scientific merit. Such considerations include the legal and social concerns about research.[28]

One example of contentious research was the Burlington Growth and Development Study.[29] In the study design, the researchers initially enrolled 75 children between the ages of 3 and 12 years, then 1 year later increased the sample to 1380 children and 312 parents. All the participants were residents of the same community, a town with a population of 5000. One of the objectives of the study was "To compile a reliable set of records on which to base extensive studies of normal growth and development and the variations that occur in malocclusion."[30] The complete set of records included annual records for 320 serial group children, as well as periodic records for all the remaining children and parents. The annual records included six cephalometric radiographs using the high voltage technique of Harvold and Cartwright, three lateral views, right and left oblique radiographs, and an anteroposterior head plate. Also taken were bite-wing radiographs and hand and wrist radiographs.

The amount of radiation was a concern, and the level of radiation was monitored throughout the longitudinal survey. However, the researchers and the board approving the study felt the levels to be acceptable. There was, nevertheless, concern about taking radiographs for research purposes. Originally the study design envisaged using a neighboring town as a control population, but this was abandoned because of the "seemingly ethical impossibility of regarding and diagnosing malocclusion without advocating treatment."[30] The control group was selected from 6-year-old children in Burlington, and they were permitted to have treatment for malocclusions.

This study was contentious on several grounds; perhaps the most immediate was the justification of exposing children to levels of risk from radiation. Given that the risks were assessed to be acceptable, we wonder whether there was sufficient expertise to assess these risks. Answering this question is difficult for two reasons: first, research has yet to adequately define the criteria for assessing risk and benefit;[31] second, it is not clear whether the moral expertise to judge a risk to be acceptable or not is available in any research setting. This may be a function of the larger problem of moral expertise.[32] Irrespective of the availability of explicit criteria, or of moral experts to judge them, judgments about research must still be made. The most rigorous justification for conducting a study is that it is scientifically and ethically acceptable. The balance of this section focuses on these issues.

Research Design

A fundamental prerequisite of ethical research is that the study is scientifically sound. Capron argues that this fulfills two ethical requirements: First, a well designed study is not wasteful of scarce resources, including institutional funding agency money, participant's time, or lab space. Second, it reduces the risk that patients will be exposed to possible harm or injury.[19] Here it is worthwhile to point out the error in assuming that all studies that are scientifically sound are also ethically acceptable. A study may be extremely well designed, but nevertheless raise several ethical problems that would prevent its activation. One could envision a study that sought to determine the effect of multiple dental x rays on pregnant women, which could be well designed and answer an important question, but nevertheless be ethically problematic. Freedman has recently argued that the scientific justification consists of two elements, *validity* and *value*:

A study is scientifically valid provided it is designed to yield reliable information according to accepted principle of research practice, concerning the hypothesis tested. The results of a study whose sample size is too small, or skewed, or poorly controlled, cannot be generalized toward confirmation or disconfirmation of the hypothesis, and the study is therefore invalid.

In contrast, a study may be evaluated on the basis of its merit quite apart from its validity:

A study may be well designed relative to its hypothesis, and therefore be scientifically valid, but nonetheless be of no value, generally because the hypothesis itself is trivial or otherwise uninteresting.[33]

No research, regardless of the elegance of its justification, may proceed without a protocol. Fundamental to research is its method, and the prevailing method of choice in clinical research is the randomized clinical trial (RCT), a device used to compare the efficacy and safety of two or more intervention regimens.[5] In a typical RCT, a group of patients is divided into two groups, one group receiving the test article (new drug, or procedure), and the other receiving a known standard treatment or placebo. "Randomization" refers to the method by which patients are assigned to either group; usually this is done by a random number generator program in a computer. Passamani has recently argued that the RCT is "the most scientifically sound and ethically correct means of evaluating new therapies" because it reduces the possibility of investigator (or patient) bias in the interpretation of results, provides accurate assessment of treatment effects, allows for careful monitoring of the safety of new drugs, procedures, or devices, and provides good explanations for why a treatment did or did not work.[34] Alternative views on the ethics of RCTs have also been discussed.[35]

Several important ethical questions emerge from this particular design.

THE NULL HYPOTHESIS VERSUS CLINICAL EQUIPOISE

It is expected that before conducting a clinical trial researchers will believe that the interventions being compared (e.g., two drugs, two surgical procedures) are scientifically equivalent. Researchers cannot have a clear preference for using one or the other intervention. This *a priori* position is known as the "null hypothesis" and presumes that researchers must believe and "reasonably maintain that the treatment and control groups will show no difference as a result of the intervention."[19] Many have recognized the difficulty in requiring that this state of genuine uncertainty (which is difficult enough to claim with complete honesty at the outset of a trial) be maintained throughout a study. In particular, it begs the question, why is the research worth doing if there is no reason to believe that the proposed intervention would be an improvement over currently accepted therapy? As an alternative, Freedman has suggested that another concept, "clinical equipoise," be adopted, in which the uncertainty necessary to justify randomizing some patients to active treatment and others either to placebo or standard treatment be held by the research community rather than the individual investigator.[36] It would be difficult, for example, to design a clinical trial to test a new fluoride because fluoride is not only widely available to the public, but clinically well accepted.

DENTIST AS RESEARCHER

The RCT has also been criticized because it places health professionals in a potential conflict of interest where they must balance the responsibility to act in the patient's best interests against the responsibility to science and society to conduct valid clinical research. Schafer explains this conflict by suggesting that the traditional ethic of patient care arising from beneficence creates a fiduciary obligation with the patient's best interests primary, whereas in the research relationship, the obligation to maximize individual patient welfare is secondary.[37] This distinction is unacceptable particularly in regard to studies where patients are prepared to accept an experimental treatment and the risks that may result, rather than accepting the chance of being randomized into a nontreatment arm. This point has been made about studies involving HIV infection,[38] where patients have argued for the right to participate in risky research because it may be their only hope of benefit. For other trials involving less exceptional circumstances, it is still unsettled whether the fact of random assignment to one or another arm of a clinical trial should be disclosed to potential participants before their enrollment[39,40] or during the study if new information becomes available.[40]

PLACEBOS

Ethical issues also arise if a study involves the use of a placebo. In contrast with the use of placebos in the clinical environment, where the ethical concern arises because patients are being deceived, placebo use in clinical research is a justifiable method for comparing the effects of an intervention against an inactive substance, and for minimizing the possibility of investigator bias.[5] Assuming that researchers hold the null hypothesis, or can at least confidently describe the existing knowledge as one of clinical equipoise, placebo use still raises two ethical questions in the research setting, both of which are discussed in more detail in the following paragraphs. The first is whether the research subject has been informed of the placebo arm of the trial. The second is whether there are some instances when it would be harmful to randomize patients to receive a placebo when there is already an effective treatment. The following hypothetical protocol was designed for discussion at the 1980

Conference on ethical and legal considerations in dental caries research[42]: Six groups were proposed, the three experimental groups as follows:

1. occlusal decay restored with amalgam plus weekly fluoride rinse
2. sealants placed over occlusal decay, plus weekly fluoride rinse
3. weekly fluoride rinse

The control groups were as follows:

4. occlusal decay restored with amalgam plus weekly placebo rinse
5. sealants placed over occlusal decay, plus weekly placebo rinse
6. weekly placebo rinse

In this study, the control group would be deprived of a known therapeutic agent, fluoride, leading one author to observe that fluoride "had already passed from the research stage to the demonstration phase and, hopefully, now to community implementation."[43] The hypothetical protocol is unacceptable because it would be unethical to deny to specific persons a proven and widely available therapy.

Identifying and Recruiting Research Subjects

Once the architecture of a study has been completed, the proper object of ethical concern in investigation involving human subjects are the subjects themselves. Which patients should be approached? How will they be selected? Can subjects be overanxious? In his elegant argument about the pace of progress in medical experimentation, Jonas argued that one of the best protections for human subjects was to recruit them using a "descending order of permissibility," in which the least vulnerable (typically, physicians and scientists who had the most knowledge about the research) would be approached first, and the most vulnerable (the sickest persons) approached last.[25] Although this argument is based on a flawed premise—that no patient would be willing to be exposed to risk, and therefore ought to be protected from participating—it highlights two important ethical questions all researchers must answer in their protocol: what is the justification for enrolling *this* group of patients in a study? and what methods are used to ensure that patients are not unfairly induced into participating? The National Commission recognized that answers to these questions devolved from the principle of distributive justice:

> . . . the selection of research subjects needs to be scrutinized in order to determine whether some classes . . . are being systematically selected simply because of their easy availability, their compromised position, or their manipulability, rather than for reasons directly related to the problems being studied.[16]

Two contrasting problems of recruitment emerge from this background: first, the protection of vulnerable subjects, and second, the problem of declining enrollment, which we call the new eligibility problem.

VULNERABLE SUBJECTS

Looking at the research protocol as a model, we can see how protection of rights and welfare may occur at many stages in the development of a study, from the generation of a testable hypothesis to offering a justification for the study, designing it, and recruiting subjects. Each of these stages may raise ethical concerns about the protection of subjects. It may be, however, that our ethics ought to be judged by the way in which we treat the most vulnerable in any environment—how we look after our homeless, those at risk of injury or illness, those who lack the opportunity for economic enjoyment, those who are most sick, in short, those who are vulnerable. This is especially true in medical-dental research involving human subjects.

What makes patients vulnerable? We take Levine's definition of vulnerable subjects to be a useful guide: vulnerable subjects are "those persons who are relatively or absolutely incapable of protecting their own interests . . . through negotiations for informed consent."[5] It is useful because, in focusing on the protection of interests, the ability to exercise choice and the welfare of patients both serve as moral constraints. Moreover, the fact of vulnerability does not entail a proscription of research involving such persons. Were a taxonomy of vulnerability to be developed, it might include persons who are relatively or absolutely incapable of protecting their interests as a result of their age (e.g., very young children); their environment, (e.g., prisoners or those who are institutionally dependent, such as individuals involuntarily committed to psychiatric hospitals); their relationship (e.g., students who are dependent upon their teachers for grades, employees who are dependent upon supervisors for employment); their capacity for comprehending information, or by medical condition (both of which may be found in certain patients with progressive dementias, but also in patients who are comatose or inebriated); and their economic status.

Two prominent examples of dental research involving vulnerable subjects are the Hopewood House[44] and Vipeholm studies,[45,46] in which adults in an asylum and children in the state's care were used as subjects without informed consent and given *ad libitum* cariogenic foods. The children residents in Hopewood House were in the state's care and had been since infancy. The Home provided a lactovegetarian diet with a high proportion of raw fruit and vegetables, a very strict nutritious diet significantly different from that of the average Australian family. In addition to living on a strict diet, these children had no organized program of oral hygiene and the majority suffered from gingivitis. However, the Home children had greatly reduced levels of dental caries. During the 15 years of the study, the children began to disperse, and this led to changing the basic diet and a deterioration in the teeth of these children.

The subjects in the Vipeholm study were mentally deficient patients who lived in departments of the hospital. Each of the 12 departments was contained so that an entire department was assigned into a specific dietary regimen. Thus subjects were assigned into the control or experimental groups based on residence only. The diets for the groups were as follows:

1. Control Group: basic diet without additional carbohydrates
2. Sucrose Group: basic diet with additional sugar in solution
3. Bread Group: basic diet plus addition of sugar in bread (sticky form)
4. Chocolate, Caramel, 8-Toffee, 24-Toffee Group: basic diet plus additional sugar in the form of candies consumed between meals.

A total of 436 subjects participated throughout the study. They had limited oral hygiene, few could use a toothbrush, and only 625 of 5.6% of the 11,238 cavities had been filled. By the end of the carbohydrate study, the number of untreated cavities had risen to 13,363.

In both these studies, the vulnerable subjects had no alternative to participation, and the regimen at Hopewood House produced shorter-than-average children with unmet dental needs, and the patients in the experimental groups at Vipeholm showed an increase in caries and unmet dental needs. The imbalance of power between the researcher or the custodian and the subjects seen in these two examples also occurred in studies on periodontal disease,[47] in which dental students were asked to be subjects for the experiment, to be conducted by one of their professors. This does not offer the subject freedom to refuse to participate without fear of negative actions. This is similar to the use of vulnerable subjects above. In the case of the dental students, they were asked to withhold normal oral hygiene procedures for 21 days. Gingivitis produced by this lack of oral hygiene was still reversible.

We have noted that different types of vulnerability exist. A further way of explaining this is to understand that vulnerability may be the result of the influence of others upon patients. Faden and Beauchamp have argued that persons can be more or less vulnerable, depending on how much of a controlling influence someone else has on them. According to the spectrum they have constructed, called the "continuum of influences," one can act in a completely or fully noncontrolled way, that is, according to their own will; and at the polar extreme, one can act in a completely controlled way, that is, being controlled by others. Between these extremes exist many types of manipulation.[48] One example is related to the possibility of economic exploitation by paying subjects to participate. Macklin clarifies what constitutes an "undue inducement," and suggests a common-sense approach to setting the level of payment.[49] Other types of inducement are less obvious, however. Because patients have been shown to believe that participating in research is expected to benefit them, it could be argued that even the invitation to participate constitutes a form of manipulation. Appelbaum and his colleagues have described this phenomenon as the "therapeutic misconception."[50]

THE NEW ELIGIBILITY PROBLEM

The science of clinical trials has become so refined that patient eligibility is often reduced because entrance and inclusion criteria are more sharply focused. Identifying persons who are eligible to participate, who have been referred by another health professional, and who ultimately agree to participate once they have been informed of the study, has been found to dramatically reduce the pool of potential participants.[51] Paradoxically, for some types of research, such as studies in oncology, the ethical concern is not on how subjects can be protected from being coerced into participating by promises of benefit (financial or therapeutic), but rather how more patients can be enrolled without compromising the scientific integrity of the study. This has led some to observe that the problem is so profound that investigators may be willing to "lie about a patient's entry criteria."[52]

We do not believe that dental research experiences the same types of recruitment challenges as oncology research, but there is some evidence that not all patients who are eligible to participate are enrolled in dental trials, and that there is interest in participation. For example, we are aware of one dental study in which prescreened subjects had an eligibility rate of 69%. This should be considered in light of the dropout rate of 39%.[53] In one longitudinal epidemiological study following the release of either baseline information gathered or from interim reports, the general public made frequent calls to one of the investigators' offices requesting that they be included in the trial.[54] In clinical trials testing new preventive or therapeutic agents for reducing or eliminating the incidence of caries, it has been reported that some patients consented to participate although their level of current disease precluded them from participation.[55]

Assessment of Harm and Benefit

Any intervention into the lives of human beings necessarily involves, at the very least, an inconvenience, and at worst, a serious risk of harm. It is imperative, therefore, to be assured that potential harms to participants do not unreasonably outweigh the potential benefits. Unlike informed consent, for which there is sophisticated literature,[18] and several comprehensive guidelines, little authoritative guidance can be found for the assessment of harm and benefit.[30] This is not surprising, given the National Commission's advice in 1978:

> It is commonly said that the benefits and risks must be "balanced" and shown to be "in a favorable ratio." The metaphorical character of these terms draws attention to the difficulty in making precise judgments. Only on rare occasions will quantitative techniques be available for the scrutiny of research protocols. However, the idea of systematic, nonarbitrary analysis of risks and benefits should be emulated insofar as possible.[16]

Little progress has been made in the ensuing 15 years towards "making precise judgments," for two reasons: *conceptually*, terms such as "harm" and "risk" are either poorly defined or not defined at all in relevant codes and guidelines; *practically*, researchers and reviews committees often lack the technical expertise to perform formal risk and benefit assessments.[30] An assessment of harm and benefit is important for two reasons: first, this information may be used as part of the *justification* for conducting the research; second, the information must be disclosed to potential research subjects as part of the informed consent process.

In the first section, we showed how the National Commission's interpretation of beneficence entails an obligation to promote well-being, and to minimize or reduce the possibility of harm. Setting aside the positive obligation to produce benefit, what do we mean by harm? Typically, harm is thought of as physical damage, such as a broken bone. Harm as "physical damage" would account for many of the possible adverse consequences from dental research, from the bruise following insertion of a needle, to the toxic reaction of an investigational drug. Unfortunately, this description will not cover all types of harm a subject might suffer including psychological, social, and economic harms.[5] Feinberg has offered a useful definition of harm: someone is harmed when his or her interests have been thwarted, defeated, or set back.[56] It is useful not only because it accounts for a diversity of negative events that could happen to patients for which physical damage makes a poor analogy (such as embarrassment), but because it also maps onto Levine's definition of vulnerable persons as being incapable of protecting or promoting their own interests.

Although researchers cannot be expected to identify all known (and unknown) threats to their patients' interests, they should be able to identify the likelihood and severity of known harms. This concept, assessing the likelihood and severity of an adverse outcome, is known as *risk*. Risk is related to but not identical with harm, because it refers to the probability and magnitude of a future harm. Both of these terms warrant more conceptual analysis than we can provide here (for example, probability has both an objective and subjective component,[57] and the severity of harm can refer not only to the amount of damage, but also to the harm's duration, the permanency of its consequences, and the extent to which it alters lifestyle[5]).

Using another hypothetical protocol from the 1980 conference described previously, involving radiographs,[58] it would appear to be a safe study (particularly if the consent form described it as "noninvasive"), and yet the radiographs and enamel biopsies contained more than minimal risk.[59] In this hypothetical protocol, or even in choosing subjects for simple clinical trials, the level of benefit can be overstated, because of enthusiasm of the researcher and the level of harm can similarly be viewed differently or even as excessive by a subject, simply because the

nature of the harm is not concrete. In the hypothetical protocol, the taking of unnecessary radiographs is considered harmful to a patient, whether they are receiving routine dental care or are part of a research project. The taking of an enamel biopsy would not produce permanent damage to a tooth because the enamel layer remineralizes with the use of proven preventive therapies such as fluoride. These observations suggest that the problems confronting the assessment of harm and benefit in biomedical research are likely to arise in dental research.

The specific ethical issues involved in the assessment of harm and benefit arise when different individuals make different assessments. It is well accepted that any of the adverse consequences from research are assessed differently by subjects than by clinicians or investigators. Moreover, we also know that the way information is framed has an important bearing on the interpretation, perception, and acceptability of risk.[60] One model for making risk judgments in medical research has been proposed[30] but not tested with researchers.

Informed Consent

Few issues in research ethics cause as much commentary as informed consent. This is probably because consent remains the single most important criterion for ensuring that research subjects are respected as persons, protected from harm, and treated fairly. Informed consent empowers individuals to decide whether and to what extent they wish to participate in research, and, should they decide to participate, to withdraw. In this sense, informed consent is more than a form that is to be completed; rather, it is the result of an ongoing process between investigator and subject, the principal purpose of which is to provide potential subjects with all the relevant information they need to decide whether or not to participate. This standard of disclosure is more rigorous in research than in therapy, a point made in the case of *Halushka v. the University of Saskatchewan*:

There can be no exception to the ordinary requirements of disclosure in the case of research as there may well be in ordinary medical practice.[61]

The concept of informed consent includes at least the following components: disclosure, comprehension, voluntariness, decision-making capacity and consent.[48] That is, research subjects have given an informed consent to participate when they have been given information, which they understand, and because they have decision-making capacity and are free of coercive constraints, actively consent to participate. Completing the first four elements and deciding not to participate is an informed refusal.

Legal commentary on informed consent, including scholarship and common or statutory law have tended to focus on disclosure requirements. Standards for disclosure to potential participants have been described in codes and regulations. The American Dental Association provides an instructive list of such requirements in its 1978 *Guidelines for the Use of Human Subjects in Dental Research*.[62] Although not directly intended for a dental research audience, one of the more comprehensive lists of such requirements is found in the Medical Research Council of Canada Guidelines for Research Involving Human Subjects:

A protocol will normally be expected to state what prospective subjects will be told; these points may include:
a) the reasons for the study;
b) research techniques which will involve the prospective subject, such as randomization of treatments;
c) the reason why the subject is being invited to take part;
d) the reasonably anticipated benefits and consequences of the study;
e) the reasonably anticipated benefits and consequences of the study for the prospective subject and society (if none, these should be stated);
f) the foreseeable risks, including discomforts and inconveniences, to the prospective subject;
g) the foreseeable risks of the study itself;
h) complete details regarding confidentiality of prospective subjects;
i) the anticipated time commitment for subjects;
j) the intent to conduct a follow-up study in the future and the retention of data;
k) the rules for stopping the study and withdrawing the subject; and
l) the right of the subject to withdraw from the study at any time and without penalty.[27]

These general disclosures can be supplemented by additional information when subjects are also patients, and their participation in a study might affect their clinical care. No list can be exhaustive; for example, many consent forms now inform subjects that the results of the study will be shared with them.

Some of the more troubling ethical issues in informed consent result from the situations in which patients with a diminished capacity to consent are eligible for enrollment in a study. Although legal requirements may change, depending on the jurisdiction, the ethical concern is whether children can be enrolled in research studies. Of particular concern is whether children can volunteer for studies from which it is unlikely that they will benefit directly. The concept of "assent" that has developed would allow children to express their willingness to participate, which approximates but does not completely satisfy the more rigorous standard of consent.[27] This concept acknowledges the differing capacities that children have as they develop and mature, irrespective of the legal age of consent in any particular jurisdiction. Central to this notion, and discussed in the previous section, is the degree of risk inherent in the proposed study. We are satisfied that children and other vulnerable persons would be adequately protected from harm, and still treated autonomously, if a sliding scale were adopted in which the quality of the consent were commensurate with the degree of risk associated with the study.[63] This would hold children (and their parents or guardians) to a higher standard of consent for studies that carried a high likelihood of a serious harm (as, for example, in a clinical trial of a new therapeutic varnish[55]), compared to epidemiologic surveys with no invasive components, such as screening questionnaires. In both instances, the standard of disclosure in research would be more rigorous than in therapy.

For a discussion of informed consent in the therapeutic context, see Chapter 5.

Privacy and Confidentiality

We have focused our comments so far on issues that tend to arise in clinical dental research involving specific interventions. Increasingly, however, epidemiological methods, such as patient record reviews, have been used to advance scientific knowledge about disease and illness. In all research, personal information is generated about patients that could be regarded as confidential. *Confidentiality* refers to the status of information about a person and the way it is managed. Information is confidential when one person discloses it to another, and the person to whom it is disclosed does not disclose the information without prior consent.[18] In contrast, *privacy* **is** a characteristic of limited accessibility to the person. As Beauchamp and Childress argue, one has privacy "if others do not have or do not use access to him or her."[18]

In the context of dental research, such access principally refers to physical accessibility to the person through the procedure or intervention, but may also refer to a patient's right to be let alone (and therefore not asked to participate in research). Because dental patients are often eligible for participation in research, dentists already have access to them by virtue of the patients coming to a dental office. Protecting against unwelcome access to this "zone of privacy" should be considered, particularly because of the potential for coercion discussed previously. Limiting access to information about a person for purposes of research is more difficult.

The particular ethical concern in epidemiologic studies is the degree to which information that a patient believes is worth protecting can reasonably be safeguarded. Consider the following hypothetical (but not unlikely) study:

> In the wake of both public and professional concern about the transmission of the Human Immunodeficiency Virus (HIV) from a Florida dentist to his patient, a study is designed to identify the seroprevalence of HIV in dentists and patients in Florida. (See the discussion of this case by Keyes and Waithe in Chapter 6.)

We are aware of sentinel population surveillance for HIV infection in more than 40 U.S. states, Great Britain, the Netherlands,[64] and some in Canada, but we are not aware of any studies involving dentists or dental patients in particular. The principal ethical concerns with such studies relate to the management of the medical information about HIV status and therefore to protection of confidentiality. Because access is necessary (whether by phone or mail surveys), privacy concerns also must be weighed. Despite precautions such as unlinked anonymous screening proposed by the World Health Organization, and a full review by a University research ethics committee, the ethical issues raised by a large Ontario study resulted in a comprehensive Ministry of Health review.[65] This suggests that promises of confidentiality may not be sufficient protection for subjects.

ETHICAL REVIEW OF RESEARCH

Capron recently observed that what made the Nazi experiments especially horrific is that they took place in a society that had promulgated strict research guidelines.[19] Indeed, not only did the Prussian government in 1900 issue a directive prohibiting any intervention that was not therapeutic in intent on a person who was not competent, who had not consented, and who had not been informed of the risks and benefits of the intervention,[66] the German government promulgated more comprehensive regulations in 1931.[67] The existence of guidelines and regulations is not a guarantee of ethical behaviour by researchers. Even though the protection of human subjects has always been and will continue to be the responsibility of individual investigators, for many of the reasons we suggested above there has been a need to develop mechanisms for assuring that research is conducted ethically.

Three levels exist for ensuring the ethics of research: (1) international approaches, evidenced by the several codes of ethics that have been adopted; (2) the promulgation of professional and governmental codes and regulations at the national level; and (3) the local institutional review board.

This latter mechanism is a relatively recent phenomenon and in many countries is part of the "national approach." At each level, we explain the relevance to dental research.

International Approaches: Codes of Ethics

Since the Second World War, many documents have been developed that offer guidance for the conduct of research involving human subjects. Four in particular have provided sources for ethical appraisal of research involving human subjects: The Nuremberg Code (1949)[68]; The Declaration of Helsinki (1964, and revised in 1975, 1983, 1989)[69]; and *two* documents prepared by the World Health Organization/Council for International Organizations of Medical Sciences (WHO/CIOMS): the Proposed International Guidelines for Biomedical Research Involving Human Subjects (1982);[70] and the International Guidelines for Ethical Review of Epidemiological Studies (1991).[71]

THE NUREMBERG CODE

Ever since the Nuremberg Code emerged from the war crimes trials after World War II, the international community has been committed to describing a set of common values that ought to govern medical research. In a sense, society has become familiar with the concern of research ethics through the Code itself. Its ten principles may seem so obvious today as to be matters of common sense. However, one need only review the account of Dr. Andrew C. Ivy, a consultant for the U.S. Department of War who helped research the War Crimes and draft the Nuremberg Code, to understand that these principles were by no means common sense in 1945.[72] The Nuremberg Code has always stood as a statement of the commitment not only to the ethical values internal to the practice of medical research, but to values external to it, namely, freedom and the inviolability of the person. This Code is perhaps the most restrictive of the international codes, primarily because its first principle, "The voluntary consent of the human subject is absolutely essential," would limit research only to those persons who are legally competent to give an informed consent.

DECLARATION OF HELSINKI

The first document to move beyond the important but largely symbolic guidance of Nuremberg was the Declaration of Helsinki, adopted at the 18th Congress of the World Medical Association in 1964 and subsequently revised in 1975, 1984, and 1989. Among the features that distinguished the 1975 revision from the Nuremberg Code was the requirement in Principle I.2 that:

> . . . the design and performance of each experimental procedure involving human subjects . . . be clearly formulated in an experimental protocol which should be transmitted to a specially appointed independent committee for consideration, comment, and guidance."[69]

This statement was the first by an international organization describing a process by which human subjects could be protected. (Such committees were empowered to review and advise research protocols, but *not* to approve, reject, or require modifications to such protocols.)

CIOMS. Other international documents have been developed. In 1981, the Council for International Organizations of Medical Sciences drafted the Proposed International Guidelines for Biomedical Research Involving Human Subjects which describes standards for applying the principles of Helsinki.[70] The requirement of ethics review was reaffirmed at the Fourth International Summit Conference on Bioethics, held in Ottawa in April 1987.[72] There, a distinguished group of delegates from Canada, the United States, the European Economic Community, the Federal Republic of Germany, France, Italy, Japan, the United Kingdom, and the World Health Organization recommended an "International Ethic" for research with human beings:

> In order to safeguard the rights and well-being of patients and research subject, research ethics committees should be established in all countries. All projects involving human subjects must be submitted for approval to a research ethics committee.[72]

Most recently, the CIOMS published guidelines on epidemiology research,[71] which are likely to have relevance for some dental research. Interestingly, the recently drafted International Code of Ethics, developed by a working group for the Federation Dentaire Internationale, contains no mention of research ethics.[73]

These documents share three characteristics. First, they are guidelines that provide general descriptions of appropriate ethical behavior. They carry moral but not legal force. Second, they tend to embrace, adopt, or affirm fundamental principles of research ethics (respect for persons/autonomy, beneficence, non-maleficence, justice). Because these principles are general, this leaves open the possibility of national, local, or institutional interpretation. Finally, with the exception of the Nuremberg Code, each specifically endorses the use of "research ethics committees" and the importance of informed consent, balancing harm and benefit, and fair selection of subjects.

It is unlikely that the four international documents will provide any specific authority for the assurance of research ethics around the world. We are also uncertain, as a matter of applied ethics, whether an "international ethic" is even desirable, let alone possible. Cultural, political, and theological factors are likely to inhibit the search for such uniformity.[74] Is uniformity a desirable value worth promoting? On the other hand, the very nature of medical research as an international enterprise will demand more collaborative work. Minimum standards will have to be set to permit such collaboration. Moreover, uniformity particularly with respect to the review of medical/dental research at the local level, may only be undesirable as an outcome attribute.

National Approaches: Regulations, Guidelines and Professional Codes

Many countries, particularly those in North America and Western Europe, have adopted useful approaches for assuring the ethics of medical research. These vary according to whether they are established by law or through guidelines established by professional or scientific organizations and societies, and whether they are to cover public research alone, or private industrial research. As a result, compliance may be voluntary or mandatory, and sanctions for noncompliance vary. They can be described as regulatory approaches and professional guidelines.

REGULATIONS

Formal mechanisms are most developed in North America, and particularly in the United States, which has an extensive regulatory history.[48] Since 1966, research conducted by institutions supported by federal funds has had to comply with various guidelines, policies, and regulations governing the conduct of research, in particular, that there be prior peer review of all research involving human subjects. A landmark policy statement, prepared by the U.S. Public Health Service and released by U.S. Surgeon General William Stewart, outlined the three topics that such committees were to consider in evaluating research: (1) the rights and welfare of subjects, (2) the appropriateness of methods used to obtain informed consent, and (3) the balance of risks and benefits.[8] Other statements of policy followed, particularly in the wake of the several cases of research abuse described above. In 1971, the U.S. Department of Health, Education and Welfare issued the "Institutional Guide to DHEW Policy on Protection of Human Subjects," the so-called "Yellow Book," which outlined the initial requirements for Institutional Review Boards, the local hospital-based committees that were charged with assuring the ethical propriety of research.

Since 1974, the conduct of research in the U.S. has been regulated by federal statute.[15] Institutions receiving federal money must sign assurances attesting to their commitment to compliance with federal regulations and principles governing research. These requirements are described in detail in the recently promulgated Federal Policy for the Protection of Human Subjects.[2] The Federal Policy brings under one umbrella several of the U.S. agencies that previously had used their own regulations, or had voluntarily complied with those set forth by the Department of Health and Human Services in 1981.[75] Additional subparts to these regulations cover research involving fetuses, pregnant women, human in vitro fertilization, prisoners, and children.[75]

CODES OF ETHICS AND ORGANIZED DENTISTRY

The American Dental Association has had a Code of Ethics since 1866. As in most professions, guidelines of the professional dental associations have quasi-legal force; the failure to comply with guidelines results in sanctions from censure to revocation of license. The ADA's *Principles of Ethics and Code of Professional Conduct* provides little guidance on research.[76] Principle-Section 4 of the 1991 *Principles* is as follows:

> **Research and Development.** Dentists have the obligation of making the results and benefits of their investigative efforts available to all when they are useful in safeguarding or promoting the health of the public.

The Code of Professional Conduct evolving from this Principle is as follows:

> "4-A **Devices and Therapeutic Methods.** Except for formal investigative studies, dentists shall be obliged to prescribe, dispense or promote only those devices, drugs and other agents whose complete formulae are available to the dental profession. Dentists shall have further obligation of not holding out as exclusive any device, agent method or technique.
>
> 4-B **Patents and Copyrights.** Patents and copyrights may be secured by dentists provided that such patents and copyrights shall not be used to restrict research or practice."

Two States have reviewed this Code and interpreted it for its members without comment on the paucity of direction for research.[77,78] Similar general guides are found in the Canadian Dental Association's *Code of Ethics*,[79] although no specific guidelines regarding research exist.

A more helpful source is the ADA's *Guidelines for the Use of Human Subjects in Dental Research*, which provides an overview of the basic ethical principles of re-

search, a classification of research into several categories, and additional considerations.[62] Approved in 1978, they mirror the guidelines prepared by the National Commission. Recognizing that some dental research may occur in environments not serviced by an IRB, these guidelines are recommended as "particularly helpful for clinical investigations conducted by private practitioners, members of the Study Clubs or others not covered by approved review committee for human research."[62] Dental research protocols will be reviewed by IRBs just like any other clinical protocol.

NATIONAL GUIDELINES

It has been suggested that the U.S. system of research ethics review is the most elaborate, sophisticated and detailed in the world.[80] This has generated some discussion regarding the applicability of less complicated systems, particularly those of Canada, Denmark, and Australia.[81] In Canada, overseeing of medical research is conducted through the use of guidelines rather than regulations. As compared with the development of guidelines by professional organizations, guidelines have been developed by the Medical Research Council, most recently in 1987, which provide advice for both investigators and research ethics boards, the Canadian equivalent of IRBs.[27] In Denmark, seven regional committees with an equal number of lay members and scientific members will advise local institutions and respond to "informal monitoring" within institutions. In addition, a national committee exists to review multicenter trials. In Australia, more than 100 research ethics committees exist, which apply criteria described in the guidelines of the National Health & Medical Research Council.[82]

Similarly, although research ethics committees are now a fixture in Europe, overseeing of research is somewhat different.[83] In the United Kingdom, the ethics review process is carried out by more than 250 different committees, mainly based within single institutions.[84] Research ethics committee review is not legally required as a prerequisite for activation of protocols. Their memberships vary in both size and specialization. In France, a permanent National Advisory Committee was established in 1983 with the authority to provide authoritative statements on different issues. In December 1988, the National Assembly passed a law governing the conduct of research involving human subjects, which requires, among other things, that research receive prior ethics approval from a regional research ethics committee. Mechanisms for assuring the ethics of research are in various stages of development in most other Western European countries.

Research ethics committees are developing outside Europe as well. For example, more than 65% of all medical schools in Japan have IRBs, and it is expected that such committees will soon be functioning in all medical schools.

Local Approaches

INSTITUTIONAL REVIEW BOARDS

The centerpiece of the U.S. regulatory framework is the Institutional Review Board (IRB), an interdisciplinary committee designed to perform a unique type of peer review. IRBs (also known as Research Ethics Committees) must review all research conducted at institutions receiving U.S. Public Health Service funding. The history of peer review of research involving human subjects has been marked by several important dates, events and publications. Although many of the well known sources have been developed in the last 40 years, it is worth mentioning that peer review has a lengthy history. For example, Thomas Percival wrote in his 1803 *Medical Ethics* what is generally regarded as the first authoritative statement on the obligation to obtain peer review when he recommended that physicians consult with their peers before proceeding with therapeutic innovation.[85]

The IRB is a unique type of committee in terms of both membership and function, regarded by some as a type of helpful bureaucratic structure.[86] Veatch has suggested that IRBs should combine the professional expertise of interdisciplinary technology assessment panel and the common sense of the reasonable person found

in juries.[41] According to the new 1991 Federal Policy (Sec. 107), the IRB must have a diverse membership with at least five members from varying backgrounds; must make "every non-discriminatory effort" to ensure that it does not "consist entirely of men or entirely of women," or entirely of one profession; must include one member "whose primary concerns are in scientific areas" and one whose primary concern is in a "nonscientific area;" and must include someone not directly affiliated with the institution or "part of the immediate family who is affiliated with the institution." The principal function of the IRB is to review, with authority to approve, require modifications in (to secure approval), or disapprove research studies presented to it.

It is worth noting that the rigor of ethics review is such that studies like the Burlington Growth and Development study described above would probably not be approved by an IRB were it submitted today. This is because of the excessive number of radiographs which were integral to the design and which were taken to assist in building an understanding of normal growth patterns and not for the good of the subjects. Because the radiographs were not principally intended to benefit the subjects themselves, IRBs would likely be reluctant to permit individuals to undertake the risk of excessive exposure to x rays. This may be because, as Veatch has noted, proposals involving potential radiation raise unique issues:

> Radiation exposure places directly at risk in addition to consenting subjects, other human beings—bystanders, lab personnel, and even future generations. Not only are potential effects not known, but most IRB members have very little understanding of the mechanisms of action of radiation and even the basic concepts underlying its effects. Because the field of radiation itself is politically and socially controversial, IRB members necessarily find themselves participating in a larger social debate.[41]

The irony is that this study has yielded a wealth of information on normal growth and development on orthodontic interventions and timing, and has resulted in a prediction model derived from computer records of these radiographs which assist in diagnosis and treatment planning for malocclusion cases.

THE CLIMATE FOR ETHICAL INVESTIGATION IN DENTISTRY

We have noted that Beecher's 1966 article has been credited with galvanizing international public interest in medical research ethics because of its expose style. Although mostly known for this extensive discussion, the real gem in the article may be found four paragraphs from the end, in a summary statement affectionately known as Beecher's Code. This was more carefully reworked in his 1970 book *Research and the Individual*, as follows:

> The ethical approach to experimentation in man has several components; two are more important than the others, the first being informed consent ... An even greater safeguard for the patient than consent is the presence of an informed, able, conscientious, compassionate, responsible investigator, for it is recognized that patients can, when imperfectly informed, be induced to agree unwisely to many things.[87]

Beecher's "Code" describes some of the character traits of the virtuous clinician/investigator. Others have added to this list.[88] More importantly, it serves to remind investigators that, irrespective of degree of sophistication in any one protocol, or the type of oversight governing the conduct of research, the final arbiter of ethical behavior in research is the investigator. This focuses attention on factors outside of the research protocol itself, and, we think, properly so. Indeed, several issues contribute to the climate for ethical investigation that are not properly "internal" to the paradigm of the research protocol we have used in this chapter. We mention only four examples of these "external" issues.

Sponsorship

Increasingly, the days of the lone investigator working in relative obscurity with a few patients are fading. Multicenter clinical trials, designed to involve large numbers of patients to show minimal differences between two or more interventions, are now the "gold standard." These studies are expensive to fund. Although a sizeable portion of clinical research is funded by public sources, industrial and otherwise privately sponsored research occurs. Two ethical issues are evident. First, given the potential for conflicts of interest, it is most important that the researcher have the responsibility and authority for collection and analysis of data, and that the relationship between the sponsoring agency and the investigator be made clear. Second, the source of sponsorship could be relevant to potential research subjects, and therefore might be disclosed in a consent form.

Fraud and Misconduct

One of us has argued elsewhere[89] that fraud is one of several categories of misconduct in research, which includes the conduct of unethical research involving human subjects; misappropriation or misuse (including waste) of research funds; conflict of interest situations. The National Institutes of Health has defined misconduct as (1) deviation from accepted practices in conducting research, or fabrication, falsification or plagiarism in research reporting and (2) failure to comply with federal requirements for research conduct, such as protecting the welfare of human or animal subjects.[90]

Examples of fraud exist and have become matters of public interest. John Darsee's publication of nearly one hundred scientific papers and abstracts in two years of cardiology research at Harvard University, and the forging of data for an upcoming paper is but one of a list of cases made known in the literature.[91,92] Fraud and misconduct are wrong because of the harms to patients, the research community, and the public that may result from publication of false information. Patients may be harmed if clinicians treat on the basis of fabricated research results; researchers may have their reputations and that of their institutions damaged, resulting in less funding and support for important research, and society is harmed by the breach of trust that it has with the research community. The potential causes of research fraud and misconduct are numerous, ranging from the multiple obligations that investigators might have to the ever-present pressure to publish. Institutional policies provide minimal criteria for behavior. There are subtle types of misconduct resulting from the reporting of data and the selection of authors for manuscripts.

Reporting Data

Reporting results of research can pose ethical problems, as in the case of prior release of data through non-peer reviewed press, or in using one study to produce several reports or even similar reports published in different journals. This activity has been termed "salami slicing."[93] Reporting of results raises a further ethical problem when multiple authors contribute to a final manuscript. Not only does the order of authorship become a matter of political importance (first or last authors receiving more academic credit than other coauthors), but so too does the inclusion of honorary authors who have not contributed directly to the manuscript. Such activities, like those involving fraud and misconduct, detract from the quality of scientific knowledge that is produced through investigation. Moreover, it threatens the integrity of the academic or scientific method.

Curriculum

No assessment of the climate for ethical investigation in any health science is complete without acknowledging the important role of the curriculum in articulating the values of ethical research. Only recently have programs in medicine implemented required courses in ethics, and the impact of teaching ethics in the medical curriculum is only now being assessed.[94] Few basic or applied science courses provide courses in research ethics, and few professional health science programs offer such courses.

CONCLUSIONS

The conduct of dental research creates ethical issues for patients, researchers, and institutions no less important or compelling than other biomedical or behavioral research. We have suggested in this chapter that these issues can be framed first by using a background in ethics to appreciate the moral content of research, and second by examining particular ethical issues that emerge using the research protocol as a paradigm. In so doing, we illuminated current areas where dentists and dental students might focus their attention when designing and conducting research, but also areas where educators can begin appraising the climate for ethical investigation in dentistry.

DISCUSSION QUESTIONS

1. Based on your understanding of the responsibilities of dentists to their patients, how do these responsibilities change when patients are also potential research subjects?
2. Assuming that informed consent is an important prerequisite for research on human subjects to proceed, how would you resolve the problem posed by pediatric dentistry: either consent is obtained from a third party, or consent is not obtained at all? Would you permit any research on children when consent was not possible?
3. Argue either in support of or in opposition to the claim that, if a dental research protocol is scientific, it must also be ethical. This requires answering the question: is scientific merit an ethical consideration in dental research?
4. If you were a member of an IRB reviewing the dental protocol for assessing seroprevalence of HIV, would you approve it outright, require modifications and then approve it, or reject it? What reasons would you give for your decision?
5. Analyze the ADA *Guidelines for the*

Use of Human Subjects in Research (1978). Are they adequate to ensure that all research subjects are both protected from harm and given an opportunity to participate in research? How would you change the guidelines?

REFERENCES

1. Dickens, B.M.: What is a medical experiment? Can. Med. Assoc. J. *114*:635, 1977.
2. Office of Science and Technology Policy. Federal Policy for the Protection of Human Subjects. *Federal Register*. Vol. 56. No. 117, June 18, 1991: 28003–28012.
3. Opinion Research Corporation.: Dental Care: What People Know. Surveying the Knowledge Gap, 1983.
4. Haraldson, T., and Zarb, G.: A 10-year follow-up study of the masticatory system after treatment with osseointegrated implant bridges. Scand. J. Dent. Res. *96*:243, 1988.
5. Levine, R.J.: Ethics and Regulation of Clinical Research. 2d. Ed. Baltimore, Urban & Schwarzenberg, 1986.
6. Lifton, R.J.: The Nazi Doctors. New York, Basic Books, 1986.
7. Rothman, D.J.: Strangers at the Bedside. New York, Basic Books, 1988.
8. U.S. Public Health Service. PPO#129, Clinical Investigations Involving Human Subjects. Bethesda, U.S. Public Health Service (February 8, 1966).
9. Beecher, H.K.: Ethics and Clinical Research. N. Engl. J. Med. *274*:1102, 1966.
10. Pappworth, M.H.: Human Guinea Pigs. London, Penguin, 1967.
11. Mill, J.S.: Utilitarianism. *In* Utilitarianism, on Liberty, Considerations on Representative Government. Edited by H.B. Acton. London, J.M. Dent, 1972.
12. Gert, B.: Morality: A New Justification of the Moral Rules. New York, Oxford, 1988.
13. Jonsen, A.R.: Do not harm. Ann. Intern. Med. *88*:827, 1978.
14. Katz, J.: Experimentation with Human Beings. New York, Russell-Sage, 1972.
15. National Research Act. Public Law 93-348. July 12, 1974.
16. National Commission for the Protection of Human Subjects of Biomedical and Behavioral research: The Belmont Report: Ethical Principles and Guidelines for the Protection of Human Subjects of Research. Washington, DHEW, 1978, p. 2.
17. Kant, as cited in reference 18, p. 71.
18. Beauchamp, T.L., and Childress, J.F.: Principles of Biomedical Ethics. 3rd Ed. New York, Oxford University Press, 1989.
19. Capron, A.M.: Human experimentation. *In* Medical Ethics. Edited by R.M. Veatch. Boston, Jones & Bartlett, 1989. p. 137.
20. Frankena, W.K.: Ethics. 2nd Ed. Englewood Cliffs, New Jersey, Prentice-Hall, 1973.
21. Branson, R.: The ethics of dental research: overview of basic principles. J. Dent. Res. *59(C)*:1214, July, 1980.
22. Walters, L.: Research with human and animal subjects. *In* Contemporary Issues in Bioethics. 3rd Ed. Edited by T.L. Beauchamp and L. Walters. Belmont, CA, Wadsworth, 1989.
23. Bernard, C.: An Introduction to the Study of Experimental Medicine [1865]. Trans. by H.C. Greene. New York, Dover Publications, 1957.
24. Eisenberg, L.: The social imperatives of medical research. Science *198*:1105, 1977.
25. Jonas, H.: Philosophical reflections in experimenting with human subjects. Daedalus *98*:219, 1969.
26. Malone, T.E.: The moral imperative for biomedical research. *In* Biomedical Research: Collaboration and Conflicts of Interest. Edited by R.J. Porter and T.E. Malone. Baltimore, The Johns Hopkins University Press, 1992.
27. Medical Research Council of Canada: Guidelines on Research Involving Human Subjects. Ottawa, MRC, 1987.
28. Prentice, E.D., Antonson, D.L.: A protocol review guide to reduce IRB inconsistency. IRB: A Review of Human Subjects Research *10*:9, 1987.
29. Popovich, F.: The Burlington Orthodontic Research Centre. Am. J. Orthod. *43*:291, 1957.
30. Burlington Orthodontic Research Centre; Progress Report Series No. 1: 1952–56; Division of Dental Research, Faculty of Dentistry, University of Toronto, 1956.
31. Meslin, E.M.: Protecting human subjects from harm through improved risk judgments. IRB: A Review of Human Subjects Research *12*:7–10, 1990.
32. Weinstein, B.: *The Possibility of Ethical Expertise.* Ann Arbor, Michigan, University Microfilms International, 1990.
33. Freedman, B.: Scientific value and validity as ethical requirements for research: A proposed explication. IRB: A review of human subjects research. *9*:174, 1987.
34. Passamani, E.: Clinical trials—are they ethical? N. Engl. J. Med. *324*:1589, 1991.
35. Hellman, S., and Hellman, D.S.: Of mice but not men: Problems of the randomized clinical trial. N. Engl. J. Med. *324*:1585, 1991.
36. Freedman, B.: Equipoise and the ethics of clinical research. N. Engl. J. Med. *317*:141, 1987.
37. Schafer, A.: The ethics of the randomized clinical trial. N. Engl. J. Med. *307*:719, 1982.
38. Salisbury, D.A., and Schecter, M.T.: AIDS trials, civil liberties and the social control of therapy: should we embrace new drugs with open arms? Can. Med. Assoc. J. *142*:1057, 1990.
39. Chalmers, T.C.: The ethics of randomization as a decision-technique, and the problem of informed consent. *In* Contemporary Issues in Bioethics. 3rd. Ed. Edited by T.L. Beauchamp and L. Walters. Belmont, CA, Wadsworth, 1989.

40. Fost, N.: Consent as a barrier to research. N. Engl. J. Med. *300*:1271, 1979.

41. Veatch, R.M.: The Patient As Partner. Bloomington, Indiana, Indiana University Press, 1987.

42. Hypothetical protocol: Clinical field trial: a comparative study of sealants, amalgam restorations, and fluoride rinsing on the progression and prevention of carious lesions. J. Dent. Res. *59(C)*: 1240, July 1980.

43. Leske, G.S., and Ripa, L.W.: Ethical and legal considerations associated with clinical field trials. J. Dent. Res. *59(C)*:1243, 1980.

44. Harris, R.: Biology of the children of Hopewood House, Bowral, Australia, IV. Observations of dental caries experience extending over five years (1957–1961). J. Dent. Res. *42*:1387, 1963.

45. Gustafsson, B.E., et al.: The Vipeholm dental caries study. Acta Odont. Scand. *11*:232, 1954.

46. McHugh, W.D.: Professional ethics in dental research. J. Am. Coll. Dent. *51*:19, 1984.

47. Linde, J., and Axelsson, P.: The effect of controlled oral hygiene and topic fluoride application on caries and gingivitis in Swedish schoolchildren. Community Dent. Oral Epidemiol. *1*:9–16, 1973.

48. Faden, R.R., and Beauchamp, T.L.: A History and Theory of Informed Consent. New York, Oxford University Press, 1986, pp. 257–260.

49. Macklin, R.: Due and undue inducements: On paying money to research subjects. IRB: A Review of Human Subjects Research *3*:1, 1981.

50. Appelbaum, P.S., et al. False hopes and best data: Consent to research and the therapeutic misconception. Hastings Cent. Rep. *17*:20–24, 1987.

51. Sutherland, H.J., Meslin, E.M., and Till, J.E.: Recruitment into clinical trials: Nature limitations and ethics of the process, 1992 (unpublished manuscript).

52. Vanderpool, H.Y., Weiss, G.B.: False data and last hopes: Enrolling ineligible patients in clinical trials. Hastings Cent. Rep. *17*:16, 1987.

53. Collins, J.F., Williford, W.O., Weiss, D.G., et al.: Planning patient recruitment: Fantasy and reality. Stat. Med. *3*:435, 1984.

54. Locker, D., et al.: Utilization of dental services by older adults in four Ontario communities. Canad. Dent. J. *57(11)*:879, 1991.

55. Sandham, H.J., et al.: Clinical trials in adults of an antimicrobial varnish for reducing *Mutans Streptococci.* J. Dent. Res. *70*:1401, 1991.

56. Feinberg, J.: Harm to Others. New York, Oxford University Press, 1984.

57. Sprent, P.: Taking Risks: The Science of Uncertainty. London, Penguin Books, 1988.

58. Hypothetical protocol: Epidemiological survey title: An epidemiologic study of dental caries and dental fluorisis. J. Dent. Res. *59(C)*:1271, July 1980.

59. Stamm, J.W.: Applying ethical guidelines in the conduct of children's dental caries surveys. J. Dent. Res. *59(C)*:1274, July 1980.

60. Slovic, R., Fischhoff, B., and Lichtenstein, S.: Facts and fears: understanding perceived risk. In Societal Risk Assessment: How Safe is Safe Enough? Edited by R. Schwing, W. Albers Jr. New York, Plenum, 1980.

61. *Halushka v. University of Saskatchewan.* (1965), 53. D.L.R. (2d) 436 at 443-444 (Sask. C.A.).

62. American Dental Association: Council on Dental Research Guidelines for the Use of Human Subjects in Dental Research. Journal of the American Dental Association. *98*:86–88, 1979.

63. Schafer, A.: Experimentation with human subjects: A critique of the views of Hans Jonas. J. Med. Ethics *9*:76–79, 1983.

64. Bayer, R., Lumey, L.H., and Wan, L.: The American, British, and Dutch response to unlinked anonymous seroprevalence studies: An international comparison. Law, Medicine, and Health Care *19*:222–230, 1991.

65. Sharpe, G.: HIV Seroprevalence Studies Report. Toronto, Ministry of Health, 1991.

66. Der Minister der geistlichen. Anweisung an die Vorsteher der Klinken, Polikliniken under sinstigen Krankensanstaken. Centralblatt der gesamten Unterrichtsverwaltung in Preussen. Berlin, Prussian Government, 1901, as cited in Capron (ref. 19), p. 128.

67. Sass, H.M.: Reichsundschreiben 1931: Pre-Nuremberg regulations concerning new therapy and human experimentation. J. Med. Philos. *8*:99, 1983.

68. The Nuremberg Code, reprinted in Annas G.J., and Grodin, M.A. (eds.): The Nazi Doctors and the Nuremberg Code. New York, Oxford University Press, 1992.

69. The Declaration of Helsinki, reprinted in Annas, G.J., and Grodin, M.A. (eds.): The Nazi Doctors and the Nuremberg Code. New York, Oxford University Press, 1992.

70. Council for International Organizations of Medical Sciences: Proposed International Guidelines for Biomedical Research Involving Human Subjects. Geneva, CIOMS, 1982.

71. Council for International Organizations of Medical Sciences: International Guidelines for Ethical Review of Epidemiological Studies. Geneva, CIOMS, 1991.

72. Ivy, A.C.: Nazi war crimes of a medical nature. Federation Bulletin *33*, 1947, reprinted *in* Bioethics. Edited by R.B. Edwards and G.C. Graber. New York, Harcourt, Brace, Jovanovich, 1988.

73. Bebeau, M.J., personal communication, January 30, 1992.

74. Fasella, P., Bertazzoni, U.: Who sets the standards for what and how? *In* Towards an International Ethic for Research with Human Beings: Documents. Ottawa, Medical Research Council, 1987, pp. 67–86.

75. U.S. Department of Health and Human Services. Title 45; Code of Federal Regulations; Part 46: Revised March 8, 1983. [45 CFR 46]

76. American Dental Association: Principles of Ethics and Code of Professional Conduct. Revised through 1991. Official Advisory Opinions of the Council on Bylaws and Judicial Affairs, Chicago, ADA, 1991.

77. California Dental Association: CDA Code of Ethics. Journal of the California Dental Association *7*:34–38, July 1989.

78. WDA's Interpretation of the ADA Principles of Ethics and Code of Professional Conduct. WDA Journal, 23–25, 84, 85, 87, 152–153, 210–212, 1989.

79. The Canadian Dental Association: Code of Ethics. Revised 1991. Ottawa, CDA, 1992.

80. Curran, W., as cited in McNeill, P.M.: Research ethics review in Australia, Europe and North America. IRB: A Review of Human Subjects Research *11*:4, 1989.

81. McNeill, P.M.: Research ethics review in Australia, Europe and North America. IRB: A Review of Human Subjects Research *11*:4, 1989.

82. [Australian] National Health & Medical Research Council: Statement on Human Experimentation and Supplementary Notes. Canberra, NH&MRC, 1985.

83. Bergkamp, L.: The rise of research ethics committees in Western Europe: Some concomitant problems. Bioethics *3*:122, 1989.

84. Nicholson, R.H., Ed.: Medical Research with Children: Ethics, Law, and Practice. Oxford, Oxford University Press, 1986.

85. Percival, T.: Percival's Medical Ethics, 1803 Reprint. Edited by Chauncey D. Leake. Baltimore, Williams & Wilkins, 1927.

86. Hall, D.: The research imperative and bureaucratic control: The case of clinical research. Soc. Sci. Med. *32*:333, 1991.

87. Beecher, H.K.: Research and the Individual: Human Studies. Boston, Little, Brown, 1970.

88. Reece, R.D., and Siegal, H.A.: Studying People: A Primer in the Ethics of Social Research. Macon, GA, Mercer, 1986.

89. Lowy, F.H., and Meslin, E.M.: Fraud in medical research. *In* Ethics in Pediatric Research. Edited by G. Koren. Melbourne, Florida, Krieger (1993).

90. Notice of Proposed rulemaking, September 19, 1988. Title 42, U.S. Code of Federal Regulations, Sec. 50; 53 Federal Register 36348.

91. Broad, W., and Wade, N.: Betrayers of the Truth: Fraud and Deceit in the Halls of Science. Simon and Schuster, New York, 1982, p. 13–14.

92. Kohn, A.: False Prophets: Fraud and Error in Science and Medicine. London, Basil Blackwell, 1986.

93. Horowitz, H.S.: Current ethical issues in research. Journal of the American College of Dentists. *57(3)*:9–12, 1990.

94. Hebert, P.C., Meslin, E.M., and Dunn, E.V.: Ethical sensitivity II: A 1991 study at the University of Toronto. J. Med. Ethics (in press).

APPENDIX 11–1. PROTOCOL REVIEW GUIDE

For research studies involving human subjects to be approved by IRBs or other institutional research ethics committees, protocols must address, at a minimum, the following issues:

- **Scientific merit,** including the validity and value of the study.
- **Justification for the study,** including the reasons for conducting the study at this time.
- **Informed consent,** including the process of obtaining informed consent from patients, and how permission will be obtained from others if the patient is not able to consent on his or her own behalf. Consent *forms* must provide adequate information, in language that subjects can understand of what is likely to occur if they agree to participate.
- **Assessment of harm and benefit,** including an objective assessment of the possible harms and benefits to the subject, including their likelihood and severity, and an appreciation of the subjective nature of the perception of risk to subjects. Although standards vary, it is expected that the risks of harm cannot be seen to outweigh the possible benefits to subjects, without good reason.

- **Selection of subjects,** including an explanation for inviting *this* group of subjects to participate, and what types of benefits they can expect.
- **Protections of privacy and confidentiality of information,** including measures for respecting the socially sensitive nature of information about persons and for ensuring that access to names and identifiers are controlled by the person.

Other protocol review guides are available, including Levine's text,[A-1] and a format to reduce inconsistency.[A-2] Meslin and Till are developing an evaluative framework for integrating science and ethics in the review of clinical trials.[A-3]

REFERENCES

A-1. Levine, R.J.: Ethics and Regulation of Clinical Research, 1986.

A-2. Prentice, E.D., and Antonson, D.L.: A protocol review guide to reduce IRB inconsistency. IRB: A Review of Human Subjects Research. *Feb*:9–11, 1987.

A-3. Meslin, E.M., and Till, J.E.: Development and evaluation of a framework for integrated ethical and scientific review of clinical trials. Strategic Grant, #806-91-0002, Social Science and Humanities Research Council of Canada (1991–1994).

APPENDIX 11–2. ADA GUIDELINES FOR THE USE OF HUMAN SUBJECTS IN DENTAL RESEARCH (1978)*

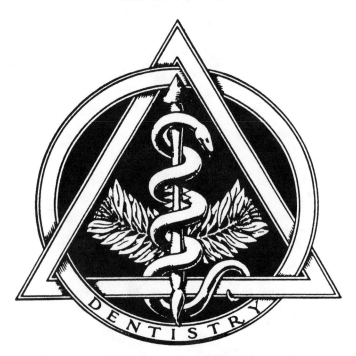

As revised and approved by the American Dental Association, the American Association for Dental Research, and the American Association of Dental Schools at their 1978 meetings.

Introduction and Background Information: Nearly all private and governmental agencies that support clinical research require written assurances from prospective investigators or institutions that the rights and welfare of participating human subjects will be protected before they approve a proposed research project.

This report contains the guidelines of the American Dental Association, the American Association for Dental Research and the American Association of Dental Schools on the use of human subjects as participants in clinical research studies. These guidelines comprise basic ethical principles that apply to all research involving humans. The guidelines may be particularly helpful for clinical investigations conducted by private practitioners, members of Study Clubs or others not covered by approved review committees for human research. However, these guidelines may

* Reprinted with permission of the American Dental Association, 1992.

serve as a basis for weighing the appropriateness of proposed research by all committees established to review the ethical propriety of research involving humans. Such review committees must be competent to evaluate a proposed study scientifically and to determine the acceptability of the study in terms of federal, state and local law, standards of professional conduct and community practice. These committees should include a variety of professional and scientific personnel as well as representatives from the community, such as clergymen, lawyers or members of consumer-interest groups who may add other dimensions to the opinion of the scientific or professional members.

I. Basic Principles of Ethics in Research Involving Human Subjects

A. Any research involving human subjects must be based upon scientific principles that offer a sound rationale for the research. The justification for the research should be supported by findings obtained from laboratory or animal experiments, scientifically established facts, or findings from other clinical studies.

B. Research involving human subjects should be conducted by or be under the supervision of clinical investigators who are scientifically qualified and experienced. The principal investigator and the sponsoring institution or organization are responsible for the conduct of all personnel in connection with an investigation.

C. Research involving human subjects should be carried out only if the rights and welfare of the participants are adequately protected. All reasonable efforts should be made to reduce possible risks to the participants, and the risks must be outweighed by the benefits to be derived or by the importance of the knowledge that will be gained. There is, of course, no justification for conducting research involving humans if the physical or mental health of any subjects is likely to be adversely altered or disturbed by either drugs or experimental procedures.

D. The informed consent of subjects who participate in a study must be obtained by methods that are adequate and appropriate. Informed consent should be obtained in writing from a subject or the subject's parents, guardian, or authorized representative only after the study and the risks involved have been fully explained. If the participants are children who have reached an age of discretion, their assent should be obtained in addition to the consent of the adults responsible for them.

All basic elements of informed consent should be in writing and should minimally consist of:

1. A general description in lay terms of the study and its purpose, followed by a fair and clear explanation of all examination and treatment procedures to be followed, including an identification of those that are experimental;

2. An explanation of why the subjects have been invited to participate and an assurance that the identity or particular findings of each subject will be held confidential by the investigator;

3. A description of any known attendant discomforts or risks that are reasonable to expect;

4. A description of the benefits that are reasonable to expect;

5. A disclosure of appropriate alternative procedures or treatments that might be advantageous for the subject in lieu of participation;

6. An offer to answer any inquiries concerning the study prior to its inception or during its course. The explanatory form should contain the name, title and telephone number of the principal investigator or his or her designee for the convenience and protection of persons who may have questions about the study before it begins or during its course;

7. An instruction that the subject is free to decline participation, withdraw consent or discontinue participation in the project or activity at any time without prejudice.

The written agreement entered into by the subject should contain no exculpatory language through which the subject waives or appears to waive any legal rights, or releases the institution, group, or individual or its agents from liability for negligence. Other items that should be contained in informed consent documents include: clear statements of whether any subjects will be deprived of usual treatment or be asked to withhold usual practices; a description of any costs or compensations to the subjects; the likelihood or chance that a subject will receive an ineffective treatment (if a placebo or untreated control group is used); and a clear statement that an affirmative response and signature indicate a decision to participate.

In essence, prospective study participants or those responsible for them should be provided with sufficient, comprehensible written information about a research project and the attendant procedures to enable them to make a rationally exercised decision about participation. Participation must be truly voluntary and not coercive in any way.

II. Classification of Research in Human Subjects

For the purpose of these guidelines, clinical research in human subjects is classified in one of three categories:

A. Research concerned with the diagnosis, control or treatment of an existing disease or condition.

B. Research concerned with the prevention of a disease or condition to which a subject is likely to be susceptible.

C. Research not concerned directly with treating an existing disease or condition of the subject, or preventing one to which the subject is likely to be susceptible, e.g., behavioral studies, plaque or saliva sampling, surveys or other descriptive research.

Although there must be concern for participants and the elements of informed consent must be adhered to for research in all these classifications, different concerns and aspects of informed consent assume particular importance in each type.

1. Research on the diagnosis, control or treatment of existing conditions

a. A clinical investigator has an obligation to ensure that subjects who have the disease or condition under investigation receive or are referred for treatment. Untreated or placebo-treated control groups are rarely justified for research in this category if the disease or condition is irreversible without treatment. Subjects who have other serious diseases or conditions should be referred or informed of the need for treatment.

b. In the treatment of a disease or condition, the clinical investigator should use a new or experimental therapeutic measure or agent only if existing evidence indicates that the new agent is likely to be at least as effective as existing measures or agents. If conventional, effective methods or agents exist to treat the same condition, one or more of these should be considered for incorporation in the design of the study as a positive control.

c. Because subjects with existing diseases or conditions are frequently in a dependent relationship to the clinical investigator or other personnel of a research project for regular therapeutic care, study personnel must exercise special caution not to exploit this dependency in soliciting consent or cooperation during the study.

d. For research in this category, the basic element of informed consent requiring disclosure of appropriate alternative procedures assumes prime importance.

2. Research on preventive measures

a. Studies of preventive agents or methods are often done in groups of students in school or in adults outside the confines of a clinical setting. The investigators are nevertheless responsible for the rights and welfare of participants with respect to these studies.

b. Although research in this category is concerned with prevention, the clinical investigator has the responsibility of informing subjects or those responsible for them of existing oral diseases or serious oral conditions. Even when there are no provisions for treating subjects in a study, subjects have the right to be informed of conditions that may affect their health or well-being and should be encouraged to seek required treatment and to continue routine dental care.

c. In order to avoid depriving subjects in control groups from receiving possibly beneficial preventive treatments, alternative designs, such as using historical base lines or comparing with reference populations, should be considered and employed when they are feasible and statistically valid.

d. Participants, their families when appropriate and pertinent institutional and health officials should be informed of a study's important findings. In addition, these persons should be informed of the extent and probable duration of the protection received by the treated subjects.

3. Research other than for treatment or prevention

a. Research in this category usually results in no therapeutic benefit to the participants, and thus may have no specific value to them. Therefore, such research should have a solid scientific foundation, expand existing knowledge and be expected to yield useful results for the good of society.

b. It is especially important that maximal confidentiality of information be maintained when behavioral research concentrates on the beliefs, practices or habits of participants. Moreover, confidentiality should be assured in studies in which demographic information of a personal nature is elicited, e.g., education and income.

c. The use of procedures in this category of research that may cause serious harm to subjects and are applied merely to gain greater general knowledge or to determine behavioral or physiologic responses to stimuli is not justified in clinical research.

III. Additional Considerations

There are special concerns about informed consent for studies that involve children, the mentally ill, or mentally retarded. Such studies should be conducted only when there is not a significant risk of physical or mental harm and when direct benefit to the subjects is anticipated, or when studying the condition that directly affects them.

There is also current concern about studies of individuals with limited civil freedom. Particular caution must be exercised in planning studies with prisoners, military personnel, students or others who may feel coerced into participating in investigations at their institutions.

Radiographs should be taken in a clinical study only when they are essential to the purposes of the study. Adequate protection should be afforded both the participants and the personnel who expose the radiographs. Every effort should be made to optimize radiographic efficiency, i.e., obtaining maximum radiographic information with minimum patient exposure. Diagnostic information from radiographs, reproductions of radiographs or duplicate films should be made available to a subject's personal dentist on request.

A research project should be terminated if serious, adverse effects develop that are associated with the treatment regimens. Moreover, consideration should be given to terminating long-term studies ahead of schedule if it becomes apparent that the answer or conclusions will be equivocal, e.g., negative interim findings or excessive loss of participants. Consideration should also be given for terminating a study ahead of schedule in unequivocal evidence of effectiveness in one or more groups is established from interim examinations and it is believed that benefits should no longer be denied to subjects in other groups.

The subjects should clearly understand that the examinations that are a part of a clinical study or survey are not a substitute for the usual examinations they may receive from their private dentists.

Laws and regulations demand that certain rules be followed or actions be avoided when conducting research in humans. Some of these laws and regulations vary from State to State. These guidelines do not cover the legal and regulatory aspects of research in humans. Investigators are cautioned, therefore, to secure competent legal opinion when planning research projects involving human subjects.

Because the possibilities for clinical research are diverse, these guidelines by necessity must be somewhat general. The interpretation and implementation of these guidelines, by acting in accordance with standards and precepts of behavior practiced in a proposed study's location, constitute the ethical and moral consideration that must be associated with research projects.

These guidelines, formulated expressly to protect the rights and welfare of human subjects involved in clinical research studies, may also serve as legal protection for the investigator. It should also be noted that a distinction between clinical research and professional practice is not always clear. For example, a practicing dentist who conducts orderly tests or trials of materials or techniques in his office in order to derive information for the eventual preparation of a clinical report, may be conducting research which requires consideration of these guidelines.

Any individual or group who is unaffiliated with an established health-related institution, but who wishes to conduct studies involving human subjects, should use a

review committee with appropriate expertise to assist in experimental design and to
assure adequate safeguards for the subjects. Advice on the scientific aspects of
clinical research may be available from
dental schools, health centers and hospitals, for example, veterans hospitals that
have a formal dental research program.

COMMENTS

*It is anticipated that certain conditions could
exist that may or may not be included or are, in
themselves, pertinent to these ethical guidelines.
The Council on Dental Research of the American Dental Association welcomes any comments
from the research community.*

Case Studies and Commentaries

SECTION SUMMARY

This final section gives you an opportunity to see how ethicists analyze a case in detail. The first two cases raise ethical questions in esthetic dentistry; the third investigates the dentist-hygienist relationship. You are invited to use these analyses, along with those from previous chapters, as models for your own commentaries on ethical issues in dentistry. You might even wish to devote portions of student, professional, or staff meetings to the ethical analysis of a challenging case as you join your colleagues in exploring what it means to be a good dentist.

Chapter 12

Esthetic Dentistry

Cases by John A. Gilbert
with Commentary by Mary Ellen Waithe

CASE I

Laura M. is a 36-year-old white woman. She has no medical problems at present, and is taking no medications. Her medical history reveals that she had a series of unexplained febrile episodes between the ages of 1 month and 6 years that were treated with tetracycline. She reports having had a hysterectomy in 1984, and is allergic to codeine. She is married and has two children aged 14 and 10. She does not smoke and reports only social alcohol consumption. Laura alternates between glasses and contact lenses for visual correction. Her weight is 103 pounds, she is 5 feet, 3 inches tall, and her blood pressure is 110/70.

Laura's occlusion is within normal limits (Class I) and she has no occlusal complaints. Her oral examination reveals no oral lesions, pink healthy tissue, and no loss of attachment, or other periodontal problems. She has 28 permanent teeth with multiple posterior conservative amalgam restorations.

There are no carious lesions. No pathology was detected in the radiographs. Her teeth display banding and marked tetracycline staining with defective amelogenesis on the labial of the maxillary anterior teeth. Where the enamel is defective, moderate abrasion has occurred.

Laura expresses marked unhappiness with the appearance of her teeth and restricts her smile to prevent a wide tooth display.

The treatment plan Laura M. accepts is porcelain veneers on teeth #6, #7, #8, #9, #10, and #11. The veneers are prepared and placed. Because of the marked contrast following placement, she also decides to have veneers placed on teeth #5 and #12. She wishes to have the lower anteriors veneered, but is restrained by financial considerations.

After placement of the veneers, Laura stops wearing her glasses (using contacts only), changes her hair color and makeup, and presents with a broad smile.

CASE 2

Carol P. is a 21-year-old white woman. She has no medical problems at present, is taking no medications, and has nothing of significance in her medical history. Carol did not finish high school, is living at home, and is an art student. She does not smoke or consume alcohol. She does report a diet high in refined carbohydrates. Her weight is 170 pounds, she is 5 feet, 9 inches tall, and her blood pressure at the time of examination is 124/82.

Carol's occlusion is Class I and she has no occlusal complaints. She has 28 teeth and has had orthodontic treatment, with a fixed lower anterior retainer still in place. Her tissue is generally healthy, with isolated areas of marginal gingivitis and bleeding. She has no loss of attachment, and no pockets greater than 4 mm. She has a moderate number of conservative anterior and posterior restorations, with no caries at present. Her teeth are normal in color with some small areas of decalcification.

Carol feels that her teeth are "dark," and has read about veneers to make them look "white." A shade analysis reveals her tooth color to be Vita B-2. She is advised that veneers are not indicated in her case. Bleaching is suggested.

She returns to the clinic 2 weeks later, insisting on the veneer treatment. She states that she hopes to become a model and needs

195

"perfect" teeth. After several consultations, the veneers are prepared and placed on teeth #5, #6, #7, #8, #9, #10, #11, and #12. Carol is very satisfied with the results and returns to have the lower anteriors veneered. Again, she is presented with arguments against such treatment. She insists and prevails, with veneers placed on #22, #23, #24, #25, #26, and #27. The measured shade change is from Vita B-2 to Vita B-1.

Two months following treatment, Carol returns to the clinic, asking that papers be signed documenting the amount and degree of tetracycline staining so that she can join in a class-action lawsuit against several drug manufacturers. The papers are not signed and Carol is informed that she shows no signs of tetracycline staining. She departs an unhappy patient, although she "loves" her "new" teeth.

Note: These cases are factual, but the names have been changed to protect confidentiality.

ETHICS AND AESTHETICS: THE MEETING OF DENTISTRY AND PHILOSOPHY

The cases of Laura M. and Carol P. appear to be unrelated except in one respect: both clients received esthetic dental treatment in the form of veneers. In the first section, I introduce the reader to the nature of the esthetic and ethical issues that esthetic dentistry faces. In the second section, I explore the issue of appropriate treatment, and in the third section I explore the issue of informed consent. In the concluding section, I suggest that, although the dentist's actions were ethically ideal in one case, they were somewhat irresponsible in the second. I offer suggestions that, had they been implemented, may have resulted in an opportunity for moral excellence on the dentist's part, with improved outcomes for all concerned.

Ethics and Esthetics in Dentistry

Theoretical inquiries into the nature of the good and the nature of the beautiful comprise the subject matters of moral philosophy (ethics) and esthetics,* respec-

* In the philosophical literature, this term is usually spelled, "aesthetics."

tively. Both fields of inquiry are traditional subspecialty areas of philosophy. In the ancient world, many, including the philosophers Pythagoras and Diotima of Mantinea, believed that the good and the beautiful were closely related.[1] More than 2000 years later, the profession of dentistry addresses ethical issues arising in the context of providing services intended to enhance esthetic qualities of the oral cavity. Nash,[2] Nasedkin,[3] and others have rightly noted that esthetic dentistry implies an improved, high-quality, lasting dental restoration that is both subjectively and objectively beautiful. Issues of ethics arise when we remember that objectively and subjectively improved beauty is a somewhat nebulous goal that might be difficult for both patient and dentist to communicate. The authors remind us that the dentist is clearly the authority on objective beauty here: questions of a tooth's anatomical structure and form, of color and translucency, of arch shape and balance, of spacing and symmetry, as well as of occlusion, are objectively specifiable by dental science and knowable by the trained, experienced esthetic dentist. It is in this purely technical sense that I use the term "objective" beauty. Moreover, two dentists may, with respect to a given patient's dentition, agree on matters of symmetry, etc., yet disagree as to whether the patient's mouth is subjectively beautiful. When it comes to subjective beauty, only the patient who has, or wants to create, an image of herself can determine whether the outcome is subjectively beautiful.

Can the dentist's purely technical criteria of the objectively beautiful be skillfully implemented in the client's mouth so that the final executed artistic production will correspond to the client's intuitive concept of what is subjectively beautiful? As philosopher Susanne Langer said in her work on esthetics:

Esthetic intuition seizes the greatest form, and therefore the main import, at once; there is no need of working through lesser ideas and serried implications first without a vision of the whole, as in discursive reasoning, where the total intuition of relatedness comes as the conclusion, like a prize. In art, it is the impact of the whole, the immediate revelation of vital import, that acts as the psychological lure to long contemplation.[4]

Clearly, the dentist has the opportunity to play a large role in informing a client's esthetic appreciation of the objectively beautiful in dentistry. The numerous technical details that the dentist specifies as contributing to the artistry of esthetic dentistry are directly perceived as a unit by anyone who sees the artistic production that is the client's mouth. That mouth is subjectively appreciated and perceived as beautiful by the client and others. The dentist might mention that the client will receive feedback from others who also subjectively appreciate such contributing factors to beauty as symmetry, shade, shape, translucency, etc.

However, sought-after results may elude the precise description of esthetic qualities that a fully informed consent process may require. The patient may not be able to describe to the dentist his or her concept of subjective beauty, and the dentist may not be able to make the patient fully grasp objective criteria of dental esthetics. Furthermore, the value to the patient of the outcome of esthetic dental treatment may not be commensurate with the time required for the procedure and with the level of difficulty involved. In addition, improved beauty is seldom the sole outcome of esthetic dentistry. Improved oral function and psychological benefits are also "goods" produced by esthetic dentistry. Conversely, damage to tooth structure may be a harm created by an esthetic procedure. Analogous issues arise with respect to the psychological benefits of improved good looks. Who can predict, let alone define, the level of emotional benefit that is worth the expense and effort of the treatment? Can the dentist? Can the client? Despite these difficulties, the assumption that improved objective beauty will be appreciated as subjective beauty by the client and will be of significant psychological benefit to the client is often an assumption of practitioner and patient alike.

Here, with the obvious and deliberate introduction of the term "client" for "patient," is perhaps the place to stress the business-like character of esthetic dentistry. Dentistry is perhaps the only health care profession that deliberately (and motivated by concerns of the public's health)[5] has endangered its own survival. Decades of persistent pressure for universal fluoridation and increased patient education efforts have resulted in less dental disease and less demand for traditional dental services. Importantly, however, it has offered consumers of dental health care the opportunity to designate dollars that would otherwise be spent for treatment of dental caries and for dental prosthetics on dental care that improves function as well as appearance. To the extent that the person seeking the services of esthetic dentistry is seeking improved oral function, or correction of handicapping esthetic problems, he or she is a patient. To the extent that the patient is seeking esthetics or improved beauty, he or she is a client, much as a dentist is to a hairdresser and interior decorator. So the esthetic dentist is as much a health care provider as a purveyor of artistry and beauty. This mixed role provides opportunity for the dentist, but also creates some ethical challenges.

Like the hairdresser and the interior decorator, the dentist, as purveyor of esthetics, has the responsibility to honestly attempt to provide the client with whatever "look" the client wants. The procedures through which a "look" is provided may be irreversible, or may have potentially serious health consequences. A client's desire for esthetic service is not usually motivated by the client's health concerns. Nevertheless, the hairdresser must not negligently spread head lice, and the interior decorator must not negligently use lead-based paint. Similarly, the practitioner of cosmetic dentistry has the responsibility to do no harm. At a minimum, that means practicing according to the ethical standards of the profession. These responsibilities are increased to the extent that the services provided significantly risk oral health and function. We want, therefore, to examine in the next section whether the alternative procedures offered to Carol and Laura are dentally sound, and, in the third section, whether each gave informed consent to them. In the fourth section, I suggest that Carol's actions show that her consent to veneers, although legally sufficient, was less than optimally informed and that, in consequence, Carol was overtreated. I will explore how additional inquiry by the dentist may have avoided the overtreatment and may have derailed her clumsy attempt to involve the dentist in fraud.

Appropriate Treatment

The range of treatment options available for improving tooth color and masking imperfections includes bleaching, direct bonding, and laminating veneers. Hypoplasia is associated with lifestyle factors such as smoking and diet, with restorations, with medications such as tetracycline and excessive fluoride, and with aging and hereditary factors.[6] Teeth are most susceptible to tetracycline staining during ondogenesis.[7] The diagnosis of hypoplasia caused by tetracycline staining is evidenced by banding and supported by Laura's history. Carol's teeth evidence some areas of decalcification.

According to Goldstein, bleaching of vital teeth to correct hypoplasia by lightening color is approximately 75% effective.[8] Poor candidates for bleaching include patients with extremely sensitive teeth, exceptionally large pulp chambers,[6] misshapen or pitted teeth, or teeth having severe loss of enamel or large restorations.[7] Bleaching does not evenly color teeth that are striated or have white spots. Bleaching is also inappropriate for discoloration caused by metallic salts, particularly silver amalgam.[7] Other contraindications that may be present in the cases we are considering, but about which the case descriptions are silent include enlargement of the pulp, and cracked or severely undermined enamel. I therefore assume that none of these contraindicative conditions are present with respect to either Carol or Laura.

Just as there are contraindications to bleaching, there are limits to what bleaching can accomplish for a client. The exact shade cannot be predicted; other restorations must be matched to the bleached tooth; incisors may not absorb as much as canines and premolars and may lighten less; and follow-up bleaching at intervals of 1 to 3 years will be needed to maintain brightness.[7] Will Carol become unhappy when her teeth are again looking "dark"?

Bleaching, a technique that has been around for a century,[6] is not effective in severe tetracycline staining. Third-degree tetracycline staining, that is, staining accompanied by banding, "usually remains even after extensive bleaching."[7] In Laura's case, bleaching alone may make the banding more evident because "the lighter stains respond more effectively to bleaching, increasing the relative contrast between the two colors."[9] The dentist appropriately advises that bleaching alone is not recommended in Laura's case because the prognosis is not good despite the fact that some lightening can be expected.[9] According to Goldstein,

> Nonetheless, bleaching alone will create considerable improvement, [in tetracycline stained teeth] sometimes after only three or four treatments. If a veneering technique is to be used, such preliminary bleaching can help make the veneered teeth appear whiter.[7]

Bleaching as a preparation to veneering Laura's teeth may be appropriate, depending upon the darkness of the stain and other factors.

In 1966, composite resin began to replace pinning and crowning of fractured teeth. With the introduction of Nuvalite in 1972 came the potential to cure resin on demand. The eighties saw the popularization of the use of visible light and microfine composite resins, creating for the first time improved color stability and high lustre. The life expectancy of composite resin bonds on etched tooth enamel was 5 to 8 years, provided that margins were properly finished.[8]

Bonds are reversible but may not cover tetracycline-stained teeth like Laura's. Can bonding mask the stain in Laura's teeth without overbuilding? How much translucency is in the teeth that requires matching? We must remember that it is difficult to incorporate translucency into a bonded tooth; translucency is much easier to achieve with veneers. A client's eating habits must also enter into the dentist's treatment recommendations. Neither Laura nor Carol is a smoker, but we do not have information about either's consumption of stain-inducers like coffee, cola, and tea.

Carol, we may infer, does not drink dark wines. We know only that Laura "drinks socially." If that social drinking is of deep colored wines, Laura can expect staining with bonds. Carol, on the other hand, has isolated areas of gingivitis, as well as a retainer. If Carol's gingivitis and pockets mean that she is a candidate for repeated professional prophylaxis, it will shorten life expectancy of bonds, and veneers would be a better choice.

Laminating, the prefabricated construction and bonding of composite resin, acrylic resin, or porcelain veneers to an etched tooth structure,[8] turned out to be the treatment provided for both Laura and Carol.

> Porcelain veneers are indicated for the esthetic correction of multiple tooth discolorations, enamel defects, diastemas and malformations. . . . Porcelain veneers offer long-term color stability; high bond strength to resist fracture and dislocation; excellent soft tissue biocompatibility; sustained abrasion resistance; and detailed surface anatomy and texture.[6]

Although individual operator's results vary with experience and technique, porcelain-fused-to-metal restorations (PFMs) on teeth with intra-enamel modification show increased resistance to stress,[3] so they might also be desirable. These are some of the numerous clinical considerations for recommending veneers to Laura and for acquiescing to the request for them by Carol. What degree of esthetic perfection is possible without significant reduction of enamel and taking into account the degree of enamel hypoplasia, the desired life expectancy of the restoration, the maintenance required, treatment time, and costs?

Veneers have some disadvantages: they are more costly than bonding, require two appointments, and are an irreversible procedure, except on the unreduced tooth.[8] In addition, there are failures in that veneers tend to chip during the contouring procedure. This is particularly true of the porcelain veneers, composites tending to permit thinner edges without chipping.[10] Carol and Laura both need to understand that porcelain veneers can chip in the future, and may need to be repaired. They also need to know that experts offer conflicting opinions as to whether porcelain

laminates can stain.[3,8] Here, the dentist's own experiences prove informative. According to Goldstein,[8] the comparative advantages and disadvantages for bonding or for laminating veneers are:

> Bonding requires no anesthesia and little or no tooth reduction. It offers immediate results that change tooth color and is a reversible, economical process. Laminating also usually requires no anesthesia because it requires little tooth reduction, it can mask dark color, and lasts longer than bonding because it wears less.

Bonding has disadvantages such as chipping and staining. Bonds may also cause the teeth to appear somewhat thicker, an unnecessary consequence with veneers unless the reduction is insufficient. Bonding to cover stained, discolored teeth gives an unesthetic appearance of marked shade contrast with adjacent teeth unless the stained tooth is first treated with opaquer, or a series of masking agents are used to help blend the restoration to the adjacent tooth structure.[8] Therefore, bonding would be a feasible alternative treatment modality for Laura, provided it was preceded by bleaching and/or by treatment with opaquers or maskers.

In sum, bonding, preceded by bleaching and/or opaquers, and veneers both appear to be appropriate esthetic dental options for Laura. Both procedures will produce for Laura comparable subjectively esthetic results. Both procedures are permanent and irreversible and in that sense morally harm Laura by foreclosing future options. Both procedures require some physical harm to underlying tooth structure, and in that sense require the dentist to "do harm" to her dentition. The harm, however does not violate the dentist's moral duty to "do no harm" because, on balance, either procedure simply corrects the harm already done by tetracycline staining. When determining which procedures to offer to the client as appropriate treatment options, it is the dentist with the greater knowledge of comparative harms to dentition, and with the greater knowledge of objective esthetics (shade, translucency, tooth thickness, etc.) who rank orders the appropriate treatments and presents them as options from which the client may choose. The dentist does not offer as an option a procedure (for example, RCT) that would not achieve the desired effect. Nor does the dentist offer as an option a procedure (for example, extractions and implants) that professional judgment indicates would cause more harm than good to the patient's oral health and function. However, once the appropriate options have been identified by the dentist and presented to the patient, the dentist has a moral duty to provide whichever option the patient decides upon or to refer the patient to another dentist if necessary. The patient has the moral right to rank-order these options based on criteria that he or she has identified as relevant, consistent with his or her own values, needs, preferences, etc. So, for example, if the need for masking and for permanent coverage of banding is of concern to Laura, or if the somewhat better life expectancy of veneers is a consideration for her, then she may consider veneers a better option. Notice that it is Laura, and not the dentist, who rank-orders subjectively esthetic and financial values.

With Carol, the situation is somewhat different. Because Carol's shade is already Vita B-2, bleaching may well provide as objectively measurable good lightening (to Vita B-1) as would bonds or veneers. Bleaching would accomplish this objectively measurable esthetic improvement at far reduced cost and with no damage to enamel. The uncertainty of Carol's gingival health and the appearance of shallow pockets, her relative youthfulness, and her diet suggest that she might not be happy with bonds. Given some objectively determinable factors such as her age, employment status, and already light tooth shade, the harm to underlying tooth structure, and the irreversibility and cost of veneers, the dentist rightly concluded that veneers were not an appropriate option for Carol. The dentist is to be commended for initially recommending against veneers and for recommending a more conservative, less harmful treatment, bleaching. In so doing, the dentist demonstrates the seriousness with which the moral requirement to "do no harm" is taken. It is Carol who calls upon the dentist to "do harm" to her enamel. What is important to reflect upon here is that selecting a treatment is not like going to your freezer and selecting tonight's dinner from among the foods you have already stocked up on. It is more like going to a restaurant and selecting from a menu designed by someone else. The client does not go to the dentist and order RCT the way that you order a BLT; the dentist, like the restauranteur, offers a choice of procedures. The dentist, as a consequence of professional duty, may only offer as options procedures that, in the dentist's judgment, are appropriate for the client. It is from this predetermined and usually very limited menu that the client may choose. As in the case with Laura, the dentist-client relationship does not morally permit the dentist to offer as a service a procedure (for example, extractions and implants) that, in the dentist's professional judgment, is inappropriate for achieving the outcome that Carol desires. The ethical difficulty for the dentist arises when a client insists that a procedure be performed and the procedure is one that, in the dentist's professional opinion, is not an appropriate option to offer this patient. If the dentist's knowledge, training, and experience leads him or her to conclude that veneers constitute unnecessarily harmful overtreatment in Carol's case, it would violate the dentist's own moral judgment to require him or her to offer as an option a procedure that he or she believes unnecessarily harms the patient. The dentist not only has no moral duty to offer the requested procedure in violation of his or her own professional moral judgment, but has no moral right to do so. From my reading of the case, Carol's situation is not the typical situation where several more or less equivalent procedures exist, *all of which* are, in the dentist's professional judgment, sound options. If Carol's were such a case, the dentist would be morally required to present at least some of those options. In Carol's case, the dentist sees no real need for any procedure (Vita B-2 is already a fairly bright shade), but because some lightening is technically possible, recommends bleaching. The dentist has neither the moral duty nor the moral right to offer options for treatments that are not in his or her judgment dentally sound options. The client may demand whatever treatment she prefers; but when the dentist believes that acquiescing to that demand requires him to violate a professional duty to do no harm, the dentist cannot morally be compelled by the client to violate that duty.

If a client is informed of the physically harmful nature of the treatment he or she is requesting, and if he or she adequately understands the information that is presented, it is difficult to turn him or her away from a treatment that will produce both objectively and subjectively esthetic results. We may be tempted to conclude that all we need do is inform the client that the procedure he or she is requesting is one that does minor yet irreversible damage to tooth structure, is expensive, and is something that he or she may ultimately regret. We may be tempted to acquiesce to the client's persistent request, provided that we are certain that he or she has given informed consent to the procedure. In the following paragraphs, I argue that, even if the dentist did believe that veneers were a viable esthetic option in Carol's case, it may be difficult to obtain truly informed consent from Carol.

Informed Consent

The primary responsibility of the dentist is to do no harm. The traditional conception of what constitutes "harm" in dentistry has been that harm is construed in terms of physical or psychological damage. However, here I want to urge that "harm" be considered more broadly to include also harms to a client's moral rights. This is the basis for claiming that a dentist harms a client if services are rendered without informed consent, if the client's autonomy is not respected, etc. Autonomy and informed consent are related concepts. A person who is an autonomous decision maker has the ethical and legal right to make an informed decision about whether to follow or reject health care recommendations made by a provider. A person is considered to be an autonomous decision maker when he or she is capable of the ordinary amount of understanding; when his or her ability to reason and make a decision is not seriously impaired by im-

maturity, ignorance or psychiatric illness; and when his or her ability to carry out a decision is likewise not seriously impaired.[11] One of the many ways in which health care providers can demonstrate respect for a client's autonomy is by engaging in mutual dialogue: the provider selecting treatment options and interpreting technical scientific information about those options for the client and the client sharing with the provider sufficient history and knowledge of his or her preferences, values, habits, level of interest in detail, etc., so that information about options can be tailored by the provider for the client. A series of exchanges occurs in which information is traded and analyzed by both parties: the dentist screening out details that are irrelevant, excessive, or otherwise unwanted by the client; the client processing information and proffering questions until he or she is satisfied that he or she has enough information to feel comfortable about reaching a decision.

We must assume that the dentist has made Carol and Laura aware of the nature of the procedures that would be dentally sound alternatives, their benefits, and the potential risks to health and/or function of each procedure. We are not told what alternatives were presented to Laura, only what recommendation was made.

Laura's unhappiness with her markedly banded maxillary anteriors may suggest that her psychological well-being would be improved by a more esthetically pleasing smile. However, the converse seems unlikely: medically significant psychological disturbance would hardly ensue were she unable to achieve a full complement of pearly whites. After all, Laura appears to have taken good care of her health. She does not engage in self-destructive behaviors like smoking or excessive alcohol consumption. She may be somewhat apprehensive about approaching 40. She may be coping with the expected difficulties of pubescent children and with the physical and psychological stresses that may attend premature hysterectomy-induced menopause. But these are routine psychological stresses, not illnesses, disorders, or dysfunctions in themselves. In someone else, these stresses might have led to serious disorder, but before making the treatment recommendation, the dentist had no reason to think that in Laura's case they would. Laura's physical and psychological health is not threatened. If she were to forego treatment, her health would not be compromised. Her self-image might well be boosted by appropriate esthetic dentistry; however, she does not seek esthetic dentistry to regain psychological or physical health. It would, I believe, be stretching the concept of "health" to suggest otherwise. What is meant here is that there is no evidence of any medical or psychological disorders that can be relieved, treated, cured, or prevented in Laura's case through the provision of esthetic dental service.

From the description given of Laura's personal as well as medical and oral health history, we get the impression of a mature, intelligent, clear-headed client whose oral health values and habits are consistent with her expressed desire for an improved appearance. Her motivation is high, her health habits are good, and, most importantly, her request for esthetic dentistry is consistent with the clinical indicators. We understand immediately the reasonableness of her desire for correction of the tetracycline staining. Nothing in her history or present interest in dental services is out of the ordinary. She appears to be an autonomous decision-maker. We must assume that the dentist's respect for her autonomy was reflected in part by the range of dentally sound alternative treatments that were presented to her. If we assume, as we must, that the treatment was competently provided and that the fee structure was within professional norms, we may safely conclude that with respect to Laura, the requirements of the "Do No Harm" principle have been met by the dentist, and additionally, Laura has given informed consent.

Like Laura, Carol is unhappy with the appearance of her teeth. Like Laura, Carol believes that she will look better with whiter teeth. Carol's situation, however, is somewhat different from Laura's and therefore poses an increased moral challenge to the dentist. On Carol's first visit, the dentist knows only her history and her (probably popular-magazine source of) desire for veneers to whiten her teeth. She walks in the door and, in a not uncommon reversal of roles, *the client informs the dentist what the list of treatment options are.* It is a one-item list. We are not told why Carol has an anterior retainer in place, nor do we know how visible it is. We do know that the dental treatment she seeks is sought because she desires to improve her appearance. On her second visit, she announces a career interest in modelling, so we feel confident that there are no health- or function-related indicators for dental treatment. Like Laura's, Carol's preference for veneers is not to relieve psychological disorder or dysfunction. In comparison to Laura's situation, however, it is not clear that a minor improvement in an already good shade (an improvement that would be imperceptible to the untrained eye) should realistically confer any psychological benefit. At least, we do not know this before completing treatment.

If the dentist has explained to Carol the dental pros and cons of bleaching versus veneers, as well as the comparative costs, and she still insists on veneers, unless (as I argued previously), one of these options is not dentally sound, the dentist may ethically provide the desired service. Carol's choice may not be the best one, and her career expectations may be overly optimistic, but she is, at least legally speaking, competent to make a choice. Morally, then, we may not refuse to provide her with the chosen treatment unless it would be unsound dentistry to do so. Informed consent cannot be obtained when a dentist fails to inform a client that an unsound procedure is not on the menu of treatment options. Unfortunately, however, the client has insisted that veneers are on the list. To help her understand why they are *not*, the dentist must follow a process that parallels that used for procedures that are menu options. The fact that Carol might continue to insist on veneers does not morally excuse the dentist for capitulating and adding them to the menu. The dentist's moral reasoning in this case is not elaborated upon, but it appears to be the case that, in the dentist's original professional judgment, the ethically more praiseworthy solution was bleaching. If I am correct in my reading of this case, the preferred solution would be to learn a bit more about Carol so that the dentist can be reassured that whatever decision Carol reaches is one that reflects a realistic assessment of what her needs really are.

Opportunity for Moral Excellence

As the case is described, we cannot determine with confidence whether the *dentist* is sufficiently knowledgeable about the relationship of the "Do No Harm Principle" to informed consent, or knows enough about Carol to be able to provide *her* with the information that she needs if she is going to make an informed choice. It is clear that, during Carol's visits, conversations took place that were necessarily omitted from the case description. We wonder, then, just what transpired during those conversations. How informed is the dentist about Carol's values, preferences, needs, and expectations? Are her esthetic values and goals clear, and is her lifestyle consistent with the pursuit of those goals? Are her subjectively esthetic preferences for a certain "look" realistically achievable, given that lifestyle? Or do her history and her present lifestyle suggest that Carol is defeating her stated goals?

If the dentist does not really understand what Carol's subjectively esthetic preferences and goals are and how they fit (or do not fit) her lifestyle, the information provided to Carol may not enable her to understand why veneers are not on the menu. Carol needs the dentist's help if she is to make a choice consistent with her values, preferences, needs, and expectations. What is worse, Carol may not learn for quite some time whether her insistence on overtreatment was consistent with her actual values, her settled preferences and her long-range needs. She may be happy for a while with her new teeth, but they are an expensive investment. The change that she wants in her appearance, if indeed one can call a change from Vita B-2 to Vita B-1 a change in appearance, is obtainable uninvasively and at far lower cost through bleaching. The harm done to Carol is not a significant physical harm in spite of the irreversibility of the procedure. It is simply that a permanent restoration has been made where an uninvasive res-

toration could have achieved the same result. The permanency of veneers precludes less invasive restorations when those veneers eventually need replacing. The harm to her enamel may not be significant, depending upon the degree of reduction needed. The harm done by unconservative treatment probably will not pose serious harm to her oral health, so I do not want to blow it out of proportion. But there is another harm, a financial harm: an immature young woman's loss of potentially better-spent savings. The savings could be applied perhaps toward completing the orthodontic treatment, some nutritional and educational counselling, or toward some other service that would be more conducive to securing Carol's long term happiness.

From the material that has been presented about Carol's personal and medical history, there is evidence that Carol does not really know what she wants. Art and modelling are similar interests of hers. Both involve objective as well as subjective standards of beauty. Carol may say that she wants to pursue modelling, but at her present weight, her career options will be limited to "large model" opportunities. It is not an unrealistic goal; many women her size are models. It is not the seeming inconsistency between her diet, her size, and her modelling aspirations that makes me wonder whether Carol knows what she really wants when she insists that veneers are on the menu.

Rather, it is that fixed lower anterior retainer that concerns me. Has Carol made other false starts at improving her smile? *Should* that retainer still be there; shouldn't the present dentist advise her that he wishes to consult with her orthodontist prior to commencing treatment? Orthodontists have reputations for being advocates for periodontal health. Faulty oral hygiene can turn successful orthodontics into an unsightly mess of gingivitis, root caries, and caries on the labial of anteriors. Carol's gingivitis and pockets suggest that her oral hygiene efforts have not supported the work begun by the orthodontist. We are not told how much of the fixed anterior is visible, nor what her smile line is; however, the reader is led to suspect that an unphotogenic smile is in the offing.

Is the retainer "still" in place because Carol quickly tires of a treatment plan, gets discouraged, and doesn't return for follow-through? Or perhaps she owes fees to the orthodontist and doesn't feel that she can return unless she can complete payment for her treatment.

The preceding observations are consistent with other indicators of habit and lifestyle-related matters. Carol is a high school dropout; when the dentist meets her, she is an art student but soon thereafter is headed toward the reputedly remunerative career of modelling. Is she making a career change, or are we to understand that her art training is preparatory to the modelling career? The dentist needs to interview her further, and to understand whether Carol's values are consistent with her choice. Carol's diet is another concern; is there a relationship between it and the decalcification, the gingivitis, the bleeding? A red flag should go up when a client insists on a treatment modality that is inconsistent with the clinical indications, and with the dentist's own professional judgment. Aren't educational, career, dietary and dental history factors multiple indicators that Carol is unhappy with her life, her appearance, and her prospects, and consistently fails to follow through on major undertakings like schooling, diet, and dental treatment?

It may just be the case that Carol's training in art is such that she *can* correctly identify Vita B-1 wherever she sees it. It may be the case that, without shade samples in front of her to compare, she can also correctly identify Vita B-2 and wouldn't mistake it for Vita B-1. However, I wonder whether she could correctly match the shade of her pre-veneered teeth on a chart. It is a shade difference so slight as to challenge even experienced operators.

I strongly suspect that further questioning would have revealed that Carol read something in a glamour magazine about what veneers can do for models' teeth. The same journalistic source may have mentioned the class action suits against a wealthy pharmaceutical manufacturer. It may have mentioned that some people (Laura comes to mind) actually had to go to the expense of having their teeth ve-

neered to cover up the unsightly stains. It may have mentioned that litigants hope to recover many times the cost of their cosmetic dentistry. So a resourceful, uneducated, unemployed, overweight, aimless young woman knocks on the dentist's door determined to walk out veneered and ready to model. She has already figured out that a litigious windfall will end up paying for the cosmetic treatment and perhaps the orthodontics too. She feeds the dentist's professional ego when she says how much she loves her new teeth as she asks the dentist to sign documents that ultimately will pay his bill and give her career its start. Admittedly, this scenario is pure speculation, but in light of what Carol really did, it is not unrealistic speculation.

Although time is needed for patients to objectively assess their esthetic dentistry needs, time alone does not suffice to ensure that a realistic choice for esthetics has been made. What is important here is the quality of the analysis of need that is done. With some appropriate interviewing by the dentist, perhaps Carol would have come to realize before demanding veneers, that the dentist knew that her teeth were not tetracycline-stained and that there would be no collusion in perpetrating a fraud upon the pharmaceutical company. Perhaps Carol would have come to understand that veneers were overkill and bleaching would suffice. Perhaps she would have realized that the pleasing appearance needed for a successful modelling career required more than whiter teeth: it required good diet, good oral hygiene, and probably the completion of her orthodontic therapy.

The constraints on a dentist's time are many. Often, and particularly when a client is new to the practice, the dentist has not had an opportunity to get to know the client. It was morally irresponsible of the dentist to acquiesce to Carol's demands. It was not a serious moral shortcoming: harm was done, but not great harm. Yet, these two seemingly unrelated cases reveal a missed opportunity for moral excellence on the part of the dentist. Further inquiry of Carol could have resulted in an improved result for her and, in an odd way, for Laura also. Perhaps if Laura had been informed by the dentist of the class-action tetracycline suit and had chosen to participate in it, the dentist could have assisted with documentation for that purpose If negligence were proven on the part of the pharmaceutical company, perhaps the settlement that Laura might receive would be used to correct tetracycline staining on her lower anteriors. But constraints on time spent with clients resulted in a lost opportunity for everyone. Perhaps the cases are not so unrelated after all.

ACKNOWLEDGEMENTS

I wish to thank Jenny Heyl, Research Assistant, Cleveland State University Bioethics Certificate Program for her capable research assistance, and for suffering through early drafts of this paper and making useful comments on them. The following members of the Professional Ethics in Dentistry Network also graciously shared their expertise: John Gilbert, DDS, School of Dentistry, University of Missouri-Kansas City provided the two cases and reassured me that I neither misinterpreted them nor misunderstood the technical foundations of esthetic dentistry described in this paper; Charles A. Clark, DDS, Case Western Reserve University School of Dentistry, my colleague as well as my student, provided insight as well as much needed guidance; Bruce D. Weinstein, Ph.D., West Virginia University Center for Health Ethics and Law, the editor of this volume, offered many useful comments and suggestions that helped me make needed clarifications to this chapter.

REFERENCES

1. Waithe, M.E.: A History of Women Philosophers, Vol 1: Ancient Women Philosophers. Dordrecht, Martinus Nijdoff, 1987.
2. Nash, D.A.: Professional ethics and esthetic dentistry. J. Am. Dent. Assoc. *117*:7E, 1988.
3. Nasedkin, J.N.: Porcelain laminates. J. Can. Dent. Assoc. *54*:249, 1988.
4. Langer, S.K.: Feeling and Form: A Theory of Art. New York, Charles Scribner's Sons, 1953.
5. Waithe, M.E.: AIDS and dentistry: conflicting rights and the public's health. Biomedical Ethics Reviews, 141–167, 1988.
6. Feinman, R.A.: A combination therapy. Can. Dent. Assoc. J. *15*:4, 10, 1987.
7. Goldstein, R.E.: Bleaching teeth: New materials—new role. J. Am. Dent. Assoc., Special Issue, December, 1987, p. 44E.
8. Goldstein, R.E.: Diagnostic dilemma: To bond, laminate or crown? Int. J. Periodont. Restor. Dentistry 7:9, 1987.
9. Goldstein, C.E., Goldstein, R.E., Feinman, R.A., and Garber, D.A.: Bleaching vital teeth: State of the art. Quintessence International *20*:729, 1989.
10. Braze, G.W.: Cosmetic laminate surgery—for better or for worse? Part III: The composite laminates. Trends Tech. Contemp. Dent. Lab. *3*: 20, 1986.
11. Waithe, M.E.: Why Mill was for paternalism. Int. J. Law Psychiatry *6*:101, 1983.

BIBLIOGRAPHY

Anitua, E., Zabalegui, B., Gil, J., and Gascon, F.: Internal bleaching of severe tetracycline discolorations: Four-year clinical evaluation. Quintessence International *21*:783, 1990.
Boksman, L., Jordan, R.E., Suzuki, M., et al.: Etched porcelain labial veneers. Ontario Dentist *62*:11, 1985.
Braze, G.W.: Cosmetic laminate dentistry—For better or for worse? Trends Tech. Contemp. Dent. Lab. *2*:12, 1985.
Braze, G.W.: Cosmetic laminate dentistry—For better or for worse? Part II: The composite laminates. Trends. Tech. Contemp. Dent. Lab. *3*:16, 1986.
Braze, G.W.: Cosmetic laminate dentistry—For better or for worse? Part III: The porcelain laminates. Trends Tech. Contemp. Dent. Lab. *3*:20, 1986.
Burgoyne, A.R., Boksman, L., Jordan, R.E., and Suzuki, M.: The conservative application of resin labial veneers: A case report. Ontario Dentist *62*: 30, 1985.
Calamia, J.R.: Etched porcelain veneers: The current state of the art. Quintessence International *16*: 5, 1985.
Calamia, J.R.: High-strength porcelain bonded restorations: Anterior and posterior. Quintessence International *20*:717, 1989.
Christensen, G.J.: Veneering of teeth, state of the art. Dent. Clin. North Am. *29*:373, 1985.
Cohen, B.D., and Abrams, B.L.: An unusual case of stained roots of unerupted third molars. Gen. Dentistry *37*:342, 1989.
Feinman, R.A.: A combination therapy. Can. Dent. Assoc. J. *15*:10, 1987.
Fleming, P., Witkop, C.J., and Kuhlmann, W.H.: Staining and hypoplasia of enamel caused by tetracycline: Case report. Pediatr. Dentistry *9*: 245, 1987.
Goldstein, C.E., Goldstein, R.E., Feinman, R.A., and Garber, D.A.: Bleaching vital teeth: State of the art. Quintessence International *20*:729, 1989.
Goldstein, R.E.: Diagnostic dilemma: To bond, laminate or crown? Internat. J. Periodont. Restor. Dentistry 7:9, 1987.
Goldstein, R.E.: Bleaching teeth: New materials—

new role. J. Am. Dent. Assoc., Special Issue, December, 44E, 1987.

Grossman, E.R.: Tetracycline and staining of the teeth (letter). JAMA 255:2442, 1986.

Jensen, O.E., Soltys, J.L.: Six months clinical evaluation of prefabricated veneer restorations after partial enamel removal. J. Oral Rehabil. 13:49, 1986.

King, N.M., and Wei, S.H.: Developmental defects of enamel: study of 12-year-olds in Hong Kong. J. Am. Dent. Assoc. 112:835, 1986.

Lackey, A.D.: Examining your smile. Dent. Clin. North Am. 33:133, 1989.

Langer, S.K.: Feeling and Form: A Theory of Art. New York, Charles Scribner's Sons, 1953.

Nasedkin, J.N.: Porcelain laminates. J. Can. Dent. Assoc. 54:248, 1988.

Nash, D.A.: Professional ethics and esthetic dentistry. J. Am. Dent. Assoc. 117:7E, 1988.

Poliak, S.C., DiGiovanna, J.J., Gross, E.G., et al. Minocycline-associated tooth discoloration in young adults. JAMA 254:2930, 1985.

Taleghani, M., and Leinfelder, K.F.: A modified technique for facial veneering. General Dentistry 33:317, 1985.

Walls, A.W.G., Murray, J.J., McCabe, J.F.: Composite laminate veneers: a clinical study. J. Oral Rehabil. 15:439, 1988.

Waithe, M.E.: A History of Women Philosophers, Vol. 1: Ancient Women Philosophers. Dordrecht, Martinus Nijhoff, 1987.

Waithe, M.E.: Why Mill was for paternalism. Int. J. Law Psychiatry 6:101, 1983.

Waithe, M.E.: AIDS and Dentistry: Conflicting Rights and the Public's Health. Biomedical Ethics Reviews, 141–167, 1988.

Wilson, C.F.G., and Seale, N.S.: Color change following vital bleaching of tetracycline-stained teeth. Pediatr. Dentistry 7:205, 1985.

Witkop, C.J., and Wolf, R.O.: Hypoplasia and intrinsic staining of enamel following tetracycline therapy. JAMA 185:1008, 1963.

Chapter 13

When the Dentist Tells the Hygienist: "Just Do It!"

B. Bizup Hawkins

SUMMARY

The goals of preventive oral health care are many. Dentists and dental hygienists screen for existing oral disease and improve patient self-care through education while maintaining oral wellness by altering the environment that fosters the disease process. One of the tools used to screen for, and likewise prevent, disease spread is the dental radiograph.

Although radiation can serve as an invaluable tool in the prevention and early detection of disease, it can also be abused. The following case illustrates a dentist's directive to take a radiograph with questionable warrant. The interprofessional conflict that ensues permeates most healthcare disciplines. For the registered dental hygienist, though, this particular moral dilemma is one of the most difficult situations to handle. This case promptly brings to our attention the conflicts associated with an order to perform an unnecessary and inappropriate procedure, with potentially harmful consequences, on a minor.

CASE 1

This incident occurred in 1983. The patient, born in 1980, was 3 years old at the time. It was his first visit to the dentist, and for purposes of confidentiality, I will refer to him as Ian. His mother was with him and was dependent upon public assistance to pay for the appointment. The child's parents are divorced, and the mother has custody of the boy.

The dental hygienist introduced Ian to the dental operatory, and began to care for him by taking a full series of pedodontic x rays which the dentist requested on all new patients. After the radiographs were developed, she polished his teeth, administered topical fluoride, and taught him how to care for his dentition. After 45 minutes, although by this time he was somewhat cranky, Ian remained a very cooperative dental patient. As the hygienist completed the caries examination and the dental charting, the dentist came into the room to examine Ian's teeth and evaluate his radiographs. Upon completion, the dentist stated that Ian had a healthy, caries-free dentition that required no further treatment. At this point, the dentist turned to the hygienist and requested that a panorex x ray be taken before the child left the office. The hygienist reminded the dentist, in a discrete manner, that a full series of films had already been taken and were found to be negative. The dentist responded by saying, "We should get one, so take it."

Because of the hygienist's mounting concern over an excess of unjustifiable radiation, and concern for the emotional stamina of a small child on his first visit to the dentist, she consulted Ian's mother. She asked how she felt about x rays on her child, hoping that the dialogue might prompt a request for more information about the necessity of the film, or even that the mother would refuse the x ray on behalf of her son. The hygienist also said that it would be necessary to make special adjustments on the equipment because this was not a routine procedure on a 3-year-old.

Ian's mother responded hesitantly, by saying that she assumed that the dentist knew what was best for her son. Her biggest concern was ensuring that her son would have good teeth. The dentist told Ian's mother that the additional film would further verify the healthy state of this child. The hygienist is concerned by the dentist's request and wonders what she should do.

Commentary

The hygienist in this case is faced with having to refuse to perform a procedure on moral grounds. The ethical question raised is this: Would the hygienist be justified in not following the dentist's request for a radiograph? Refusing to reply to a demand for action, for moral reasons, is called a *conscientious objection*. For example, many young men and women in the 1960s refused to participate in the Vietnam War because they held that the war was morally wrong. Although it was *illegal* for them to so abstain, those persons believed they were morally justified in doing so. They held that there was an authority higher than the law, which required them to refuse to participate in the war. It is important to consider what the relevant laws are, however, before reaching a moral conclusion about what the hygienist in the case ought to do. Thus I begin my analysis by considering some of the applicable regulations. I continue by identifying other relevant facts that play a role in the case, as well as some important moral considerations, before identifying options open to the hygienist and defending one from a moral point of view.

Dental hygienists, like registered nurses, have legal restrictions placed upon their professional autonomy, but unlike nurses, registered dental hygienists do not have the privilege to set the standards that guide their education, licensure, and scope of practice.[1] At the time of the writing of this text, the self regulation of dental hygiene by dental hygienists is nonexistent in the United States. Dental hygiene is the only remaining licensed occupation whose members must pass both national, regional and state board exams, but who are legislatively denied the freedom to regulate the conditions under which they must work.

Clarification over regulatory conflicts can be noted in the rules and regulations established by the following state's Dental Boards: Georgia, Illinois, Massachusetts, New Hampshire, New Jersey, Pennsylvania, Virginia. For example, although hygienists are responsible for obtaining radiographs, in some states they are not allowed to determine the need for them. One example of a specific state in which the need for radiographs must be prescribed under the direct supervision of dentist is Pennsylvania. In this state, because dental hygienists cannot prescribe this need, neither can they legitimately refuse its recommendation. Also, conscientious refusals by nurses to carry out work orders are often supported by the professional guidelines for the license under which they practice, because nurses set the standards for the practice of nursing. Without such self-regulated guidelines, dental hygienists are forced to comply with an occupational environment often grossly inconsistent with their capabilities and with the knowledge required to pass dental hygiene licensing board examinations. Although nurses experience various kinds of interprofessional conflict, they do not experience regulatory conflicts to the degree that dental hygienists do.[2] According to current legislation, if directives given to dental hygienists by dentists are dictated according to poor or careless judgement, there is little to protect the hygienist from advancing or withholding a particular action.

The hygienist in this case is considering making a conscientious objection because she believes that taking a radiograph may harm the patient. What is the nature of this harm? Are there any benefits to taking the radiograph? In other words, what are the *consequences* of the panorex radiograph that the dentist orders? Among the hazardous effects of exposing young children to panorex x rays are the increased susceptibility of immature tissue to the long-term effects of radiation exposure; an increased concentration of radiation exposure to children relative to adults because of decreased head size, which may heighten the risk of thyroid cancer. Additional tissues that are particularly radiosensitive in young dental patients are the lenses of the eyes, the occipital and temporomandibular regions, and the bone marrow of the mandible.[3] The cumulative effect of ionizing radiation is unknown.[4,5] Although the Occupational Safety and Health Administration (OSHA) provides no guidelines for radiation safety for the dental patient, some believe that the safest level of radiation is no radiation at all.[6,7] Another nontrivial risk is the possibility of exhausting the child from yet another dental procedure.

The dentist in the case is using the panorex radiograph as a preventive measure. He may hold that his duty to detect potential problems includes protecting his patients from asymptomatic pathology or occult osseous malignancies that might be potentially life-threatening.[4,6,8] However, research on the efficacy of the panorex as a screening device on preschool children suggests that, of the small percentage of pathoses that might be detected in this age group, none of the findings would be considered life-threatening. It is for this reason, along with the potential dangers of the procedure outlined, that many in the academic community believe that the panorex as a diagnostic tool yields a poor risk/benefit ratio,[8] and that panographic screening in pedodontic patients is too harmful to justify its utilization.[3,7,9]

Ian's mother trustingly depends on the educated advice of the dentist to help her make decisions for her son. Her willingness to abide by the dentist's recommendation is based on the assumption that the radiograph is taken because it will be beneficial to her son's welfare. In this case, that turns out to be a questionable assumption. As with the majority of the general public, Ian's mother is unaware of the contraindications or electiveness of certain procedures. Likewise, under such circumstances, she is unable to provide informed consent based on an intelligent assessment of all the consequences, and this makes the likelihood of her making an autonomous decision for her son very remote. We are getting closer to deciding whether the hygienist is obligated to respect a decision that is based upon an incomplete understanding of the treatment.

Other factual considerations play a role in our ethical analysis of the case. Because Ian is a minor, he does not have the capacity to make treatment decisions on his own behalf. Who, then, has the authority to do so? Even though the state is subsidizing the child's oral health care, it is the child's mother to whom society defers to make the relevant treatment decisions (and most others, for that matter). While a parent's right to make such decisions is not absolute (e.g., parents who are Jehovah's Witnesses may refuse blood transfusions for themselves but not for their children), the presumption in our society is that parents will make decisions that are truly in the best interests of their dependents. Thus it is Ian's mother who has the moral authority to provide or refuse consent to dental procedures.

We are now in a position to consider what is morally at stake in the case. Because Ian is too young to make an autonomous decision for himself, the principle of respect for autonomy does not play a role in this case. However, the hygienist does have a duty to respect the right of her patient's proxy decision maker to make informed choices on her son's behalf. Another category of moral responsibility is the hygienist's obligation of fidelity to her employer. In other words, it is appropriate to use the language of ethics in framing the dentist-hygienist relationship, and to say that the hygienist has a moral duty of faithfulness toward the dentist to do what he in good faith asks of her. (If we were addressing the question of what the dentist ought to do, moral language would be appropriate in discussing what he owes to her as well.) Thus, the essential conflict is between the hygienist's duty to protect Ian from harm and her obligation of fidelity to the dentist. If we could decide which of these ethical responsibilities takes precedence, we would be able to determine what the hygienist ought to do.

There is one final moral consideration that deserves mention. The hygienist might reason that, because the costs of the unnecessary radiographs will be absorbed by public funds, those funds would be deflected from other social services deserving higher priority. There are approximately five primary occult malignancies of the adult jawbones per one million

people per year.[10] The expense of detect-
ing just one of these malignancies would
not be cost-effective and could not possibly
justify the use of the panorex for screening
purposes, when valuable funds are des-
perately needed in other areas of health
care. In terms of this particular case, the
panorex merely serves the purpose of cur-
iosity rather than function as an early
detection device because pedodontic patients tend not to be at risk for such
malignancies. In other words, the hygienist
might consider her duty to *other patients* in
her deliberation about what she should do.
In so doing, she would be reflecting upon
how resources ought to be allocated to
distribute with fairness scarce social benefits like health care funds.

With an understanding of the facts of
the case, as well as what moral considerations play a role therein, we are now in a
position to identify options open to the
hygienist. One thing the hygienist could
do would be simply to take the radiograph
as the dentist requested. She could reason
that Ian's mother is financially incapable
of bringing him to a general dentist who
was not a participant in the programs
available to those persons who depend on
public assistance for their care. If there
are few other dentists in their locale who
were willing to treat these patients, any
action the hygienist takes to steer her away
from the present dentist might make the
mother reluctant to return to this office
with her son. With no alternative choices
for gaining access to treatment, Ian may
not be provided with preventive dental
care at all. The hygienist might conclude
that the consequences of overtreatment are
preferable to the harmful outcome of
treatment unavailability. In the desperate
attempt to avoid jeopardizing Ian's access
to care, one unnecessary panorex seems a
small price to pay for ensuring continuity
in caries examinations, routine prophylaxis, and fluoride treatments.

This option reveals the moral limitations
of doing a cost/benefit analysis for other
people. The preceding calculation presumes that Ian's mother (and, later, Ian
himself) would place the same relative
weight on the harm of unnecessary radiation and the benefit of continued treatment by the dentist. It may be, however,
that Ian's mother would believe Ian would
be better off without dental treatment at
all than with procedures that are being
taken merely to advance the interest of the
dentist. Because the hygienist cannot be
sure that Ian's mother would make the
same moral calculation that she would, she
would not be ethically justified in making
the decision to withhold information about
the radiograph and complete the procedure.

A second option is to pretend to take
the x ray. This appears to satisfy the hygienist's obligations to both the dentist and
the patient, but there are ethical as well as
practical objections to it. An act of deception would postpone, not eliminate the
need for a frank discussion with the dentist, because there is no reason to believe
that this will be the last time the dentist
treats a patient this way. The dentist might
discover that a sham procedure had been
performed and order it again, perhaps at
the expense of the hygienist's job. Regardless of these practical objections, however,
lies or acts of deception are rarely the most
ethically defensible solutions to a moral
problem.

A third option is to dismiss the patient
by ushering him and his mother out of the
operatory without comment or explanation. It is difficult to see how the hygienist
would be fulfilling *any* of her moral duties
by choosing this course of action, because
the patient is unlikely to get further care,
and the relationship with the dentist will
be compromised. The best option from a
moral point of view is to speak with the
dentist privately about her concerns, and
to strongly urge him to reconsider ordering the radiograph. Although there are
obstacles to the success of this option (such
as the dentist's current lack of respect for
the hygienist's professional judgment as
well as the patient's welfare), only this
course of action allows the hygienist to
fulfill her multiple responsibilities before
having to choose to whom she ultimately
owes allegiance. (It also avoids having to
take into account allocational decisions,
which many believe is a task properly
falling to society, not to clinicians at chairside.) Only if the dentist insists on ordering
the radiograph does the hygienist have to
decide whether her primary moral respon-

sibility is to her patient and the patient's mother or to the dentist. Given the nature of professions in general and dental hygiene in particular, it is difficult to hold otherwise.

Although various state rules and regulations limit the professional autonomy of dental hygienists, they do not eliminate it. Hygienists are independent moral agents, and this means that their obligation to carry out the dentist's orders is but one of several obligations that they have. If the hygienist's primary moral responsibility is to do for patients what the patients would want to have done for themselves, it is difficult to hold that their *primary* responsibility is to do whatever the dentist tells them to do, especially when, in so doing, they are placing their patient at risk of harm, and/or failing to respect a patient's (or proxy's) right to self-determination.

DISCUSSION QUESTIONS

1. Does a dentist have an ethical responsibility to provide enough information about the necessity of specific dental procedures regardless of whether or not the patient is personally responsible for reimbursing the cost of such procedures?
2. If a patient is psychologically comforted by having elective diagnostic procedures performed for the verification of a disease free state, does the hygienist have an obligation to see to this need of the patient, even if the procedure is clinically not justifiable?
3. Do dentists have the obligation to perform only those procedures which are absolutely necessary on DPA patients regardless of the cost ineffectiveness of the DPA coverage?
4. What responsibilities do patients have in critically questioning their dentists and dental hygienists with regard to the necessity of specific procedures?
5. Given that there are often multiple approaches toward treating dental patients, what obligation do dental hygienists and dentists have in responding defensively on behalf of the patient, when patients cannot intelligently discriminate between necessary and unnecessary treatment?
6. Suppose the dental hygienist in this case were to follow the directive advanced by the dentist, but intentionally take the panorex with the radiation switch turned off. Would it be wrong for her to do this to protect the child, and then tell the dentist that this action occurred by mistake? Would taking the film without radiation protect the child in the same manner as not taking the film at all?
7. According to Kant, a person is not morally responsible for an action that they are incapable of carrying out. For example: a deaf mute is incapable of screaming "fire" in a burning movie theater, and is therefore not held morally accountable for alerting others with a scream. The hygienist in this case is physically capable of withholding the action of taking the x ray. Can the hygienist's act of taking the film be justified according to Kant's reasoning?

REFERENCES

1. Harrison, B., et al.: Rules and Regs: Who needs them? J. Am. Dent. Assoc. *122*:155, 1991.
2. Cotton, F.: Quality control or just control. J. Dent. Hyg. *64*:322, 1990.
3. Meyers, D.R., et al.: Radiation exposure during panoramic radiography in children. Oral Surg. *46*:588, 1978.
4. Brooks, S.L., et al.: Benefits and risks of dental radiography: Putting them into perspective. J. Mich. Dent. Assoc. *64*:471, 1982.
5. Kaugers, G.E., et al.: An evaluation of the risks of dental radiology. Va. Dent. J. *67*:19, 1990.
6. Jones, G.A., et al.: Dental radiographs and oral cancer. Gen. Dentistry *37*:218, 1989.
7. Barrett, A.P., et al.: A critical evaluation of panoramic radiography as a screening procedure in dental practice. Oral Surg. *57*:673, 1984.
8. Miles, D.A., et al.: Radiographs and the responsible dentist. Gen. Dentistry *37*:201, 1989.
9. Ignelzi, M.A., et al.: Screening panoramic radiographs in children: Prevalence data and implications. Pediatr. Dentistry *11*:■■, 1989.
10. Zeichner, S.J., et al.: Dental radiography: Efficacy

in the assessment of intraosseous lesions of the face and jaws in asymptomatic patients. Radiology *162*:691, 1987.

BIBLIOGRAPHY

Beauchamp, T.L., and Childress, J.F.: Principles of Biomedical Ethics, 3rd ed. New York, Oxford University Press, 1989.

Childress, J.F.: Priorities in Biomedical Ethics. Philadelphia, Westminster Press, 1981.

Daniels, N.: Just Health Care. New York, Cambridge University Press, 1988.

Held, V.: Rights and Goods: Justifying Social Action. Chicago, University of Chicago Press, 1989.

Larson, M.S.: The Rise of Professionalism: A Sociological Analysis. Los Angeles, University of California Press, 1979.

Kant, I.: Foundations of the Metaphysics of Morals. 1785. Trans. by Lewis White Beck. New York, Bobbs-Merrill, 1959.

Lock, J.: Second Treatise of Government. New York, Bobbs-Merrill, 1952.

Niebuhr, R.: Moral Man in Immoral Society: A Study of Ethics and Politics. New York, Charles Scribners Sons, 1960, Chap. 10.

Pennsylvania State Dental Board: Rules and regulations for the Practice of Dental Hygiene. Harrisburg, PA, 1992.

Rawls, J.: A Theory of Justice. Cambridge, Mass., Harvard University Press, 1971.

Raz, J.: The Morality of Freedom. Oxford, Claredon Press, 1989, Section I.

Singer, P.: Practical Ethics. New York, Cambridge University Press, 1980, pp. 158–220.

Veatch, R.M.: A Theory of Medical Ethics. New York, Basic Books, 1981. pp. 141–126.

SUGGESTED FURTHER READING

Beauchamp, T.L., and Walters, L. (eds.): Contemporary Issues in Bioethics, 3rd ed. Belmont, CA, Wadsworth, 1989.

Bell, J.M., and Mendus, S.: Philosophy and Medical Welfare. New York, Cambridge University Press, 1988.

Childress, J.F.: Who Should Decide? Paternalism In Health Care. New York, Oxford Univ. Press, 1982.

Davis, A., and Aroskar, M.: Ethical Dilemmas in Nursing Practice. New York, Appleton-Century-Crofts, 1978.

Dworkin, R.: Taking Rights Seriously. Cambridge, Massachusetts, Harvard University Press, 1977.

Feinberg, J.: Social Philosophy. Englewood Cliffs, N.J., Prentice-Hall, 1973.

Levine, C. (ed.): Cases in Bioethics: Selections from the Hastings Center Report. New York, St. Martin's Press, 1989.

Mill, J.S.: Utilitarianism and Other Writings. Cleveland, Meridian, 1962. (originally published in 1863).

Motley, W.E.: History of the American Dental Hygienists' Association. Chicago, American Dental Hygienists' Association, 1986.

Wright, R.A.: Human Values in Health Care: The Practice of Ethics. New York, McGraw-Hill, 1987. pp. 1–64, 105–125, 157–168.

Dental and dental hygiene students are taught to strive for perfection with the expectation that mistakes are never made. Dentists and dental hygienists, like all human beings, are imperfect and capable of error. What happens when human infallibility results in harmful mistakes or accidents in the provision of care? How are the consequences of failure to be handled in an ethical manner by those who are responsible or by those who happen to observe such incidents? Consider the following true case history. Again, the names have been changed to protect the confidentiality.

CASE 2: Doctor's mistake

Mildred is a frail elderly woman with a personality that is meek-mannered and dependent. Because of her thin veneer of emotional security, her husband routinely accompanies her to all medical and dental appointments. Apparently she has been experiencing extreme sensitivity following a series of periodontal surgeries and has been directed to the periodontist's hygienist for maintenance care, desensitization, home care instructions, and special patient management. The immediate concern is to relieve her of her daily pain from tactile and thermal sensitivity.

Throughout a series of appointments with the dental hygienist, Mildred's husband continues to question the hygienist as to the cause of her extreme pain and sensitivity in one particular quadrant. The hygienist is aware that the periodontist for whom she works, and in whom she has great confidence, had recently begun active periodontal therapy on Mildred, and that a complication had occurred after one of the surgeries. In fact, it was Mildred's third periodontal surgery, and the hygienist vividly recalls the incident.

The day after this particular surgery, Mildred began to experience generalized pain and swelling in the quadrant treated. She complained to her husband, but neither one of them knew whether or not what she was experiencing was within the normal range of postoperative discomfort. They did know that the two previous surgeries had not posed any similar complication. The periodontist was contacted by telephone, symptoms were explained, and she returned to the office later that day with her husband.

The periodontist examined her mouth and was perplexed as to why she was in so much pain, and why there was so much swelling. A complete activity history was taken, and the periodontist remained mystified. It was not until the dental assistant pointed to the patient's written records that the periodontist realized that the surgery just performed was in a quadrant previously completed 2 weeks earlier.

DISCUSSION QUESTIONS

1. If dentists or dental hygienists answer questions from patients in a misleading way, are they directly responsible for the misinterpretations made by the patient?

2. Being truthful with other persons is an important duty. This case study, however, calls into question the circumstances under which this duty holds exceptions, particularly in terms of role-specific professional parameters. How would you rationalize having the duty to withhold the truth from another person, as a consequence of assuming the role of a dental hygienist?

3. Suppose the patient discovers that this dental hygienist has responded to her in a deceptive manner, in her attempt to protect both herself and the periodontist. What justification might the hygienist need to offer in defending her actions?

4. If this dental hygienist was not discriminatingly aware of how her responses to the patient's questions might result in further harm, can she still be held morally liable if she relies upon a plea of ignorance, after answering the patient truthfully?

5. Withholding the truth, in this case, can be considered a form of secrecy, both in terms of record keeping and in terms of interprofessional collaboration. This secret is maintained for the purposes of protecting an emotionally fragile person. How might this unusual form of professional confidentiality cause a moral injustice to be done to employees who are forced to act in a deceptive way in their occupational roles?

BIBLIOGRAPHY

Beauchamp, T.L., and Childress, J.F.: Principles of Biomedical Ethics, 3rd ed. New York, Oxford University Press, 1989.

Bok, S.: Lying: Moral Choice in Public and Private Life. New York, Pantheon, 1978.

Bok, S.: Secrets: On the Ethics of Concealment and Revelation. New York, Vintage Books, 1984.

Bosk, C.L.: Forgive and Remember: Managing Medical Failure. Chicago, University of Chicago Press, 1979.

Childress, J.F.: Who Should Decide? Paternalism in Health Care. New York, Oxford University Press, 1982.

Hare, R.M.: Moral Thinking: Its Levels, Method and Point. Oxford, Clarendon Press, 1981.

Kant, I.: Fundamental Principles of the Metaphysics of Morals. Trans. by Abbott, T.K. Buffalo, Prometheus, 1987.

Levine, C. (ed.): Cases in Bioethics: Selections from the Hastings Center Report. New York, St. Martin's Press, 1989.

MacIntyre, A.: After Virtue, 2nd ed. Notre Dame, IN, Notre Dame Press, 1984.

Mackie, J.L.: Ethics: Inventing Right and Wrong, New York, Penguin, 1986.

Sidgwick, H.: Methods of Ethics, 7th ed. London, Macmillan & Co. Ltd., 1962.

Veatch, R.M.: A Theory of Medical Ethics. New York, Basic Books, 1981. pp. 141–189.

Vogel, J. and Delgado, R.: To Tell the Truth: Physician's Duty to Disclose Medical Mistakes. UCLA Law Review 28:55, 1980.

Wright, R.A.: Human Values in Health Care: The Practice of Ethics. New York, McGraw-Hill, 1987. pp. 84–104.

American Dental Association: Principles of Ethics and Code of Professional Conduct (Revised May 1992).

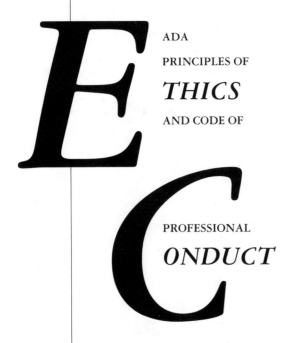

American Dental Association

ADA

PRINCIPLES OF

THICS

AND CODE OF

PROFESSIONAL

ONDUCT

*T*he ethical statements which have historically been subscribed to by the dental profession have had the benefit of the patient as their primary goal. Recognition of this goal, and of the education and training of a dentist, has resulted in society affording to the profession the privilege and obligation of self-government. The Association calls upon members of the profession to be caring and fair in their contact with patients. Although the structure of society may change, the overriding obligation of the dentist will always remain the duty to provide quality care in a competent and timely manner. All members must protect and preserve the high standards of oral health care provided to the public by the profession. They must strive to improve the care delivered – through education, training, research and, most of all, adherence to a stringent code of ethics, structured to meet the needs of the patient.

With official advisory opinions
revised to May 1992.

Principle – Section 1

SERVICE TO THE PUBLIC AND QUALITY OF CARE.

The dentist's primary professional obligation shall be service to the public. The competent and timely delivery of quality care within the bounds of the clinical circumstances presented by the patient, with due consideration being given to the needs and desires of the patient, shall be the most important aspect of that obligation.

Code of Professional Conduct

1-A. PATIENT SELECTION.

While dentists, in serving the public, may exercise reasonable discretion in selecting patients for their practices, dentists shall not refuse to accept patients into their practice or deny dental service to patients because of the patient's race, creed, color, sex, or national origin.

Advisory Opinion

1. A dentist has the general obligation to provide care to those in need. A decision not to provide treatment to an individual because the individual has AIDS or is HIV seropositive, based solely on that fact, is unethical. Decisions with regard to the type of dental treatment provided or referrals made or suggested, in such instances, should be made on the same basis as they are made with other patients, that is, whether the individual dentist believes he or she has need of another's skills, knowledge, equipment or experience and whether the dentist believes, after consultation with the patient's physician if appropriate, the patient's health status would be significantly compromised by the provision of dental treatment.

1-B. PATIENT RECORDS.

Dentists are obliged to safeguard the confidentiality of patient records. Dentists shall maintain patient records in a manner consistent with the protection of the welfare of the patient. Upon request of a patient or another dental practitioner, dentists shall provide any information that will be beneficial for the future treatment of that patient.

Advisory Opinions

1. A dentist has the ethical obligation on request of either the patient or the patient's new dentist to furnish, either gratuitously or for nominal cost, such dental records or copies or summaries of them, including dental X-rays or copies of them, as will be beneficial for the future treatment of that patient.

2. The dominant theme in Code Section 1-B is the protection of the confidentiality of a patient's records. The statement in this section that relevant information in the records should be released to another dental practitioner assumes that the dentist requesting the information is the patient's present dentist. The former dentist should be free to provide the present dentist with relevant information from the patient's records. This may often be required for the protection of both the patient and the present dentist. There may be circumstances where the former dentist has an ethical obligation to inform the present dentist of certain facts. Dentists should be aware, however, that the laws of the various jurisdictions in the United States are not uniform, and some confidentiality laws appear to prohibit the transfer of pertinent information, such as HIV seropositivity. Absent certain knowledge that the laws of the dentist's jurisdiction permit the forwarding of this information, a dentist should obtain the patient's written permission before forwarding health records which contain information of a sensitive nature, such as HIV seropositivity, chemical dependency or sexual preference. If it is necessary for a treating dentist to consult with another dentist or physician with respect to the patient, and the circumstances do not permit the patient to remain anonymous, the treating dentist should seek the permission of the patient prior to the release of data from the patient's records to the consulting practitioner. If the patient refuses, the treating dentist should then contemplate obtaining legal advice regarding the termination of the dentist/patient relationship.

1-C. COMMUNITY SERVICE.

Since dentists have an obligation to use their skills, knowledge, and experience for the improvement of the dental health of the public and are encouraged to be leaders in their community, dentists in such service shall conduct themselves in such a manner as to maintain or elevate the esteem of the profession.

Advisory Opinion

1. A dentist who becomes ill from any disease or impaired in any way shall, with consultation and advice from a qualified physician or other authority, limit the activities of practice to those areas that do not endanger the patients or members of the dental staff.

1-D. EMERGENCY SERVICE.

Dentists shall be obliged to make reasonable arrangements for the emergency care of their patients of record.

Dentists shall be obliged when consulted in an emergency by patients not of record to make reasonable arrangements for emergency care. If treatment is provided, the dentist, upon completion of such treatment, is obliged to return the patient to his or her regular dentist unless the patient expressly reveals a different preference.

1-E. CONSULTATION AND REFERRAL.

Dentists shall be obliged to seek consultation, if possible, whenever the welfare of patients will be safeguarded or advanced by utilizing those who have special skills, knowledge, and experience. When patients visit or are referred to specialists or consulting dentists for consultation:

1. The specialists or consulting dentists upon completion of their care shall return the patient, unless the patient expressly reveals a different preference, to the referring dentist, or if none, to the dentist of record for future care.

2. The specialists shall be obliged when there is no referring dentist and upon a completion of their treatment to inform patients when there is a need for further dental care.

Advisory Opinion

1. A dentist who has a patient referred by a third party for a "second opinion" regarding a diagnosis or treatment plan recommended by the patient's treating dentist should render the requested second opinion in accordance with this Code of Ethics.

In the interest of the patient being afforded quality care, the dentist rendering the second opinion should not have a vested interest in the ensuing recommendation.

1-F. USE OF AUXILIARY PERSONNEL.

Dentists shall be obliged to protect the health of their patient by only assigning to qualified auxiliaries those duties which can be legally delegated. Dentists shall be further obliged to prescribe and supervise the work of all auxiliary personnel working under their direction and control.

1-G. JUSTIFIABLE CRITICISM.

Dentists shall be obliged to report to the appropriate reviewing agency as determined by the local component or constituent society instances of gross or continual faulty treatment by other dentists.

Patients should be informed of their present oral health status without disparaging comment about prior services.

Dentists issuing a public statement with respect to the profession shall have a reasonable basis to believe that the comments made are true.

Advisory Opinion

1. A dentist's duty to the public imposes a responsibility to report instances of gross or continual

faulty treatment. However, the heading of this section is "Justifiable Criticism." Therefore, when informing a patient of the status of his or her oral health, the dentist should exercise care that the comments made are justifiable. For example, a difference of opinion as to preferred treatment should not be communicated to the patient in a manner which would imply mistreatment. There will necessarily be cases where it will be difficult to determine whether the comments made are justifiable. Therefore, this section is phrased to address the discretion of dentists and advises against disparaging statements against another dentist. However, it should be noted that where comments are made which are obviously not supportable and therefore unjustified, such comments can be the basis for the institution of a disciplinary proceeding against the dentist making such statements.

1-H. EXPERT TESTIMONY.

Dentists may provide expert testimony when that testimony is essential to a just and fair disposition of a judicial or administrative action.

Advisory Opinion

1. It is unethical for a dentist to agree to a fee contingent upon the favorable outcome of the litigation in exchange for testifying as a dental expert.

1-I. REBATE AND SPLIT FEES.

Dentists shall not accept or tender "rebates" or "split fees."

1-J. REPRESENTATION OF CARE.

Dentists shall not represent the care being rendered to their patients in a false or misleading manner.

Advisory Opinions

1. Based on available scientific data the ADA has determined through the adoption of Resolution 42H-1986 (Trans. 1986:536) that the removal of amalgam restorations from the non-allergic patient for the alleged purpose of removing toxic substances from the body, when such treatment is performed solely at the recommendation or suggestion of the dentist, is improper and unethical.

The Council reminds constituent and component societies that before a dentist can be found to have breached any ethical obligation the dentist is entitled to a fair hearing.

2. A dentist who represents that dental treatment recommended or performed by the dentist has the capacity to cure or alleviate diseases, infections or other

conditions, when such representations are not based upon accepted scientific knowledge or research, is acting unethically.

1-K. REPRESENTATION OF FEES.

Dentists shall not represent the fees being charged for providing care in a false or misleading manner.

Advisory Opinions

1. A dentist who accepts a third party* payment under a copayment plan as payment in full without disclosing to the third party* that the patient's payment portion will not be collected, is engaged in overbilling. The essence of this ethical impropriety is deception and misrepresentation; an overbilling dentist makes it appear to the third party* that the charge to the patient for services rendered is higher than it actually is.

2. It is unethical for a dentist to increase a fee to a patient solely because the patient has insurance.

3. Payments accepted by a dentist under a governmentally funded program, a component or constituent dental society sponsored access program, or a participating agreement entered into under a program of a third party* shall not be considered as evidence of overbilling in determining whether a charge to a patient, or to another third party* in behalf of a patient not covered under any of the aforecited programs constitutes overbilling under this section of the Code.

4. A dentist who submits a claim form to a third party* reporting incorrect treatment dates for the purpose of assisting a patient in obtaining benefits under a dental plan, which benefits would otherwise be disallowed, is engaged in making an unethical, false, or misleading representation to such third party.*

5. A dentist who incorrectly describes on a third party* claim form a dental procedure in order to receive a greater payment or reimbursement or incorrectly makes a non-covered procedure appear to be a covered procedure on such a claim form is engaged in making an unethical, false, or misleading representation to such third party.*

6. A dentist who recommends and performs unnecessary dental services or procedures is engaged in unethical conduct.

*A third party is any party to a dental prepayment contract that may collect premiums, assume financial risks, pay claims, and/or provide administrative services.

1-L. PATIENT INVOLVEMENT.

The dentist should inform the patient of the proposed treatment, and any reasonable alternatives, in a manner that allows the patient to become involved in treatment decisions.

Principle – Section 2

EDUCATION.

The privilege of dentists to be accorded professional status rests primarily in the knowledge, skill, and experience with which they serve their patients and society. All dentists, therefore, have the obligation of keeping their knowledge and skill current.

Principle – Section 3

GOVERNMENT OF A PROFESSION.

Every profession owes society the responsibility to regulate itself. Such regulation is achieved largely through the influence of the professional societies. All dentists, therefore, have the dual obligation of making themselves a part of a professional society and of observing its rules of ethics.

Principle – Section 4

RESEARCH AND DEVELOPMENT.

Dentists have the obligation of making the results and benefits of their investigative efforts available to all when they are useful in safeguarding or promoting the health of the public.

Code of Professional Conduct

4-A. DEVICES AND THERAPEUTIC METHODS.

Except for formal investigative studies, dentists shall be obliged to prescribe, dispense, or promote only those devices, drugs, and other agents whose complete formulae are available to the dental profession. Dentists shall have the further obligation of not holding out as exclusive any device, agent, method, or technique.

4-B. PATENTS AND COPYRIGHTS.

Patents and copyrights may be secured by dentists provided that such patents and copyrights shall not be used to restrict research or practice.

Principle – Section 5

PROFESSIONAL ANNOUNCEMENT.

In order to properly serve the public, dentists should represent themselves in a manner that contributes to the esteem of the profession. Dentists should not misrepresent their training and competence in any way that would be false or misleading in any material respect.*

5-A. ADVERTISING.

Although any dentist may advertise, no dentist shall advertise or solicit patients in any form of communication in a manner that is false or misleading in any material respect.*

1. If a dental health article, message, or newsletter is published under a dentist's byline to the public without making truthful disclosure of the source and authorship or is designed to give rise to questionable expectations for the purpose of inducing the public to utilize the services of the sponsoring dentist, the dentist is engaged in making a false or misleading representation to the public in a material respect.

2. The Council on Ethics, Bylaws and Judicial Affairs believes it would be of service to the members to provide some insight into the meaning of the term "false or misleading in a material respect." Therefore, the following examples are set forth. These examples are not meant to be all-inclusive. Rather by restating the concept in alternative language and giving general examples, it is hoped that the membership will gain a better understanding of the term. With this in mind, statements shall be avoided which would: a) contain a material misrepresentation of fact, b) omit a fact necessary to make the statement considered as a whole not materially misleading, c) contain a representation or implication regarding the quality of dental services which would suggest unique or general superiority to other practitioners which are not susceptible to reasonable verification by the public, and d) be intended or be likely to create an unjustified expectation about results the dentist can achieve.

3. The use of an unearned ōr nonhealth degree in any general announcements to the public by a dentist may be a representation to the public which is false or misleading in a material respect. A dentist may use the title Doctor, Dentist, DDS, or DMD, or any additional earned advanced degrees in health service areas. The use of unearned or nonhealth degrees could be misleading because of the likelihood that it will indicate to the public the attainment of a specialty or diplomate status. It may also suggest that the dentist using such is claiming superior dental skills.

For purposes of this advisory opinion, an unearned academic degree is one which is awarded by an educational institution not accredited by a generally recognized accrediting body or is an honorary degree.

Generally, the use of honorary degrees or nonhealth degrees should be limited to scientific papers and curriculum vitae. In all instances state law should be consulted. In any review by the council of the use of nonhealth degrees or honorary degrees, the council will apply the standard of whether the use of such is false or misleading in a material respect.

4. A dentist using the attainment of a fellowship in a direct advertisement to the general public may be making a representation to the public which is false or misleading in a material respect. Such use of a fellowship status may be misleading because of the likelihood that it will indicate to the dental consumer the attainment of a specialty status. It may also suggest that the dentist using such is claiming superior dental skills. However, when such use does not conflict with state law, the attainment of fellowship status may be indicated in scientific papers, curriculum vitae, third party payment forms, and letterhead and stationery which is not used for the direct solicitation of patients. In any review by the council of the use of the attainment of fellowship status, the council will apply the standard of whether the use of such is false or misleading in a material respect.

5. There are two basic types of referral services for dental care: not-for-profit and the commercial.

The not-for-profit is commonly organized by dental societies or community services. It is open to all qualified practitioners in the area served. A fee is sometimes charged the practitioner to be listed with the service. A fee for such referral services is for the purpose of covering the expenses of the service and has no relation to the number of patients referred.

In contrast, experience has shown that commercial referral services generally limit access to the referral service to one dentist in a particular geographic area. Prospective patients calling the service are referred to the single subscribing dentist in the geographic area and the respective dentist is commonly billed for each patient referred. Commercial referral services often advertise to the public stressing that there is no charge for use of the service and the patient is not informed of the referral fee paid by the dentist. There is a connotation to such advertisements that the referral that is being made is in the nature of a public service.

A dentist is allowed to pay for any advertising permitted by the Code, but is generally not permitted to make payments to another person or entity for the referral of a patient for professional services. While the particular facts and circumstances relating to an individual commercial referral service will vary, the council believes that the aspects outlined above for commercial referral services violate the Code in that it constitutes advertising which is false or misleading in a material respect and violate the prohibitions in the Code against fee splitting.

6. An advertisement which omits a material fact or facts necessary to put the information conveyed in the advertisement in a proper context can be misleading in a material respect. An advertisement to the public of HIV negative test results, without conveying additional information that will clarify the scientific significance of this fact, is an example of a misleading omission. A dental practice should not seek to attract patients on the basis of partial truths which create a false impression.

5-B. NAME OF PRACTICE.

Since the name under which a dentist conducts his or her practice may be a factor in the selection process of the patient, the use of a trade name or an assumed name that is false or misleading in any material respect is unethical.

Use of the name of a dentist no longer actively associated with the practice may be continued for a period not to exceed one year.*

Advisory Opinion

1. Dentists leaving a practice who authorize continued use of their names should receive competent advice on the legal implications of this action. With permission of a departing dentist, his or her name may be used for more than one year, if, after the one year grace period has expired, prominent notice is provided to the public through such mediums as a sign at the office and a short statement on stationery and business cards that the departing dentist has retired from the practice.

5-C. ANNOUNCEMENT OF SPECIALIZATION AND LIMITATION OF PRACTICE.

This section and Section 5-D are designed to help the public make an informed selection between the practitioner who has completed an accredited program beyond the dental degree and a practitioner who has not completed such a program.

The special areas of dental practice approved by the American Dental Association and the designation for ethical specialty announcement and limitation of practice are: dental public health, endodontics, oral pathology, oral and maxillofacial surgery, othodontics, pediatric dentistry, periodontics, and prosthodontics.

Dentists who choose to announce specialization should use "specialist in" or "practice limited to" and shall limit their practice exclusively to the announced special area(s) of dental practice, provided at the time of

the announcement such dentists have met in each approved specialty for which they announce the existing educational requirements and standards set forth by the American Dental Association.

Dentists who use their eligibility to announce as specialists to make the public believe that specialty services rendered in the dental office are being rendered by qualified specialists when such is not the case are engaged in unethical conduct. The burden of responsibility is on specialists to avoid any inference that general practitioners who are associated with specialists are qualified to announce themselves as specialists.

GENERAL STANDARDS.

The following are included within the standards of the American Dental Association for determining the education, experience, and other appropriate requirements for announcing specialization and limitation of practice:

1. The special area(s) of dental practice and an appropriate certifying board must be approved by the American Dental Association.

2. Dentists who announce as specialists must have successfully completed an educational program accredited by the Commission on Dental Accreditation, two or more years in length, as specified by the Council on Dental Education, or be diplomates of an American Dental Association recognized certifying board. The scope of the individual specialist's practice shall be governed by the educational standards for the specialty in which the specialist is announcing.

3. The practice carried on by dentists who announce as specialists shall be limited exclusively to the special area(s) of dental practices announced by the dentist.

STANDARDS FOR MULTIPLE-SPECIALTY ANNOUNCEMENTS.

Educational criteria for announcement by dentists in additional recognized specialty areas are the successful completion of an educational program accredited by the Commission on Dental Accreditation in each area for which the dentist wishes to announce.

Dentists who completed their advanced education in programs listed by the Council on Dental Education prior to the initiation of the accreditation process in 1967 and who are currently ethically announcing as specialists in a recognized area may announce in additional areas provided they are educationally qualified or are certified diplomates in each area for which they wish to announce. Documentation of successful completion of the educational program(s) must be submitted to the appropriate constituent society. The documentation must assure that the duration of the program(s) is a minimum of two years except for oral and maxillofacial surgery which must have been a minimum of three years in duration.*

Advisory Opinion

1. A dentist who announces in any means of communication with patients or the general public that he or she is certified or a diplomate in an area of dentistry not recognized by the American Dental Association or the law of the jurisdiction where the dentist practices as a specialty area of dentistry is engaged in making a false or misleading representation to the public in a material respect.

5-D. GENERAL PRACTITIONER ANNOUNCEMENT OF SERVICES.

General dentists who wish to announce the services available in their practices are permitted to announce the availability of those services so long as they avoid any communications that express or imply specialization. General dentists shall also state that the services are being provided by general dentists. No dentist shall announce available services in any way that would be false or misleading in any material respect.*

*Advertising, solicitation of patients or business, or other promotional activities by dentists or dental care delivery organizations shall not be considered unethical or improper, except for those promotional activities which are false or misleading in any material respect. Notwithstanding any ADA *Principles of Ethics and Code of Professional Conduct* or other standards of dentist conduct which may be differently worded, this shall be the sole standard for determining the ethical propriety of such promotional activities. Any provision of an ADA constituent or component society's code of ethics or other standard of dentist conduct relating to dentists' or dental care delivery organizations' advertising, solicitation, or other promotional activities which is worded differently from the above standard shall be deemed to be in conflict with the ADA *Principles of Ethics and Code of Professional Conduct.*

Interpretation and Application of 'Principles of Ethics and Code of Professional Conduct'

The preceding statements constitute the *Principles of Ethics and Code of Professional Conduct* of the American Dental Association. The purpose of the *Principles and Code* is to uphold and strengthen dentistry as a member of the learned professions. The constituent and component societies may adopt additional provisions or interpretations not in conflict with these *Principles of Ethics and Code of Professional Conduct* which would enable them to serve more faithfully the traditions, customs, and desires of the members of these societies.

Problems involving questions of ethics should be solved at the local level within the broad boundaries established in these *Principles of Ethics and Code of Professional Conduct* and within the interpretation by the component and/or constituent society of their respective codes of ethics. If a satisfactory decision cannot be reached, the question should be referred on appeal to the constituent society and the Council on Ethics, Bylaws and Judicial Affairs of the American Dental Association, as provided in Chapter XII of the *Bylaws* of the American Dental Association. Members found guilty of unethical conduct as prescribed in the American Dental Association *Code of Professional Conduct* or codes of ethics of the constituent and component societies are subject to the penalties set forth in Chapter XII of the American Dental Association *Bylaws.*

The 1992 PEDNET Bibliography

David T. Ozar
John A. Gilbert
Margaret Welch

This bibliography is the work of the Professional Ethics in Dentistry Network (PEDNET). PEDNET is a national network of dental school faculty, dental hygiene faculty, ethicists, dental association officers, practicing dentists and dental hygienists, social scientists, and other persons who are concerned about professional and ethical issues in dentistry and education regarding them. PEDNET was originally conceived at a meeting on the teaching of professional ethics in dental schools at the University of Minnesota in November, 1982. Since then, PEDNET has grown to more than 200 members, including those who teach professional ethics in almost every dental school in the United States and Canada, as well as representatives of many of the major dental professional organizations, and many other practicing dentists and other interested parties. PEDNET holds two national meetings each year, one in the fall in conjunction with the meetings of the Society for Health and Human Values, and a shorter meeting in the spring in conjunction with (as a "Special Interest Group" at) the meetings of the American Association of Dental Schools. It also publishes a twice-yearly Newsletter; surveys of materials used in teaching dental professional ethics in the dental schools, and, more recently, in continuing education programs; and *The PEDNET Bibliography*.

This bibliography compiles three earlier bibliographies prepared by members of PEDNET (Ozar and Hockenberry's in 1985, published in the Journal of Dental Education, *49*:244; Ozar's 1987 additions, published by PEDNET for its members; and Gilbert's 1989 bibliography, prepared as an interim step toward this more comprehensive effort). To this composite have been added a large number of additions through the end of 1991 and the most recent results of our continuing effort to develop a comprehensive bibliography of earlier literature on dental professional ethics.

It is impossible to draw a clean line between writing on ethics, which is essentially hortatory in nature, and work in which the reasoning behind the positions that an author takes is carefully articulated. But it is the latter contributions to reflections on dental professional ethics that have been the principal focus of the compilers of this bibliography. That is, materials designed principally to encourage good deeds, rather than to explain the reasons for judging them correct, have not ordinarily been included, important though they are to the life of the dental community.

In addition, this is not a bibliography of materials in dental law. Although many issues connect the ethical and legal aspects of dental practice and dental education, and so some discussion of legal matters will be found among these works, the bibliography does not include materials that focus narrowly on the law or legal aspects of dentistry.

Finally, although some important works on professional ethics as a general topic are included, the bibliography does not include materials from the broader literature of health care ethics unless those materials explicitly examine practice or education in dentistry or dental hygiene. A number of excellent bibliographies of that larger literature are already available for those who wish to apply them to dental ethics to consult.

The authors welcome readers' additions and corrections for future editions of *The PEDNET Bibliography*.

THE 1992 PEDNET BIBLIOGRAPHY

1. Ahlberg, J.E.: The development of ethics in dentistry. Scand. J. Dent. Res. *89:*1, 1981.
2. Albino, J.E.: Insuring informed review of proposed behavioral science research. J. Dent. Res. *59C:*1327, 1980.
3. Allen, D.L.: Factors revealed by the dental curriculum study which influence professionalism in dental practice. J. Am. Coll. Dent. *46:*35, 1979.
4. Alman, J.: Statistical and ethical considerations in clinical trials. Community Dent. Oral Epidemiol. *5:*261, 1977.
5. Alper, M.N.: Ethics and the dental hygiene profession. J. Am. Dent. Hyg. Assoc. *40:*157, 1966.
6. Alstadt, W.R.: Ethics—of what value? J. Am. Dent. Hyg. Assoc. *41:*15, 1967.
7. Amenta, C.A., Jr.: The evolution and ethics of dentistry's dilemma. C.D.S. Rev. *84:*50, 1991.
8. Amorosi, P.C.: The history of dental malpractice litigation in America. Bull. Hist. Dent. *19:*12, 1971.
9. Anderson, C.: Values and ethics—A perspective on long term prosperity. Can. Dent. Assoc. J. *55:*695, 1989.
10. Anonymous: 1866 Code of dental ethics. Trans. Am. Dent. Assoc. *6:*401, 1866.
11. Anonymous: 1947 Code of ethics. Digest of Official Actions: 1922–1946. Chicago, American Dental Association, 1947.
12. Anonymous: A history of dentistry. Trans. Calif. State Dent. Assoc. *1872:*84.
13. Anonymous: A history of dentistry—protest concerning. Trans. Calif. State Dent. Assoc. *1872:*84.
14. Anonymous: ADA Principles of ethics and code of professional conduct, with official advisory opinions. (American Dental Association, Council on Ethics, Bylaws, and Judicial Affairs). Chicago, American Dental Association, 1991 or most recent.
15. Anonymous: AIDS and dentistry: The legal and ethical issues. Dent. Management *27:*38, 1987.
16. Anonymous: Chemical dependency and dental practice. ADA Council on Dental Practice. J. Am. Dent. Assoc. *114:*509, 1987.
17. Anonymous: Chemical dependency: The road to recovery. J. Am. Dent. Assoc. *115:*18, 1987.
18. Anonymous: Child abuse: Recognition and reporting. Spec. Care Dent. *6:*62, 1986.
19. Anonymous: The control of transmissable disease in dental practice: a position paper of the American Association of Public Health Dentistry. J. Public Health Dent. *46:*13, 1986.
20. Anonymous: Curriculum guidelines on ethics and professionalism in dentistry. J. Dent. Educ. *53:*144, 1989.
21. Anonymous: The delivery of dental care: An assessment of five alternative systems. J. Am. Dent. Assoc. *109:*131, 1982.
22. Anonymous: Dentistry rejects advertising. Ontario Dent. *60:*34, 1983.
23. Anonymous: Dentist's professional and ethical responsibilities for HIV-positive patients and patients with AIDS. J. Irish. Dent. Assoc. *33:*11, 1987.
24. Anonymous: The dentists' responsibility in identifying and reporting child abuse. Ill. Dent. J. *58:*26, 1989.
25. Anonymous: Duties of dentists infected with human immunodeficiency virus (HIV) or suffering from AIDS [editorial]. Br. Dent. J. *164:*61, 1988.
26. Anonymous: Enforcement of the principles of ethics. J. Am. Dent. Assoc. *73:*1352, 1966.
27. Anonymous: Ethical and legal considerations associated with behavior and social science research studies: discussion. J. Dent. Res. *59C:*1335, 1980.
28. Anonymous: Ethical and legal considerations associated with clinical field trials: Discussion. J. Dent. Res. *59C:*1267, 1980.
29. Anonymous: Ethical and legal considerations associated with epidemiological surveys: discussion. J. Dent. Res. *59C:*1299, 1980.
30. Anonymous: Ethical guidelines. J. Dent. Child. *42:*74, 1975.
31. Anonymous: Ethics. Digest of Official Actions, 1946–1953. Chicago, American Dental Association, 1954.
32. Anonymous: Enforcement of the principles of ethics. J. Am. Dent. Assoc. *73:*1353, 1966.
33. Anonymous: A focus on the American Association of Oral and Maxillo-facial Surgeons Commission on Professional Conduct. J. Oral Maxillofac. Surg. *42:*276, 1984.
34. Anonymous: Human subjects in dental research: Coping with the regulations. ADA Council on Research. J. Am. Dent. Assoc. *110:*243, 1985.
35. Anonymous: Informed consent—A risk management view (ADA Council on Insurance). J. Am. Dent. Assoc. *115:*630, 1987.
36. Anonymous: The liability issue: Protecting the profession. J. Am. Dent. Assoc. *112:*607, 1986.
37. Anonymous: The mercury scare. J. Dent. Que. *25:*139, 1988.
38. Anonymous: The mercury scare—If a dentist

wants to remove your fillings because they contain mercury, watch your wallet. Can. Dent. Assoc. J. *59:*902, 1986.

39. Anonymous: National Dental Association Code of Ethics—Report of the Committee. Transactions of the NDA *3:*481, 1899.

40. Anonymous: The patient and profession at risk . . . alternative delivery systems. Can. Dent. Assoc. J. *53:*447, 1987.

41. Anonymous: Principles of Ethics [pamphlet]. Chicago, American Dental Association, 1958.

42. Anonymous: Principles of Ethics. Chicago, American Dental Hygiene Association, 1975.

43. Anonymous: Response to "60 Minutes." J. Am. Dent. Assoc. *122:*10, 1991.

44. Anonymous: Rules defining unprofessional conduct. N.Y. State Dent. J. *44:*274, 1978.

45. Anonymous: Toward a broader understanding of ethics, self-regulation, and quality assurance. ADA Office of Quality Assurance. J. Am. Dent. Assoc. *114:*246, 1987.

46. Anonymous: Undermining the ethics of dentistry. Ontario Dent. *65:*38, 1988.

47. Anonymous: The use of human subjects in clinical research. Br. Dent. J. *135:*501, 1973.

48. Anonymous: The use of patients in clinical board examinations. J. Am. Dent. Assoc. *110:*164, 1985.

49. Anonymous: What is professionalism? (WDA Ethics and Dental Relations Committee). Wis. Dent. Assoc. J. *64:*78, 1988.

50. Asher, R., and Milana, T.: Division of professional conduct investigates advertising complaints from DSSNY. N.Y. State Dent. J. *46:*138, 1980.

51. Axelsson, P.: Ethical and legal considerations associated with clinical field trials: The views of discussant. J. Dent. Res. *59C:*1262, 1980.

52. Bailey, B.L.: Informed consent in dentistry. J. Am. Dent. Assoc. *110:*709, 1985.

53. Bailit, H.L.: Issues in regulating quality of care and containing costs within private sector policy. J. Dent. Educ. *44:*530, 1980.

54. Bailit, H.: Symposium on ethical issues related to social and behavioral sciences research in dentistry. Community Dent. Oral Epidemiol. *5:*257, 1977.

55. Barber, R.L.: Treatment for patients having communicable diseases: Ethical problems, issues, controversies. Ky. Dent. J. *41:*11, 1989.

56. Barish, N.H., and Barish, A.M.: The ethical dilemma of the dental hygienist. J. Am. Coll. Dent. *39:*169, 1972.

57. Barlow, W.R.: Ethics—Life blood of a profession. Univ. Toronto Undergrad. Dent. J. *1:*11, 1964.

58. Barmes, D.: The impact of ethical and legal consideration on future epidemiology of dental caries. J. Dent. Res. *59C:*1335, 1980.

59. Barnett, P.R., and Kowal, L.S.: Professionalism, ethics, and corporate dental care. Compendium *9:*156, 1988.

60. Barr, C.S.: Promoting interrelated care. Spec. Care Dent. *6:*203, 1986.

61. Barry, V.J.: "I won't accept AIDS patients. . . " [editorial]. GMDA Bull. *55:*64, 1989.

62. Barzun, J.: The professions under seige: private practice versus public need. J. Am. Dent. Assoc. *98:*672, 1979.

63. Batey, A.: Guidelines for professional ethics. J. Am. Coll. Dent. *41:*259, 1974.

64. Baxter, M.P. Interplay between dental and legal ethics during a professional liability case. Ohio Dent. J. *64:*28, 1990.

65. Bayles, M.D.: Professional Ethics. 2nd Ed. Belmont, CA, Wadsworth, 1989.

66. Beauchamp, T.L.: Principles of ethics. J. Dent. Educ. *49:*214, 1985.

67. Beazley, B.J.: Dentistry and the dental trade working together. J. Am. Coll. Dent. *55:*22, 1988.

68. Bebeau, M.J.: Ethics for the practicing dentist. Can ethics be taught? A look at the evidence. J. Am. Coll. Dent. *58:*5, 1991.

69. Bebeau, M.J.: Professional responsibility curriculum report. J. Am. Coll. Dent. *50:*20, 1983.

70. Bebeau, M.J.: Teaching ethics in dentistry. J. Dent. Educ. *49:*236, 1985.

71. Bebeau, M.J.: Teaching professional ethics. Encounters (The Science Museum of Minnesota). Sept–Oct, 1983, p. 19.

72. Bebeau, M.J., Oberle, M., and Rest, J.R.: Developing alternate cases for the Dental Ethical Sensitivity Test (DEST). J. Dent. Res. *63:*196 [Abstract #228], 1984.

73. Bebeau, M.J., Reifel, N., and Speidel, T.M.: Measuring the type and frequency of professional dilemmas in dentistry. J. Dent. Res. *60:*532 [Abstract #891], 1981.

74. Bebeau, M.J., Rest, J.R., Speidel, T.M., and Yamoor, C.M.: Assessing student sensitivity to ethical issues in professional problems. J. Dent. Res. *61:*208 [Abstract #266], 1982.

75. Bebeau, M.J., Rest, J.R., and Yamoor, C.M.: Measuring dental students ethical sensitivity. J. Dent. Educ. *49:*225, 1985.

76. Bebeau, M.J., Spidel, T.M., and Yamoor, C.M.: A Professional Responsibility Curriculum for Dental Education. Minneapolis, MN, University of Minnesota Press, 1982.

77. Beck, F.: Placebos in dentistry: Their profound potential effects. J. Am. Dent. Assoc. *95:*1122, 1977.

78. Beck, J.D.: Dentists and the elderly: Attitudes and behaviors. *In* Clinical Geriatric Dentistry: Biomedical and Psychological Aspects. Edited by H.H. Chauncey. Chicago, American Dental Association, 1985.

79. Bentley, J.M., and Barnett, P.R.: Advertising in dentistry. J. Am. Coll. Dent. *48:*227, 1981.

80. Bergamo, F.C.: Ethics in the 80's. Spec. Care Dent. *5:*204, 1985.

81. Bergamo, F.C., and Bird, L.P.: A Personal Probe: Ethical Problems in Dental Practice. Richardson, TX, Christian Medical Society, 1980.

82. Bergsrud, M., and Furey, M.: Advertise or not? Ethics under fire. Dent. Stud. *59:*54, 1981.

83. Berns, J.D.: Reducing blame through group treatment. Dent. Survey *55:*40, 1979.

84. Berry, J.H.: Questionable care: What can be done about dental quackery? J. Am. Dent. Assoc. *115:*679, 1987.

85. Biddington, W.R.: The dental policy perspective. J. Am. Coll. Dent. *57:*20, 1990.

86. Biddington, W.R., and Nash, D.A.: A person within a community of persons. J. Am. Coll. Dent. *51:*12, 1984.

87. Bird, L.P.: Dental ethics: Where science and sensitivity touch. Spec. Care Dent. *5:*198, 1985.

88. Birge, J.J.: Professional ethics. Trans. Calif. State Dent. Assoc. 1879, p. 257.

89. Black, D.: Ethics and research. Aust. Dent J. *31:*53, 1986.

90. Blaikie, D.C.: Cultural barriers to preventative dentistry. Aust. Dent. J. *24:*398, 1979.

91. Blair, K.P.: Importance of principles. Can. Dent. Assoc. J. *16:*31, 1988.

92. Blauch, L.E.: The professional man in our time. J. Am. Coll. Dent. *18:*216, 1951.

93. Block, L.E.: Advertising and dentistry. J. Bergen Cty. Dent. Soc. *46:*11, 17, 1979.

94. Block, L.E.: The advertising of dental services. Dent. Survey *54:*12, 1978.

95. Block, M.J.: An overview: The need to change the attitude of students of the helping professions toward the aged through education. Spec. Care Dent. *2:*212, 1982.

96. Boerschinger, T.H.: Dentists' advertising. Patient welfare or caveat emptor. Dentistry *9:*5, 1989.

97. Bonkowski, J.H., Farman, A.G., and Scheible, L.: A master of professional conscience: maximizing patient radiation safety. J. Mich. Dent. Assoc. *70:*525, 1988.

98. Bonner, P.: Public relations as an ethical marketing tool. Dent. Econ. *75:*77, 1985.

99. Boucher, L.J.: The professional person. J. Wis. Dent. Assoc. *60:*14, 1984.

100. Boundy, S.S., and Reynolds, N.J.: Changing role of the dental hygienist. *In* Current Concepts in Dental Hygiene. Vol II. Edited by S. Styers-Boundy and N.J. Reynolds, St. Louis, C.V. Mosby, 1977.

101. Bowers, D.F.: Ethics in dentistry: Devising a code for all reasons. J. Kans. Dent. Assoc. *68:*34, 1984; Ohio Dent J. *58:*26, 1985.

102. Boyer, E.M., and Nielson-Thompson, N.J.: Legality and dental hygienists' performance of expanded functions. Dent. Hyg. (Chicago) *60:*104, 1986.

103. Brahams, D.: Interpretation of "serious professional misconduct": Changing the rules. Lancet *2(8569):*1159, 1987.

104. Branson, R.: The ethics of dental research: An overview of basic principles. J. Dent. Res. *59C:*1214, 1980.

105. Brown, M.: Ethics. Contact Point *65:*11, 1987.

106. Brown and Solyman: Remarks on professional morality. Am. J. Dent. Sci. *1:*1, 1839.

107. Brown, M.: Ethics. Contact Point *65:*11, 1987.

108. Brown, S.: Remarks on professional morality. Am. J. Dent. Sci. *1:*1, 1839.

109. Bruce, H.W.: Time to change. J. Dent. Educ. *44:*639, 1980.

110. Burnell, F.E.: Dental ethics. Trans. Calif. State Dent. Assoc., 1873, p. 204.

111. Burns, C.: Dentistry: Professional codes in American dentistry. *In* Encyclopedia of Bioethics. Vol. I. Edited by W. Reich. New York, The Free Press, 1978.

112. Burns, C.: The evolution of professional ethics in American dentistry. Bull. Hist. Dent. *22:*59, 1974.

113. Burt, B.A.: Ethical considerations in dental epidemiological studies. J. Dent. Res. *59C:*1289, 1980.

114. Cagle, L. The role of ethics in the profession of dentistry. Ill. Dent. J. *47:*601, 1978.

115. Cain, M.J., Silberman, S.L., Mahan, J.M., and Meydrech, E.F.: Changes in dental students' personal needs and values. J. Dent. Educ. *47:*604, 1983.

116. Camenisch, P.F.: Grounding Professional Ethics in a Pluralistic Society. New York, Haven, 1983.

117. Campbell, P.M.: Ethics for the eighties. Tex. Dent. J. *103:*10, 1986.

118. Carlson, M.H.: Keeping dentistry on the professional track. Oper. Dent. *11:*117, 1986.

119. Chantrell, S.B.: Excuse me, sir, I thought I was worth something. Am. Dent. Stud. Assoc. News. *18:*2, 1988.

120. Cheney, E.: Professional responsibility and the orthodontist. Am. J. Orthod. *57:*615, 1970.

121. Church, L.E. Dental malpractice and dental discipline. J. Md. State Dent. Assoc. *23:*91, 1980.

122. Church, T., Moretti, R., and Ayer, W.A.: Issues and concerns in the development of the dentist-patient relationship. New Dentist *10:*20, 1980.

123. Chiodo, G.T., and Tolle, S.W.: Doctor-patient confidentiality and the adolescent patient. J. Am. Dent. Assoc. *120:*126, 1990.

124. Chiodo, G.T., and Tolle, S.W.: Doctor-patient confidentiality and the potentiality HIV-positive patient. J. Am. Dent. Assoc. *119:*652, 1989.

125. Chiodo, G.T., and Tolle, S.W.: Patient death and bereavement: What is the dentist's role? Spec. Care Dent. *8:*198, 1988.

126. Christensen, G.J.: Esthetic dentistry and ethics. Quintessence International *20:*747, 1989.

127. Ciesielski, C., Gooch, B., Hammetterr, T., and Metler, R.: Dentists, allied professionals with AIDS. J. Am. Dent. Assoc. *122:*42, 1991.

128. Clark, C.A., and Vanek, E.P.: Meeting the health care needs of people with limited access to care. J. Dent. Educ. *48:*213, 1984.

129. Cohen, K.: Social sciences research: Ethical and policy implications. Community Dent. Oral Epidemiol. *5:*261, 1977.

130. Cohen, L.A., and Grace, E.G., Jr.: Attitudes of dental faculty toward individuals with AIDS. J. Dent. Educ. *53:*199, 1989.

131. Cohen, L.A., and Grace, E.G., Jr.: Attitudes of dental students toward individuals with AIDS. J. Dent. Educ. *53:*542, 1989.

132. Cohen, L.A., and Grace, E.G., Jr.: Dentists' attitudes toward mandatory screening of dental personnel for infectious diseases and the continued practice of infected dental personnel. J. Law Eth. Dent. *2:*199, 1989.

133. Cohen, L.A., and Grace, E.G., Jr.: Infection control practices related to treatment of AIDS patients. J. Dent. Pract. Adm. *7:*108, 1990.

134. Cohen, D.W.: Supply and demand: lessons from dental medicine? J. Med. Educ. *63:*108, 1988.

135. Cole, L.A.: Dentistry and ethics: A call for attention. J. Am. Dent. Assoc. *109:*559, 1984.

136. Cole, L.A.: The influence of "busyness" on attitudes about fluoridation and oversupply. J. N.J. Dent. Assoc. *Fall, 1985*, p. 22.

137. Cole, L.A.: A new look in American dentistry. The New York Times Magazine, April 5, 1981, 86.

138. Collins, P.J.: A commitment to accountability. New Zeal. Dent J. *86:*2, 1990.

139. Colman, H.L., and Dedmon, W.W.: Educational goals versus patient needs: Workshop report. J. Dent. Educ. *48:*25, 1984.

140. Colwell, E.B.: Ethics and human relations. J. Am. Coll. Dent. *23:*300, 1956.

141. Comer, R.W., et al. Management considerations for an HIV positive dental student. J. Dent. Educ. *55:*187, 1991.

142. Conley, J.F.: Settings standards. C.D.A. J. *17:*9, 1989.

143. Conrad, D.A., and Emerson, M.L.: State dental practice acts: Implications for competition. J. Health Policy Law. *5:*610, 1981.

144. Conrad, D.A., and Sheldon, G.C.: The effects of legal constraints on dental care prices. Inquiry *19:*51, 1982.

145. Cons, N. Interpreting ethical guidelines for dental epidemiological surveys. J. Dent. Res. *59C:*1292, 1980.

146. Conway, B.J.: The ethics of dental practice. J. Tenn. State Dent. Assoc. *39:*95, 1959.

147. Conway, B.J., and Rutledge, C.: The ethics of our profession. J. Am. Dent. Assoc. *62:*333, 1961.

148. Corah, N.L., O'Shea, R.M., and Bissell, G.D.: The dentist-patient relationship: Mutual perceptions and behaviors. J. Am. Dent. Assoc. *113:*253, 1986.

149. Corah, N.L.: Behavioral science research: Ethical and policy implications. Community Dent. Oral Epidemiol. *5:*265, 1977.

150. Cormier, P.P.: Who is handicapped: Patient or provider? J. Dent. Educ. *46:*166, 1982.

151. Cote, E.F.: The crystallizing professionalism. Am. J. Orthod. Dentofacial Orthop. *94:*525, 1989.

152. Coury, V.M.: Professional ethics in dental education. J. Tenn. Dent. Assoc. *65:*34, 1985.

153. Coury, V.M., et al.: Ethics curriculum identifies ethical conflicts. J. Am. Coll. Dent. *55:*31, 1988.

154. Coury, V.M., Slagle, W.F., Jr., and Fields, W.T.: Ethics curriculum identifies ethical conflicts. J. Am. Coll. Dent. *55:*31, 1988.

155. Cummings, J., and Vergo, T.J., Jr.: Traditional dentistry versus retail dentistry: A sociological pilot study of the dental profession. Quintessence International *169:*651, 1985.

156. Cussler, M., and Gordon, E.W.: Dentists, Patients, and Auxiliaries. Pittsburgh, University of Pittsburgh Press, 1968.

157. D'Anton, D.: The dilemma of dental advertising. Dent. Assist. *55:*17, 1986.

158. Davis, M.: Dentistry and AIDS: An ethical opinion. J. Am. Dent. Assoc. *119(Supplement):*9S, 1989.

159. Davis, T.B.: Ethics and drug abuse [editorial]. Tex. Dent. J. *105:*5, 1988.

160. Dean, M.S.: Dental ethics. Dent. Cosmos. *13:* 412, 1867.

161. Dean, G.: Professional ethics. Dent. Cosmos. *35:* 505, 1983.

162. DeMartino, B.K.: Commitment to the safe administration of dental anesthesia: The moral obligation. Dent. Clin. North Am. *31:*17, 1987.

163. Deuben, C.J., Sumner, W.L., and Johns, R.M.: Expanded functions: Future roles for dental hygienists. Dent. Hyg. (Chicago). *54:*29, 1980.

164. Devine, J.A.: If you don't care, who will? J. Am. Dent. Assoc. *51:*8, 1984.

165. Dewell, B.F.: The oath and the code revisited. Am. J. Orthod. *69:*587, 1976.

166. Dewhirst, F.E.: Dental education's responsibility and accountability. J. Dent. Educ. *41:*499, 1977.

167. De Angelis, A.J.: Quality assurance: definitions and directions for the 1980s. J. Dent. Educ. *48:* 27, 1984.

168. Diesendorf, M.: Diet and caries: Human experiments [letter]. J. Dent. Res. *67:*1538, 1988.

169. DiLullo, S.A., and Sanchez, P.M.: At what cost a free market: A review of antitrust laws versus professional ethics. J. Dent. Pract. Adm. *6:*16, 1989.

170. Donahue, T.J.: Patient autonomy and the bad result. J. Am. Dent. Assoc. *120:*478, 1990.

171. Dodes, J.E.: Greed and gullibility—A dental cataclysm. J. Colorado Dent. Assoc. *65:*4, 1987.

172. Doerr, R.: Enforcement: Every dentist's responsibility. J. Mich. Dent. Assoc. *58:*263, 1976.

173. Dolinsky, E.H., and Dolinsky, H.B.: Infantilization of elderly patients by health care providers. Spec. Care Dentist *4:*150, 1984.

174. Dougherty, H.L.: Progress with intellectual integrity. J. Charles H. Tweed Int. Found. *13*19, 1985.

175. Dove, S.B., and Cottone, J.A.: Knowledge and attitudes of Texas dentists concerning AIDS. Am. J. Dent. *3:*5, 1990.

176. Dummett, C.O.: Bioethics in dentistry: Birth . . . demise . . . renaissance. J. Indiana Dent. Assoc. *62:*17, 1983.

177. Dummett, C.O.: The influences of bioethics and history on the future of prosthodontics. Internat. J. Prosthod. *1:*241, 1988.

178. Dummett, C.O.: Dentistry: Ethical issues in dentistry. *In* Encyclopedia of Bioethics. Vol. 1. Edited by W. Reich. New York, The Free Press, 1978.

179. Dummett, C.O.: Year 2000: Community dentistry. J. Am. Dent. Assoc. *82:*280, 1971.

180. Dummett, C.O., and Dummett, L.D.: The Hillenbrand Era: Organized Dentistry's Glanzperiode. Bethesda, MD, American College of Dentists, 1986.

181. Dunn, W.G.: Leadership and the Professional Ethic. J. Am. Coll. Dent. *42:*74, 1976.

182. Dunn, W.J.: The dental professional: A historical review of developments . . . for testing and licensure. J. Can. Dent. Assoc. *52:*402, 1986.

183. Dunn, W.J.: Dentistry rejects advertising. Ontario Dentist *60:*34, 1983.

184. Dunn, W.J.: Third party coverage and ethical implications in dentistry. Compend. Contin. Educ. Dent. *6:*751, 1985.

185. Durand, R.W., and Morgan, D.: The Law and Ethics of Dental Practice. London, Hodder & Stoughton, 1950.

186. Durante, S.J.: Fallacy and danger of "public service." C.D.S. Review 83:33, 1990; also in J. Dent. Pract. Adm. 6:144, 1989.

187. Durard, R.W.: The Law and Ethics of Dental Practice. London, Hodder and Stoughton, 1950.

188. Ehrlich, A.B.: Ethics and Jurisprudence. Champaign, IL, Colwell, 1978.

189. Ehrlich, D.: Professional misconduct of organizations and agencies. J. Am. Coll. Dent. 41: 62, 1974.

190. Eli, I., and Shuval, J.T.: Professional socialization in dentistry. A longitudinal analysis of attitude changes among dental students toward the dental profession. Soc. Sci. Med. 16:951, 1982.

191. Enarson, H.L.: Dental education's responsibility and accountability. J. Dent. Educ. 41:489, 1977.

192. Engleheardt, H.T.: Humanism and the profession(al). J. Dent. Educ. 49:202, 1985.

193. Epstein, J.M.: Dental jurisprudence: Informed consent. J. Colorado Dent. Assoc. 57:25, 1979.

194. Epstein, J.M.: Dental jurisprudence: The nonpaying patient: Can services be terminated? J. Colorado Dent. Assoc. 57:43, 1978.

195. Evans, S.: Ethics and malpractice. Bull. Ninth Dist. Dent. Soc. (White Plains, NY) 54:9, 1970.

196. Fain, C.W.: The pursuit of excellence: President elect's address. J. Am. Coll. Dent. 52:4, 1985,

197. Federal Trade Commission: The final order on ethical restrictions against advertising by dentistry. J. Am. Dent. Assoc. 99:927, 1979.

198. Feldman, C.A., Saporito, R.A., and Martin, J.A.: Teaching ethics, jurisprudence, and risk management at the New Jersey Dental School. J. Law Ethics Dent. 2:101, 1989.

199. Feldman, S.M., and Sheetz, J.P.: Motivating dental auxillaries: Theories and applications. J. Am. Coll. Dent. 46:162, 1979.

200. Ferris, R.T.: What the responsibilities of a dentist who discovers sub-standard dentistry performed by another dentist? J. Dent. Pract. Adm. 2:186, 1985.

201. Fitch, C.P.: Professional ethics. Dent. Cosmos 3:60, 1862.

202. Flint, R.T.: Professionalism and the health occupations. J. Am. Dent. Hyg. Assoc. 41:190, 1967.

203. Fontana, V.J.: A physician's view of responsibility in reporting child abuse. Spec. Care Dentist 6:55, 1986.

204. Ford, R.T.: The dentist's responsibility in providing acceptable masticatory function. J. Dent. Pract. Adm. 5:174, 1988.

205. Formicola, A.J.: Educational goals versus patient needs. J. Dent. Educ. 48:20, 1984.

206. Fowlie, J.P.: Ethics and the component dental society. Arizona Dent. J. 22:25, 1976.

207. Fowler, M.D. Acquired immunodeficiency syndrome and refusal to provide care. Heart Lung 17:213, 1988.

208. Frazier, P.: Provider expectations and consumer perceptions of the importance and value of dental care. Am. J. Public Health Jan. 1977, p. 37.

209. Fredericks, M.A., Lobene, R.R., and Mundy, P.: Dental Care in Society: The Sociology of Dental Health. Jefferson, NC, McFarland, 1980.

210. Friedman, J.W.: Peer review—friend or foe? N. Engl. Dent. J. 77:85, 1981.

211. Friedson, E. The future of the professions. J. Dent. Educ. 51:140, 1987.

212. Gairola, G., and Skaff, K.O.: Ethical reasoning in dental hygiene practice. Dent. Hyg. (Chicago) 57:16, 1983.

213. Gaston, M.A., Brown, D.M., and Waring, M.B.: Survey of ethical issues in dental hygiene. J. Dent. Hygiene 64:217, 1990. [Published erratum appears in 64:352, 1990.]

214. George, W.A.: Factors affecting professional orientation in the delivery of oral health care: The pre-dental student. J. Am. Coll. Dent. 46: 29, 1979.

215. Gerbert, B.: AIDS and infection control in dental practice: Dentists' attitudes, knowledge, and behavior. J. Am. Dent. Assoc. 114:311, 1987.

216. Gerbert, B., et al.: Dental care experience of HIV-positive patients. J. Am. Dent. Assoc. 119: 601, 1989.

217. Gervasi, R.: Powerplay: Sexual harassment on the job. Dent. Assist. 51:6, 1982.

218. Gervasi, R.: Sexual harassment in the dental office: Results of ADAA's nationwide survey. Dent. Assist. 53:25, 1984.

219. Gervasi, R.: Sexual harassment and the politics of power. Dent. Assist. 53:30, 1984.

220. Giangreco, E.: Child abuse: Recognition and reporting. Spec. Care Dent. 6:62, 1986.

221. Giangrego, E.: Ethics of everyday practice. J. Dent. Hygiene 64:208, 1990.

222. Gibson, J.M.: Dentists, lawyers, and values: Suggestions for professional rapprochement. Dent. Clin. North Am. 26:229, 1982.

223. Gibson, W.A.: Human subjects in dental research: Coping with the regulations. J. Am. Dent. Assoc. 110:243, 1985.

224. Gift, H.C., Newman, J.F., and Loewy, S.B.: Attempts to control dental health care costs: The U.S. experience. Soc. Sci. Med. 15A:767, 1981.

225. Gilberg, S.L.: Are ethical dentists ethical? J. Am. Dent. Assoc. 86:34, 1973.

226. Gilbert, B.: AIDS and infection control in dental practice—dentists' attitudes, knowledge, and behavior. J. Am. Dent. Assoc. 114:311, 1987.

227. Gilbert, J.A.: Posterior composites: An ethical issue. Oper. Dent. 12:79, 1987.

228. Gilbert, J.A.: Ethics and esthetics. J. Am. Dent. Assoc. 117:490, 1988.

229. Gillett, G.: Giving ethics some teeth. N. Zeal. Dent. J. 87:2, 1991.

230. Glenn, R.E., and Kerber, P.E.: Measurement and evaluation of professional attitudes in dental students in remote site training programs. J. Am. Coll. Dent. 48:92, 1981.

231. Glick, M.: HIV-testing. More questions than answers. Dent. Clin. North Am. 34:45, 1990.

232. Glover, J.J., Ozar, D.T., and Thomasma, D.C.: Teaching ethics on rounds: The ethicist as teacher, consultant, and decision-maker. Theor. Med. 7:13, 1986.

233. Gluck, G., Aroskar, M., and Nezu, A.: Cost containment in dentistry and its impact on the distribution of service. Theor. Med. 4:207, 1983.

234. Gold, S.L.: Holistic dentistry: Disease is a result of social, psychological, and physical factors. Dent. Stud. 56:48, 1978.

235. Goldberg, A.: Ethics in the professions. J. Am. Coll. Dent. 42:218, 1975.

236. Goldberg, M.H.: Preoperative surgical judgment [letter]. J. Oral. Maxillofac. Surg. 46:636, 1988.

237. Goldhaber, P.: Ethics in Academe. J. Am. Coll. Dent. 55:10, 1988.

238. Goldman, A.H.: The Moral Foundations of Professional Ethics. Totowa, NJ, Rowan and Littlefield, 1980.

239. Gondela, L.: The delivery of dental care: An assessment of five alternative systems. J. Am. Dent. Assoc. 105:431, 1982.

240. Gondela, L.: Dentistry in the marketplace: An economic forecast. J. Am. Dent. Assoc. 104:18, 1982.

241. Gorovitz, S.: Dental school-industry relations: Areas of concern. J. Dent. Res. 61:743, 1982.

242. Gosselin, C.E.: The use and transfer of patient records. J. Dentaire Quebec 26:472, 1989.

243. Green, A.E., and Jong, A.: The role and responsibilities of hygienists and their association. Dent. Hygiene (Chicago) 54:377, 1980.

244. Green, D.: Can peer review be made to work? Dent. Manage. 17:31, 1977.

245. Green, D.: Dental advertising: Where in the world will it end? Dent. Manage. 17:33, 1977.

246. Green, T.G.: Dental student response to moral dilemmas. J. Dent. Educ. 45:137, 1981.

247. Greenwood, I.J.: Early history of dentistry. Dent. Reg. 15:29, 1861.

248. Griffiths, R.: What is ethics in practice? J. Am. Coll. Dent. 50:9, 1983.

249. Guralnick, W.: Ethics and the Board of Registration in dentistry. J. Mass. Dent. Soc. 39:11, 1990.

250. Gurenlian, J.R., and Forrest, J.L.: Recognizing professional responsibility. R.D.H. 5:24, 1985.

251. Gurley, J.E.: The Evolution of Professional Ethics in Dentistry: Report of the Historian. St. Louis, American College of Dentists, 1961.

252. Gryfe, J.: We've got substandard standards. Can. Dent. Assoc. J. 55:326, 1989.

253. Haffner, A.N.: Professionalism endures through dentistry is changing: Societal pressures affect traditional concepts of professionalism. J. Am. Coll. Dent. 48:151, 1981.

254. Halsband, E.R.: An introduction to the problems of dental ethics. Med. Law 3:377, 1984.

255. Halsband, E.R.: Dental ethics in practice. Med. Law 5:499, 1986.

256. Hamilton, J.: Child abuse: The dentist's responsibility. C.D.S. Rev. 83:18, 1990.

257. Hamrick, F.N.: What is a professional? Dentistry 7:8, 1987.

258. Hankin, R.: Retail store dentistry. J. Am. Dent. Assoc. 105:434, 1982.

259. Harrell, J.A.: It there a moral majority in dentistry? J. Am. Dent. Assoc. 112:148, 1986.

260. Harrington, M.S.: Accountability within dental hygiene. Educ. Dir. Dent. Aux. 3:19, 1978.

261. Harrison, R.L., and Feigal, R.J.: Challenges and dilemmas in behaviour guidance of the pediatric dental patient. Can. Dent. Assoc. J. 55:793, 1989.

262. Hartley, M.: Dental discrimination? Dentist 66: 1, 1988.

263. Hartley, M.: Dentists wear gloves, balk at treating victims. Dentist 66:46, 1988.

264. Harvey, W.L., and Gearhart, H.C.: The battle against denturism is both professional and moral. Dental Student 56:64, 1977.

265. Hasegawa, T.K., Jr.: Professional ethics instruction at Baylor College of Dentistry. J. Law Ethics Dent. 1:230, 1988.

266. Hasegawa, T.K., Jr., Lange, B., Bower, C.F., and Purtilo, R.B.: Ethical or legal perceptions by dental practitioners. J. Am. Dent. Assoc. 116: 354, 1988.

267. Hatasaka, H.: Informed consent—defense orthodontics. Am. J. Orthod. 76:448, 1979.

268. Hazelkorn, H.M.: The reaction of dentists to members of groups at risk of AIDS. J. Am. Dent. Assoc. 119:611, 1989.

269. Healy, J.M.: Ethical and legal aspects of dental medicine: perspectives for the practitioner. J. Conn. State Dent. Assoc. 60:27, 1986.

270. Heermance, E.L.: Codes of Ethics. New York, Free Press, 1924.

271. Heifitz, S.B.: Ethical considerations and study design. J. Dent. Res. 63(Spec):719, 1984.

272. Heifetz, S.B., and Kingman, A.: The impact of ethical considerations on future dental caries research: Clinical field trials. J. Dent. Res. 59(C): 1337, 1980.

273. Hein, J.W.: Dental education in a capitalistic society. J. Dent. Educ. 46:523, 1982.

274. Hein, J.W.: Implications of ethical and legal considerations on dental caries research—present and future. J. Dent. Res. 59C:1353, 1980.

275. Hesselberg, M.I.: Advertising and ethics. Br. Dent. J. 155:80, 1983.

276. Hickey, J.C.: Denturism—we must make an ethical choice. J. Prosthet. Dent. 38:360, 1977.

277. Hidey, M.J.: Professionalism: The conduct, aims, or qualities that characterize or mark a professional or professional person. Dent. Assist. 45:27, 1976.

278. Hillenbrand, H.: The necessity for trained advanced dental professionals. J. Dent. Educ. 45: 76, 1981.

279. Hine, M.K.: History of the modern ethical dental society. Bull. Hist. Dent. 14:1, 1966.

280. Hine, M.K.: The professional concept—its history and meaning to health service. J. Am. Coll. Dent. 37:19, 1970.

281. Hirsch, A.C., and Gert, B.: Ethics in dental practice. J. Am. Dent. Assoc. 113:599, 1986.

282. Hirschi, R.G.: The dentist and the nuclear debate: Search for solutions. J. Okl. Dent. Assoc. 75:18, 1985.

283. Hitchcock, R.C.: AIDS, Hepatitis B and the problems of confidentiality [letter]. Br. Dent. J. 159:243, 1985.

284. Hodges, L.W.: Toward a rekindled professionalism. Va. Dent. J. 64:6, 1987.

285. Hodish, M.T.: Advertising, ethics, and the free market. J. Am. Dent. Assoc. 118:353, 1989.

286. Hollaway, J.A., McNeal, D.R., and Lotzkar, S.: Ethical problems in dental practice. J. Am. Coll. Dent. 52:12, 1985.

287. Holz, F.M., and Johnson, D.W.: Legal Provisions on Expanded Functions for Dental Hygienists and Assistants Summarized by State. Rockville, Md., National Institutes of Health, 1974.

288. Hook, C.R.: The four commandments: A code to ethical dentistry. Dentistry 7:6, 1987.

289. Horowitz, H.S.: Current ethical issues in research. J. Am. Coll. Dent. 57:9, 1990.

290. Horowitz, H.S.: Ethical considerations in human experimentation. J. Dent. Res. 56C:C154, 1977.

291. Horowitz, H.: Ethical considerations of study participants in dental caries clinical trials. Commun. Dent. Oral Epidemiol. 4:43, 1976.

292. Horowitz, H.S.: Ethical issues in research [editorial]. J. Dent. Res. 69:1345, 1990.

293. Horowitz, H.S.: Overview of ethical aspects of clinical studies. Commun. Dent. Oral Epidemiol. 5:258, 1977.

294. Horowitz, H.S.: Overview of ethical issues in clinical studies. J. Public Health Dent. 38:35, 1978.

295. Horseman, R.E.: A code of ethics for dentistry. Dental Econ. 78:70, 1988.

296. Huntley, P.: Professional misconduct and mitigating circumstances [letter]. Br. Dent. J. 160:113, 1986.

297. Hynson, G.B.: Truth is truth. Oral Hygiene 9:1398, 1919. Ingle, I.I., and Blair, P., (eds.): International Dental Care Delivery Systems: Issues in Dental Health Policies. Cambridge, MA, Ballinger, 1978.

298. Jackson, E.: Managing dental fears: A tentative code of practice. J. Oral Med. 29:96, 1974.

299. Jacobs, A.D.: The commercialization of dentistry [editorial]. Int. J. Orthod. 20:5, 1982.

300. Jacobson, R.L.: Junk vs. ethical advertising—one doctor's discovery. Dent. Econ. 72:67, 1982.

301. Jenkins, J.J.: Legal implications of infectious disease control in the dental office. J. Indiana Dent. Assoc. 64:31, 1986.

302. Jenny, J.: Basic social values, structural elements in oral health systems and oral health status. Internat. Dent. J. 30:276, 1980.

303. Jhala, R.M.: Medico-legal aspects of dental practices. News Bull. Indiana Dent. Assoc. 5:27, 1974.

304. Johnson, D.L., and Hess, R.E.: In a crisis, give assistance, not advice. J. Okl. Dent. Assoc. 78:59, 1987.

305. Johnson, E.P.: An FTC view on codes of ethics. J. Am. Coll. Dent. 50:10, 1983.

306. Johnson, K.A.: The dilemma discussion: A strategy for teaching professional decision-making to dental hygienists. Educ. Dir. Dent. Aux. 9:4, 1984.

307. Jones, L.B., 3d.: Professionalism and ethics. J. Am. Dent. Assoc. 57:40, 1990.

308. Jong, A.W.: Dental advertising: A help or a hindrance? New patients use advertising to find dental care. Dentistry 7:9, 1987.

309. Jong, A.W.: Dental care for the cognitively impaired: An ethical dilemma. Gerodontics 4:172, 1988.

310. Jong, A.W.: Ethical issues in dental care. In Community Dental Health. 2nd Ed. Edited by A.W. Jong. St. Louis, Mosby-Yearbook, 1988.

311. Jong, A.W., and Heine, C.: The teaching of ethics in the dental hygiene curriculum. J. Dent. Educ. 46:699, 1982.

312. Jordan, W.K.: Advertising—is it a dirty word? J. Okl. Dent. Assoc. 75:12, 1985.

313. Jorgenson, R.J.: The role of the dentist in genetic counseling. Birth Defects 16:139, 1980.

314. Judy, K.W.: Implantology as a dental speciality: A moral and an educational focus. Implantologist 4:15, 1986.

315. Kaldenberg, D.O., Hallan, J.B., and Becker, B.W.: Continued treatment of an AIDS patient. J. Dent. Pract. Adm. 7:103, 1990.

316. Kassel, V.: On the criticism of colleagues. N.Y. State Dent. J. 41:210, 1975.

317. Kaplan, R.I.: The decline of ethical standards. J. Am. Coll. Dent. 44:78, 1977.

318. Keenan, P.A.: The ethical framework of medical/dental malpractice litigation. Dent. Clin. North Am. 26:245, 1982.

319. Kennedy, J.E.: Dental education and the objectives of the American College of Dentists. J. Am. Coll. Dent. 51:10, 1984.

320. Kennedy, J.E.: The case of dentistry, a harbinger for the profession? J. Dent. Educ. 51:145, 1987.

321. Kennedy, L.M.: The health professional as citizen. J. Am. Coll. Dent. 56:19, 1989.

322. Kennemer, C.E.: The ethics of consent [letter]. J. Am. Dent. Assoc. 113:864, 1986.

323. Knobel, G.J.: AIDS in dental practice: Hazards, infection control, medico-legal and ethical aspects. J. Forensic Odontostomatol. 4:15, 1986.

324. Koelbl, J.J.: AIDS at the Medical College of Georgia—A study in institutional ethics. J. Dent. Educ. 55:235, 1991.

325. Kohn, D.W.: Twenty-one years of child advocacy: An editorial retrospective of the Teuscher years. A.S.D.C. J. Dent. Child. 57:18, 1990.

326. Konvalinka, K.R.: Child abuse: Ethical and practical considerations for the dental team. J. Mich. Dent. Assoc. 70:139, 1988.

327. Konvalinka, K.R.: Setting the bounds of treatment: How to choose, refuse and dismiss patients. Dentistry 7:19, 1987.

328. Koot, A.C., and Darby, M.L.: Values: A review of the literature and implications for dental hygiene. Dent. Hyg. (Chicago). 52:381, 1978.

329. Koot, A.C., and Darby, M.L.: Values of dental hygienists in three different occupational settings. Educ. Dir. Dent. Aux. 4:13, 1978.

330. Kramer, M.G.: Professionalism and principles of ethics: changing concepts for dentistry. Pediatr. Dent. 2:245, 1980.

331. Kratenstein, D.I.: Periodontal ethics and referral modes. N.Y. State Dent. J. 55:46, 1989.

332. Kress, G.C.: The impact of professional education on the performance of dentists. In Social Sciences in Dentistry: A Critical Bibliography. Vol. 2. Edited by L.K. Cohen and P.S. Bryant. London, Quintessence, 1984.

333. Krol, A.J.: The professional man's sense of responsibility. Contact Point 45:246, 1967.

334. Krol, A.J.: Professional man and his search for truth. Contact Point 45:211, 1967.

335. Kulick, A.A.: The legal and professional responsibilities of the implantodontist. Newslet. Am. Acad. Implant. Dent. *Jan, 1969*, p. 8.

336. Kultgen, J.: Ethics and Professionalism. Philadelphia, University of Pennsylvania Press, 1988.

337. Laird, M.R.: The professional man. J. Am. Dent. Assoc. *77:*1052, 1968.

338. Lange, A.L., Loupe, M.J., and Meskin, H.L.: Professional satisfactions in dentistry. J. Am. Dent. Assoc. *104:*619, 1982.

339. Larkin, G.V.: Professionalism, dentistry, and public health. Soc. Sci. Med. *14A:*223, 1980.

340. Laskin, D.M.: Access to health care: A right or privilege? [editorial]. J. Oral Maxillofac. Surg. *45:*297, 1987.

341. Laskin, D.M.: Choosing your treatment with care [editorial]. J. Oral Maxillofac. Surg. *47:*1, 1989.

342. Laskin, D.M.: Ethical aspects of professional practice [editorial]. J. Oral Maxillofac. Surg. *37:*234, 1979.

343. Laskin, D.M.: The ethics of expert testimony [editorial]. J. Oral Maxillofac. Surg. *47:*1131, 1989.

344. Laskin, D.M.: Holism not "hole-ism" in oral and maxillofacial surgery [editorial]. J. Oral Maxillofac. Surg. *36:*753, 1978.

345. Laskin, D.M.: The "hypocritic" oath [editorial]. J. Oral Maxillofac. Surg. *48:*335, 1990.

346. Laskin, D.M.: Keeping our professional promises [editorial]. J. Oral Maxillofac. Surg. *49:*671, 1991.

347. Laskin, D.M.: Keeping the boundaries of specialization [editorial]. J. Oral Maxillofac. Surg. *43:*480, 1985.

348. Laskin, D.M.: The plight of the plaintiff [editorial]. J. Oral Maxillofac. Surg. *43:*402, 1985.

349. Laskin, D.M.: Treatment of patients with AIDS: A matter of professional ethics [editorial]. J. Oral Maxillofac. Surg. *46:*719, 1988.

350. Laskin, D.M.: Truth or consequences [editorial]. J. Am. Coll. Dent. *41:*9, 1984.

351. Laskin, D.M.: Who's cheating whom? J. Oral Maxillofac. Surg. *38:*89, 1980.

352. Laster, J.: The research imperative. J. Dent. Res. *59C:*1225, 1980.

353. Latimer, C.E.: Ethics—a discussion. Am. Dent. Assoc. Trans. 1871, p. 62.

354. Lawrence, S., et al.: Parental attitudes toward behavior management techniques used in pediatric dentistry. Pediatr. Dent. *13:*151, 1991.

355. Lawton, F.: President's address to the General Dental Council. Br. Dent. J. *165:*385, 1988.

356. Legler, D.W.: Relationships: Tending the garden in a high tech society. J. Am. Coll. Dent. *54:*4, 1987.

357. Lehman, J.P.: The spirit of obligation. Can. Dent. Assoc. J. *16:*27, 1988.

358. Lentchner, E.W.: Emergency dental care: The responsibility of the dental society. N.Y. State Dent. J. *42:*213, 1976.

359. Leske, G.S.: Ethical and legal considerations associated with clinical field trials. J. Dent. Res. *59C:*1243, 1980.

360. Levenson, C.A.: When you make an honest error. Dent. Manage. *8:*44, 1968.

361. Lewis, J.: The role of ethics in the profession of dentistry. Ill. Dent. J. *47:*598, 1978.

362. Linn, E.L.: Service to others and economic gain as professional objectives of dental students. J. Dent. Educ. *32:*75, 1968.

363. Loader, C.F., and Kishi, S.R.: Legacy: The Dental Profession. Bakersfield, CA, Loader/Kishi, 1990.

364. Logan, H., Hayden, H., and Jakobsen, J.: Role expectations of dental hygienists. Dent. Hyg. (Chicago). *54:*321, 1980.

365. Logan, M.K.: The HIV-infected dental professional. A challenge to law, ethics, and the dental profession. J. Dent. Pract. Adm. *6:*162, 1989.

366. Logan, M.K.: Informed consent: Does the doctrine apply to HIV, amalgam, fluoride? J. Am. Dent. Assoc. *122:*18, 1991.

367. Logan, M.K.: Legal, ethical issues for dentists. J. Am. Dent. Assoc. *115:*402, 1987.

368. Logan, M.K.: Legal implications of infectious disease in the dental office. J. Am. Dent. Assoc. *115:*850, 1987.

369. Loupe, M.J., Meskin, H.L., and Mast, T.A.: Change in the values of dental students and dentists over a ten year period. J. Dent. Educ. *43:*170, 1979.

370. Lovett, E.: An Approach to Ethics. 2nd ed. Baltimore, Waverly Press, 1963.

371. Luks, S.: The endodontic stabilizer and the patient's bill of rights. N.Y.J. Dent. *44:*44, 1974.

372. Lundberg, J.F.: Legal and ethical aspect of the AIDS crisis. J. Dent. Educ. *53:*515, 1989.

373. Luoma, H.: Ethics of experiments involving human subjects. Scand. J. Dent. Res. *89:*5, 1981.

374. Lyons, K.J., and Leonhardt, R.D.: Patient records: Who has access to them? Greater Milw. Dent. Bull. *47:*263, 1980.

375. MacDonald, S.K.: Parental needs and professional responses: a parental perspective. Cleft Palate J. *16:*188, 1979.

376. Macklin, R., Sadowsky, D., and Kunzel, C.: Consultants' advice and professional responsibility: An ethical analysis. J. Law Eth. Dent. *1:*113, 1988.

377. Maihofer, G.: Principles of ethics and code of professional conduct. G.M.D.A. Bull. *55:*144, 1988.

378. Maloney, J.D.: Current challenges to the professions in America. J. Am. Coll. Dent. *41:*52, 1974.

379. Mandel, I.D.: Changing dental images—from stone tablets to comic strips. J. Am. Dent. Assoc. *118:*695, 1991.

380. Mappes, T.A., and Zembaty, J.S.: Case—the dentist and patient autonomy. *In* Biomedical Ethics. 3rd Ed. Edited by T.A. Mappes and J.S. Zembaty. New York, McGraw-Hill, 1991.

381. Marbach, J.J.: Malpractice and temporomandibular joint dysfunction syndrome. N.Y. State Dent. J. *53:*37, 1987.

382. Marbach, J.J.: The solid gold placebo. N.Y. State Dent. J. *51:*278, 1985.

383. Marshall, P., Thomasma, D., and O'Keefe, P.: Disclosing HIV status. J. Am. Dent. Assoc. *122:*11, 1991.

384. Martin, J.G.: The new professionalism. J. Am. Dent. Hyg. Assoc. *45:*182, 1971.

385. Martin, M.D., Danner, F., and McNeal, D.R.: Ethical concerns of practicing dentists. Gen. Dent. 34:277, 1986.

386. May, W.: The physician's covenant. J. Am. Coll. Dent. 51:16, 1984.

387. McCall, L., Kennedy, L.M., and Zinman, E.J.: What are the responsibilities of a dentist who discovers sub-standard dentistry performed by another dentist? J. Dent. Pract. Admin. 2:186, 1985.

388. McCardy, T.R.: Utilization review: PSRO and the oral surgeon. Oral Surg. 42:271, 1976.

389. McCarthy, F.M.: The protopappas anesthesia deaths. J. Am. Dent. Assoc. 110:26, 1985.

390. McCullough, L.B.: Ethics in dental medicine: A framework for moral responsibility in dental practice. J. Dent. Educ. 49:219, 1985.

391. McCullough, L.B.: Moral dimensions of leadership. J. Am. Coll. Dent. 56:19, 1989.

392. McCullough, L.B.: Ethical Issues in Dentistry. In Clinical Dentistry. Revised ed. Vol. One. Edited by J.W. Clark. Philadelphia, Harper and Row, 1983.

393. McCurdy, T.R., and Chase, D.C.: Utilization review: PSRO and the oral surgeon. Oral Surg. Oral Med. Oral Pathol. 42:271, 1976.

394. McDonald, R.E., and Barton, P.: Activities by the schools to improve the distribution of dentists: An AADS report. J. Dent. Educ. 44:246, 1980.

395. McHugh, W.D.: Professional ethics in dental research. J. Am. Coll. Dent. 51:19, 1984.

396. McIntosh, S.R.: AIDS . . . dentistry's concern in Missouri. Mo. Dent. J. 68:14, 1988.

397. McIvor, J.: A lay member's perspective. Br. Dent. J. 167:96, 1989.

398. McMahan, E.L.: Summary from group discussions: what should dental public health be? The issues, constituencies, and priorities of the future and how to get to the "should"—strategies and interventions using the community approach. J. Public Health Dent. 50(Spec):139, 1990.

399. Melcher, A.H.: An ancient oath? [editorial]. Int. J. Oral Maxillofac. Implants. 2:123, 1987.

400. Meskin, L.H.: Societal and professional forces affecting graduate dental education .J. Dent. Educ. 44:714, 1980.

401. Milgrom, P.: Continuing education and the prospect for a national standard of dental care. J. Dent. Educ. 8:482, 1974.

402. Milgrom, P.: Quality control of end results: identifying avoidable adverse events. J. Am. Dent. Assoc. 90:1282, 1975.

403. Milgrom, P.: Regulation and the Quality of Dental Care. Rockville, MD, Aspen Systems Corp., 1978.

404. Milgrom, P., and Ingle, J.I.: Patient consent procedures for dental care. J. Oral Maxillofac. Surg. 33:515, 1975.

405. Miller, S.L., Ramirez, A., and Pelton, W.J.: Programmed course in dental ethics compared with two other methods of instruction. J. Public Health Dent. 30:229, 1970.

406. Mills, J.C. Dentistry: An art, a science or a profession? J. Ala. Dent. Assoc. 73:12, 1989.

407. Mitsis, F.J.: Hippocrates in the golden age: His life, his work and his contributions to dentistry. J. Am. Coll. Dent. 58:26, 1991.

408. Moniz, D.M.: Terminating the doctor-patient relationship: How to have a graceful exit. Hawaii Dent. J. 19:18, 1988.

409. Moody, P.M., Van Tassel, C., and Cash, D.M.: Cynicism, humanitarianism, and dental career development. J. Dent. Educ. 38:645, 1974.

410. Moore, J.R.: The Webb-Johnson lecture—ethics and experiment. Br. Dent. J. 162:360, 1987.

411. More, D., and Kahn, N.: Some motives for entering dentistry. Am. J. Sociology. 66:48, 1960.

412. Moretti, R.J., Ayer, W.A., and Derefinko, A.: Attitudes and practices of dentists regarding HIV patients and infection control. Gen. Dent. 2:144, 1989.

413. Morris, R.T., and Sherlock, B.J.: Decline of ethics and the rise of cynicism in dental school. J. Health Soc. Beh. 12:290, 1971.

414. Morris, W.O.: Ethical and legal duties of a parent to provide dental treatment to a minor. J. Law Eth. Dent. 1:194, 1988.

415. Morgenstein, W.: Informed consent—the doctrine evolves. J. Am. Dent. Assoc. 93:637, 1976.

416. Moskowitz, D.P., and Farrell, V.D. Professional disciplinary proceedings and the licensed dental practitioner. N.Y. State Dent. J. 50:437, 1984.

417. Motley, W.E.: Ethics, Jurisprudence, and History for the Dental Hygienist. 3rd Ed. Philadelphia, Lea & Febiger, 1983.

418. Mozer, J.E.: Frustration and values. J. Am. Coll. Dent. 52:17, 1985.

419. Mulcahy, D.F.: Special facilities for dental treatment of patients with AIDS? [letter]. Can. Dent. Assoc. J. 56:27, 1990.

420. Mumma, R.D., Jr.: Institutional survival versus social responsibility: finances as a driving force—a dental education perspective. J. Dent. Educ. 52:287, 1988.

421. Mundie, G.E.: The importance of a team approach when identifying and treating child maltreatment: A personal view. Spec. Care Dent. 6:58, 1986.

422. Murphy, W.J.: Development of the concept of informed consent. Dent. Clin. North Am. 26:287, 1985.

423. Nash, D.A.: Ethics . . . and the quest for excellence in the profession. J. Dent. Educ. 49:1981, 1985.

424. Nash, D.A.: The ethics of profession in dental medicine. Health Matrix 2:3, 1984.

425. Nash, D.A.: Ethics in dentistry: Review and critique of Principles of Ethics and Code of Professional Conduct. J. Am. Dent. Assoc. 109:597, 1984.

426. Nash, D.A.: Professional ethics and esthetic dentistry. J. Am. Dent. Assoc. 117E:7E–9E, 1988.

427. Nash, D.A.: Professional ethics in dentistry. Ky. Dent. J. 40:11, 1988.

428. Nash, P.J., Nash, D.A., and Hutton, J.L.: Moral reasoning and clinical performance of student dentists. J. Dent. Educ. 46:721, 1982.

429. Neidle, E.: Dentistry, ethics, and the humanities: A three-unit bridge. J. Dent. Educ. *44:*963, 1980.
430. Neidle, E.A.: A matter of policy. J. Am. Dent. Assoc. *122:*45, 1991.
431. Neidle, E.A.: On the brink—will dental education be ready for the future? J. Dent. Educ. *54:* 564, 1990.
432. Nelsen, R.J.: The nature of professionalism—its value to society. J. Am. Coll. Dent. *41:*37, 1974.
433. Nelsen, R.J.: Economic and philosophical factors in fee structuring. J. Am. Coll. Dent. *44:* 215, 1977.
434. Nelsen, R.J.: The student becomes a professional—an important metamorphosis. Odontol. Bull. *55:*9, 1975.
435. Newell, K.J., Young, L.J., and Yamoor, C.M.: Moral reasoning in dental hygiene students. J. Dent. Educ. *49:*79, 1985.
436. Nordstrom, N.K., Soller, H., and Odom, J.: Hygiene practice ethics. Can. Dent. Assoc. J. *16:*27, 1988.
437. Norris, C.: The dental hygienist: Will she carve a separate slice of the pie? Dent. Manage. *19:* 19, 1979.
438. Noyes, E.: Ethics and Jurisprudence for Dentists. Chicago, Conkey Co, 1923.
439. Odom, J.G.: A dental ethics institute for Ohio State University dental students and practitioners. Ohio Dent. J. *59:*11, 1985.
440. Odom, J.G.: Ethics and dental amalgam removal. J. Am. Dent. Assoc. *122:*69, 1991.
441. Odom, J.G.: Ethics and the cognitive development of the dentist. Med. Law *6:*565, 1987.
442. Odom, J.G.: Ethics: Who makes the treatment decision? J. Dent. Pract. Adm. *3:*57, 1986.
443. Odom, J.G.: Formal ethics instruction in dental education. J. Dent. Educ. *46:*553, 1982.
444. Odom, J.G.: Making a commitment to teaching ethics. J. Am. Coll. Dent. *53:*4, 1986.
445. Odom, J.G.: Parameters and goals for teaching ethics. Ohio Dent. J. *58:*36, 1984.
446. Odom, J.G.: The practical ramifications of cheating. J. Dent. Educ. *55:*272, 1991.
447. Odom, J.G.: Recognizing and resolving ethical dilemmas in dentistry. Med. Law *4:*543, 1985.
448. Odom, J.G.: The status of dental ethics instruction. J. Dent. Educ. *52:*306, 1988.
449. Odom, J.G.: Teaching dental students to solve ethical problems. Dentistry *7:*16, 1987.
450. Odom, J.G.: Who makes the treatment decision? J. Dent. Pract. Adm. *3:*57, 1986.
451. Odom, J.G., and Messina, M.: Treatment decision making: Student choices of autonomy versus paternalism. J. Law Eth. Dent. *4:*12, 1991.
452. Odom, J.G., and Morris, W.O.: The autonomy of the practitioner. J. Dent. Practice Adm. *6:*12, 1989.
453. Oler, K.D.: Redefining our purposes, redirecting our efforts. J. Am. Coll. Dent. *52:*10, 1985.
454. Oler, K.D.: Winds of change. Can. Dent. Assoc. J. *16:*201, 1988.
455. Olsen, E.D.: Ethical conduct in professional administration. J. Am. Dent. Assoc. *55:*11, 1988.
456. Olsen, N.H.: Professionalism and ethics: Their place in modern society. Chicago Dent. Soc. Rev. J, 1986, 11.
457. Orzack, L.H.: New profession by fiat: Italian dentistry and European Common Market. Soc. Sci. Med. *15A:*807, 1981.
458. O'Shea, R.M., and Cohen, L.K., (eds): Toward a Sociology of Dentistry [special issue]. Milbank Mem. Fund. *49:*3, 1971.
459. Ozar, D.T.: AIDS, ethics, and dental care. *In* Clark's Clinical Dentistry. Edited by J. Hardin. Philadelphia, J.B. Lippincott Co., 1992.
460. Ozar, D.T.: AIDS, risk, and obligations of health professionals. *In* AIDS and Ethics: Biomedical Ethics Reviews—1988. Edited by J.M. Humber and R.F. Almeder. Clifton, NJ, Humana, 1989.
461. Ozar, D.T.: Dentistry. *In* Encyclopedia of Bioethics. Revised edition. Edited by Warren Reich. New York, Macmillan, 1993 (forthcoming).
462. Ozar, D.T.: Ethical issues at chairside. Bull. Soc. Health Hum. Values. *19:*4, 1989.
463. Ozar, D.T.: Ethical issues in dental care for the compromised patient. Spec. Care Dent. *16:*206, 1990.
464. Ozar, D.T.: Ethical issues in pediatric dentistry. Pediatr. Dent. *13:*374, 1991.
465. Ozar, D.T.: The ethical ramifications of cheating. J. Dent. Educ. *55:*276, 1991.
466. Ozar, D.T.: Ethics for the practicing dentist. A framework for studying professional ethics. J. Am. Coll. Dent. *58:*4, 1991.
467. Ozar, D.T.: Ethics of management techniques and therapeutic approaches. *In* Behavior Management for the Pediatric Dental Patient. Edited by J. Bogert and R. Creedon. Chicago, American Academy of Pediatric Dentistry, 1989.
468. Ozar, D.T.: Formal instruction in dental professional ethics. J. Dent. Educ. *49:*696, 1985.
469. Ozar, D.T.: A Framework for Studying Professional Ethics, J. Am. Coll. Dent. *58:*4, 1991.
470. Ozar, D.T.: On ethics of chairside. J. Am. Dent. Assoc. *116:*697, 1988.
471. Ozar, D.T.: Teaching ethics in the professions. *In* Educating Professionals. Edited by L. Curry and J. Wergin. San Francisco, Josse Bass, 1993.
472. Ozar, D.T.: The Joe Shovich case. N.C. Dent. G. *11:*19, 1989.
473. Ozar, D.T.: Three models of professionalism and professional obligations in dentistry. J. Am. Dent. Assoc. *110:*173, 1985.
474. Ozar, D.T.: The values of geriatric dentistry. Spec. Care Dentist *7:*44, 1987.
475. Ozar, D.T., and Hockenberry, K.L.: Professional ethics in dentistry: The PEDNET bibliography. J. Dent. Educ. *49:*244, 1985.
476. Ozar, D.T., Schiedermayer, D.L., and Siegler, M.: Value categories in clinical dental ethics. J. Am. Dent. Assoc. *116:*365, 1988.
477. Ozar, D.T., and Sokol, D.J.: Dental Ethics at Chairside: Professional Principles and Practical Applications. St. Louis, Mosby-Yearbook, 1993 (forthcoming).
478. Pallasch, T.J.: The patient: First, last, always. Can. Dent. Assoc. J. *16:*23, 1988.
479. Palmer, B.B.: The philosophy of dental health service: Its relation to the changing social order. J. Am. Coll. Dent. *48:*179, 1981.

480. Parish, J.: Professional conduct in dental school and after. J. Dent. Educ. *32:*326, 1968.

481. Pavalko, R.M.: Social background and occupational perspectives of predental students. J. Dent. Educ. *28:*253, 1964.

482. Perich, M.L.: Maintaining ethical standards in today's dental practice—a perspective of the American Dental Association. J. Am. Coll. Dent. *55:*18, 1988.

483. Perich, P.: The ethical marketing of dentistry: Is it a misnomer? J. Am. Coll. Dent. *50:*.12, 1983.

484. Perry, H.T., Jr.: The dentists' responsibility to health care delivery. J. Am. Coll. Dent. *52:*12, 1985.

485. Perry, H.T., Jr.: Professional liability [editorial]. J. Craniomandib. Disord. *1:*83, 1987.

486. Peterson, L.M.: AIDS: The ethical dilemma for surgeons. J. Law Eth. Dent. *2:*78, 1989.

487. Petterson, E.O.: Ethics courses in the dental curriculum. J. Am. Coll. Dent. *41:*249, 1974.

488. Pindborg, J.J.: Ethics of publishing results from research. Scand. J. Dent. Res. *89:*12, 1981.

489. Plunk, P.L.: From the moral majority [letter]. J. Am. Dent. Assoc. *112:*596, 1986.

490. Pollack, B.R.: A case of questionable ethics, or fulfilling professional responsibility. J. Law Eth. Dent. *2:*130, 1989.

491. Pollack, B.R.: Teaching law, ethics, and risk management at the School of Dental Medicine State University of New York at Stony Brook. J. Law Eth. Dent. *2:*32, 1989.

492. Pollack, B.R., and Marineli, R.D.: Ethical, moral, and legal dilemmas in dentistry: The process of informed decision making. J. Law Ethics Dent. *1:*27, 1988.

493. Pollick, H.F.: Ethics and geriatrics. Spec. Care Dentist *1:*7, 1981.

494. Poupard, J.: California's dental health: What role does government play? J. Calif. Dent. Assoc. *8:*39, 1980.

495. Powell, D.: The dentist's perspective as a member of an interdisciplinary health team. Birth Defects *16:*125, 1980.

496. Press, B.H.: Ethics in the practice of dentistry. J. Am. Coll. Dent. *51:*9, 1984.

497. Prout, R.W.: Morality and insurance. Dent. Dimens. *9:*2, 1975 and *10:*7, 1976.

498. Quarantelli, E.: Career choice patterns of dental students. J. Health Human Behavior *2:*124, 1961.

499. Quinlan, L.W.: How's your ethics I.Q.? Dent. Manage. *16:*41, 1976.

500. Quinn, N.K., and Capron, M.A.: Expert witness testimony. J. Oral Maxillofac. Surg. *46:*1086, 1988.

501. Randolph, K.V.: Dental ethics—fact or fancy. J. Am. Coll. Dent. *49:*217, 1982.

502. Randolph, K.V.: What role should ethics play in the education of professionalism? The Nebraska Humanist *7:*55, 1984.

503. Rankin, J.A., and Harris, M.B.: Patient's preferences for dentists' behaviors. J. Am. Dent. Assoc. *110:*323, 1985.

504. Rau, C.F.: Positive reinforcement in clinical teaching and evaluation. J. Am. Coll. Dent. *51:*22, 1984.

505. Redcliffe-Maud, L.: Professional responsibility. Br. Dent. J. *143:*125, 1977.

506. Reeves, J.F.: Standards in dentistry. Br. Dent. J. *156:*123, 1984.

507. Reynolds, R.J.: Health care: Changes, challenges. J. Am. Coll. Dent. *51:*35, 1984.

508. Reynolds, R.J.: A positive view. J. Am. Coll. Dent. *49:*11, 1982.

509. Reynolds, R.J.: Professional ethics. J. Am. Coll. Dent. *55:*41, 1988.

510. Robinson, H.B.: Maintaining professional ethics: A challenge of the times. Dent. Survey *52:*13, 1976.

511. Robinson, J.B.: Report of the committee on conduct. J. Am. Coll. Dent. *25:*37, 1958.

512. Robinson, J.B.: History of the American Dental Association—1859–1897. J. Am. Dent. Assoc. *58:*21, 1959.

513. Robinson, J.B.: Dental history as a subject of undergraduate instruction. N.Y.J. Dent. *39:*228, 1969.

514. Robinson, W.H.: Our ethical code. Dental Jairus *1*, 1880.

515. Rogers, V.C.: Dentistry and AIDS: ethical and legal obligations in provision of care. Med. Law *24:*326, 1987.

516. Rogers, V.C.: Ethical considerations of appropriate versus comprehensive dental care for patients in nursing homes. J. Law Eth. Dent. *1:*82, 1988.

517. Rosen, A.C., Marcus, M., and Johnson, N.: Changes in role perceptions by first year dental students. J. Dent. Educ. *41:*507, 1977.

518. Rosenblum, A.B., Goldstein, C.M., and Crawford, C.C.: Ethics by case analysis. J. Calif. Dent. Assoc. *17:*35, 1989.

519. Rosenburg, J.L.: Attitude changes in dental and medical students during professional education. J. Dent. Educ. *49:*399, 1985.

520. Rosner, J.F.: Self-regulation in the dental profession. J. Am. Dent. Assoc. *98:*919, 1979.

521. Ross, I.F.: Committee on ethics. J. Periodont. *47:*299, 1976.

522. Rostoff, A.J.: Informed Consent: A Guide for Health Care Providers. Rockville, MD, Aspen, 1981.

523. Rovelstad, G.H.: Some historical perspectives on dentistry, the Americal College of Dentists, and professionalism. J. Am. Coll. Dent. *44:*93, 1977.

524. Rozovsky, L.E.: When does the dentist have to tell? Guidelines to confidentiality. Oral Health *77:*37, 1987.

525. Rudd, T.: The ethics of ease. J. Okl. Dent. Assoc. *79:*28, 1988.

526. Rule, J., and Veatch, R.: Ethical Questions in Dentistry. Chicago, Quintessence, 1993.

527. Runnells, R.R.: Infection control answers issues surrounding AIDS in ethical way. Dentist *67:*28, 1989.

528. Rydman, R.J., et al.: Preventive control of AIDS by the dental profession: a survey of practices in a large urban area. J. Public Health Dent. *50:*7, 1990.

529. Sachs, R.H., Zullo, T.G., and Close, J.M.: Concerns of entering dental students. J. Dent. Educ. *45:*133, 1981.

530. Sadowsky, D.: Moral dilemmas of the multiple prescription in dentistry. J. Am. Coll. Dent. *46:* 245, 1979.

531. Sadowsky, D., and Kunzel, C.: Are you willing to treat AIDS patients? J. Am. Dent. Assoc. *122:* 28, 1991.

532. Saddoris, J.A.: Preserve our commitment to professionalism. J. Am. Coll. Dent. *57:*16, 1990.

533. Saha, P.S., and Saha, S.: Clinical trials of medical devices and implants—ethical concerns. IEEE Engineering Med. Biol. *6:*85, 1988.

534. Saha, P.S., and Saha, S.: Ethical responsibilities of the clinical engineer. J. Clin. Eng. *11:*17, 1986.

535. Saha, P.S., and Saha, S.: The need of biomedical ethics training in bioengineering. *In* Biomedical Engineering I: Recent Developments. Edited by S. Saha. New York, Pergamon, 1982.

536. Sakumura, J.S.: Values of dental hygiene faculty and students: A cross sectional study. Educ. Dir. Dent. Aux. *3:*610, 1978.

537. Sakumura, J.S.: Values of dental hygiene faculty and students: A longitudinal study. Educ. Dir. Dent. Aux. *5:*13, 1980.

538. Sakumura, J.S.: Values of dental hygiene practioners, faculty and seniors. Educ. Dir. Dent. Aux. *6:*21, 1981.

539. Savage, T.J.: Ethics everywhere everyday: A perspective. J. Am. Coll. Dent. *57:*23, 1990.

540. Schafer, A.: Dental ethics—Part I: What ethics is not. Can. Dent. Assoc. J. *55:*125, 1989.

541. Schafer, A.: Dental ethics—Part II: Getting the balance right. Can. Dent. Assoc. J. *55:*189, 1989.

542. Schafer, A.: Dental ethics—Part III. Challenge and crisis. Can. Dent. Assoc. J. *55:*283, 1989.

543. Scheutz, F., and Pindborg, J.J.: Dentists professional and ethical responsibilities for HIV-positive patients and patients with AIDS. Aust. Dent. J. *32:*298, 1987; and J. Mass. Dent. Society. *36:*6, 1987.

544. Schicke, R.K.: Prevention and the demand for dental care in an international perspective. Internat. Dent. J. *31:*320, 1981.

545. Schiedermayer, D.L.: The process of deprofessionalization: getting down to business in dentistry: The effect of advertising on a profession. J. Am. Coll. Dent. *55:*10, 1988.

546. Schissel, M.J.: As long as the patient gets well. Dent. Econ. *79:*21, 1989.

547. Schissel, M.J.: Innovative marketing or unfair competition? Dent. Econ. *77:*19, 1987.

548. Schmidt, D.A.: Why welfare patients are welcome. Dent. Manage. *20:*40, 1980.

549. Schoen, M.H.: Dental care in a socialized health system. J. Public Health Dent. *39:*195, 1979.

550. Scholle, R.H.: Caries prevention: Second thoughts. J. Am. Dent. Assoc. *102:*602, 1981.

551. Scholle, R.H.: The privilege of practice. J. Am. Dent. Assoc. *98:*159, 1979.

552. Schuman, S.K.: Ethics and the patient with dementia. J. Am. Dent. Assoc. *119:*747, 1989.

553. Schuman, N.J., and Hamilton, R.L.: Discovery of child abuse with associated dental fracture in a hospital-affiliated clinic: Report of a case with four year follow up. Spec. Care Dent. *2:*250, 1982.

554. Schwartz, B.: Should selling products be a part of your practice? Dent. Manage. *29:*28, 1989.

555. Schwartz, H.C.: Professional responsibility—more than just treatment [letter]. J. Oral Maxillofac. Surg. *45:*750, 1987.

556. Schwartzseid, E.E.: Ethics as an important determinant of success of orthopaedic dental care for debilitated and elderly patients. Gerodontology *8:*83, 1989.

557. Secrest, B.G.: Report poor work. J. Am. Dent. Assoc. *91:*1141, 1975.

558. Seear, J.: Consent to treatment. Dent. Update. *1:*265, 1974.

559. Seear, J.: Law and Ethics in Dentistry. 2nd ed. Boston, Bristol, 1981.

560. Segal, H., and Warner, R.: Origins of paternalism. Med. Law *4:*269, 1985.

561. Segal, H., and Warner, R.: The rationale for a philosopher in a dental school. Quintessence International *14:*573, 1983.

562. Seigal, M., et al.: Treating persons with AIDS—report of a survey of Ohio dentists' knowledge, attitudes, and practices in 1989. Ohio Dent. J. *64:*8, 1990.

563. Senseman, C.: Ethics—why? Dent. Hyg. (Chicago) *52:*74, 1978.

564. Sfikas, P.M.: Maintaining ethical standards in today's dental practice—a historical perspective. J. Am. Coll. Dent. *55:*19, 1988.

565. Shahan, D.D.: Malpractice: Medical abandonment. J. Dent. Pract. Adm. *4:*76, 1987.

566. Shapira, E.Z.: Professionalism and ethics. Can. Dent. Assoc. J. *16:*55, 1988.

567. Sheehan, T.J., et al.: Moral judgement as a predictor of clinical performance. Eval. Health Prof. *3:*393, 1980.

568. Shefrin, A.P.: The use of role-playing for teaching professionalism and ethics. J. Dent. Educ. *42:*150, 1978.

569. Sheiham, A.: Discussion of symposium on ethical issues in dentistry. Commun. Dent. Oral Epidemiol. *5:*269, 1977.

570. Sherlock, B.J., and Cohen, A.: The strategy of occupational choices: recruitment to dentistry. Social Forces *44:*303, 1966.

571. Sherlock, B.J., and Morris, R.T.: Becoming a Dentist. Springfield, IL, Charles C Thomas, 1972.

572. Shipman, B., and Teitelman, J.L.: Learned helplessness and the older dental patients. Spec. Care Dent. *5:*261, 1985.

573. Shira, R.R.: The ethical, legal, and moral responsibilities of the practicing dentist. J. Hosp. Dent. Pract. *10:*35, 1976.

574. Shuman, S.K.: Ethics and rationing health care. J. Am. Dent. Assoc. *121:*639, 1990.

575. Shuman, S.K.: Ethics and the patient with dementia. J. Am. Dent. Assoc. *119:*747, 1989.

576. Siegal, M.D.: Dentists' reported willingness to treat disabled patients. Spec. Care Dent. *5:*102, 1985.

577. Siegler, M., Bresnahan, J.F., Schiedermayer, D.L., and Roberson, D.: Exploring the future of clinical dental ethics: A summary of the Odontographic Society of Chicago Centennial Symposium. J. Am. Coll. Dent. *56:*13, 1989.

578. Siegler, M., and Schiedermayer, D.L.: Clinical

dental ethics: Defining an ethic for practicing professionals. J. Am. Coll. Dent. *55:*4, 1988.

579. Silberman, S.L.: Standardization of value profiles of dental students and dental faculty. J. Dent. Res. *55:*939, 1976.

580. Silberman, S.L., Cohen, L.A., and Runyon, H.: Values clarification in dental education. J. Am. Coll. Dent. *46:*224, 1979.

581. Silversin, J.B., and Moody, P.M.: Dentists and the oral health behavior of patients: a sociological perspective. J. Behav. Med. *4:*283, 1981.

582. Simonsen, R.J.: AIDS—a question of informed consent [editorial]. Quintessence International *21:*857, 1990.

583. Simpson, R.B., and Crabb, L.: Ethics: Developing your professional principles. Dent. Stud. *59:*18, 1981.

584. Simpson, R.B., Hall, D., and Crabb, L.: Decision-making in dental practice. J. Am. Coll. Dent. *48:*238, 1981.

585. Singer, J.L., Cohen, L., and LaBelle, A.: Dental hygienists in nontraditional settings: practice and patient characteristics. J. Public Health Dent. *46:*86, 1986.

586. Slagle, W.F.: Ethical professionalism. J. Tenn. Dent. Assoc. *67:*24, 1987.

587. Smith, C.: Ethics—is it time for dentists to reexamine their ethical guidelines? AGD Impact *Nov. 1990,* p. 10.

588. Smith, C.J.: The dental implications of HIV infection. Br. Dent. J. *166:*136, 1989.

589. Smith, J.: The dentist's role in combating child abuse. Va. Dent. J. *53:*18, 1978.

590. Smith, R.T.: A Study of the Professional Role of Dentists. Ann Arbor, MI, University Microfilms, 1960.

591. Smith, T.J.: Informed consent doctrine in dental practice: A current case review. J. Law Eth. Dent. *1:*159, 1988.

592. Sniderman, M.: Preservation of private practice and fee-for-service. Pa. Dent. J. *42:*7, 1976.

593. Soble, R.K.: A research summary: A study of student value change and congruency with faculty values in professional education. J. Baltimore Coll. Dent. Surg. *34:*11, 1980.

594. Soh, G.: Institutional advertising: Boon or bane? Singapore Dent. J. *15:*20, 1990.

595. Sokol, D.J.: Endodontic intervention—is it paternalism? J. Am. Dent. Assoc. *117:*205, 1988.

596. Sokol, D.J.: Informed consent in dentistry. J. Dent. Pract. Adm. *6:*157, 1989.

597. Springstead, C.: Professional ethics in dental auxiliary education. Educational Directions *1:*28, 1976.

598. Squeglia, E.A.: Terminating a dentist-patient relationship without creating legal or ethical problems. Ohio Dent. J. *64:*25, 1990.

599. Stamm, J.W.: Applying ethical guidelines in the conduct of children's dental caries surveys. J. Dent. Res. *59(Spec):*1274, 1980.

600. Stamm, J.W.: Types of clinical caries studies: Epidemiological surveys, randomized clinical trials and demonstration programs. J. Dent. Res. *63(Spec):*701, 1984.

601. Steinberg, D.N.: Change in attitude of dental students during their professional education. J. Dent. Educ. *37:*36, 1973.

602. Stevenson, R.B.: Ethics and patient initiative. J. Am. Dent. Assoc. *118:*414, 1989.

603. Stimson, P.G.: Professional responsibility (malpractice). Dent. Clin. North Am. *21:*137, 1977.

604. Strauss, R.P.: Ethical and social concerns in facial surgical decision making. Plast. Reconstr. Surg. *72,* 1983.

605. Strauss, R.P.: Surgery, activism, and esthetics: A sociological perspective on treating facial disfigurement. *In* Psychological Aspects of Facial Form. Edited by J.A. McNamara. Ann Arbor, MI, 1981.

606. Strauss, R.P., Claris, S.M., Lindahl, R.L., and Parker, P.: Patients' attitudes toward quality assurance in dentistry. J. Am. Coll. Dent. *47:* 1980.

607. Strauss, R.P., and Davis, J.U.: Prenatal detection and fetal surgery of clefts and craniofacial abnormalities in humans: Social and ethical issues. Cleft Palate J. *27:*176, 1990.

608. Strauss, R.P., Lindahl, R.L., and Barksdale, M.B.: A study of dentists' perceptions of a quality assurance project conducted in their private offices. Qual. Rev. Bull.: J. Qual. Assur. *8:* 1982.

609. Strauss, R.P., Lindalh, R.L., and Barksdale, M.B.: Patient response to participation in a quality review program conducted in private dental offices. J. Am. Dent. Assoc. *105:* 1982.

610. Strevel, D.W.: Consumer choice between dental delivery systems. J. Am. Dent. Assoc. *104:*157, 1982.

611. Tanner, T.P.: On ethics at chairside [letter]. J. Am. Dent. Assoc. *117:*10, 1988.

612. Tattersall, W.R.: The Dentist's Handbook on Law and Ethics. 2nd Ed. London, Eyre and Spottiswoode, 1962.

613. Ter Horst, G., et al.: AIDS and infection control: Amsterdam dentists surveyed. J. Public Health Dent. *49:*201, 1989.

614. Teuscher, G.W.: Ethics and the professional environment. J. Dent. Child. *41:*428, 1974.

615. Thordarson, G.R.: Moral and ethical issues related to infectious diseases in the dental practice. Can. Dent. Assoc. J. *53:*677, 1987.

616. Thornberg, A.F.: When goals become responsibilities. R.I. Dent. J. *23:*8, 1990.

617. Tillis, B.: Ethics—their origins and insertions. N.Y. State Dent. J. *45:*375, 1979.

618. Tremayne-Lloyd, T.: Do our dentists enjoy freedom of speech and expression? Can. Dent. Assoc. J. *54:*807, 1988.

619. Tryon, A.F.: Informed consent patient records and the doctor/patient relationship. J. Am. Coll. Dent. *51:*15, 1984.

620. Unger, R.M.: And lead me not into temptation. J. Am. Coll. Dent. *50:*8, 1983.

621. Van Hassel, H.J.: Ethics and objectives in advanced dental education. J. Endodont. *1:*318, 1975.

622. Vann, W.F.: Factors affecting professional orientation in the delivery of oral health care: the dental student. J. Am. Coll. Dent. *46:*42, 1979.

623. Veatch, R.M.: The relationship of the profession(al) to society. J. Dent. Educ. *49:*207, 1985.

624. Verrusio, A.C.: Risk of transmission of the human immunodeficiency virus to health care

workers exposed to HIV-infected patients—a review. J. Am. Dent. Assoc. *118:*339, 1989.

625. Verrusio, A.C., et al.: The dentist and infectious diseases: A national survey of attitudes and behavior. J. Am. Dent. Assoc. *118:*553, 1989.

626. Waite, F.C.: Ethics in administration of dental schools. Trans. Inst. Dental Teachers, *1923*, p. 29.

627. Waithe, M.E.: AIDS and dentistry: Conflicting right and the public's health. *In* AIDS and Ethics: Biomedical Ethics Reviews—1988. Edited by J.M. Humber and R.F. Almeder. Clifton, NJ, Humana, 1989.

628. Waldman, H.B.: Closed panels, professionalism, and the American Dental Association. Med. Care *11:*156, 1973.

629. Waldman, H.B.: Dentistry and peer review—sham, smoke screen or reality. J. Am. Coll. Dent. *43:*164, 1976.

630. Waldman, H.B.: The ethical obligation. J. Kansas State Dent. Assoc. *59:*22, 1975.

631. Waldman, H.B.: A new ethical obligation: Is peer review informing? J. Am. Coll. Dent. *42:* 147, 1975.

632. Waldman, H.B., and Schlissel, E.: Honor codes and peer review—is peer review really possible? J. Dent. Educ. *41:*126, 1977.

633. Waldman, H.M., and Shakun, M.L.: Variations in the practice of dentistry and the supply of dentists. J. Am. Coll. Dent. *51:*24, 1984.

634. Walsh, J.: The profession's responsibility. Int. Dent. J. *17:*75, 1967.

635. Warner, R., and Hansen, J.: The legal and moral implications of consent—free vs. informed consent. Dentistry *7:*13, 1987.

636. Warner, R., and Segal, H.: Ethical Issues of Informed Consent in Dentistry. Chicago, Quintessence, 1980.

637. Warner, R., and Segal, H.: Informed consent in dentistry. J. Am. Dent. Assoc. *99:*957, 1979.

638. Warren, K.L.: Increasing access to dental care for the older patient—a special challenge. Spec. Care Dent. *2:*248, 1982.

639. Wasinger, J.L.: A personal approach to dental care for patients with handicapping conditions. Spec. Care Dent. *6:*156, 1986.

640. Wathen, W.F.: The patient's interest [editorial]. J. Am. Dent. Assoc. *116:*600, 1988.

641. Weber, F.N.: Professionalism in dentistry: One man's opinion. J. Am. Coll. Dent. *55:*44, 1988.

642. Wei, S.H.: Ethics: What can editors do? Int. Dent. J. *41:*124, 1991.

643. Weinstein, B.D.: Dental ethics and the role of experts. J. Law Eth. Dent. *4:*4, 1991.

644. Weinstein, B.D.: Ethics and its role in dentistry. Gen Dent. *40:*414, 1992.

645. Weinstein, B.D., and Keyes, G.G.: Management considerations for an HIV positive dental student; ethical and legal commentary. J. Dent. Educ. *55:*238, 1991. [Published erratum appears in *55:*348, 1991.]

646. Wentworth, E.T.: Is DSSNY ethical behavior declining? N.Y. State Dent. J. *54:*24, 1988.

647. Wetle, T.: Ethical issues in geriatric dentistry. Gerodontology, *6:*73, 1987.

648. Whinery, J.G.: What to do about ethics. Tex. Dent. J. *103:*12, 1986.

649. Whitehouse, N.: Freedom of movement in the European community. Int. Dent. J. *40:*237, 1990.

650. Wigdor, H.: More about lasers [letter]. J. Am. Dent. Assoc. *122:*12, 1991.

651. Willens, S.H.: Marketing, advertising and ethics, the dental profession's dilemma of today. J. Am. Coll. Dent. *50:*29, 1983.

652. Williams, C.H.: Factors affecting professional orientation in the delivery of oral health care: the dental practice. J. Am. Coll. Dent. *46:*49, 1979.

653. Wimer, G.L.: Just how professional are you? Dent. Econ. *67:*46, 1977.

654. Winspear, W.J.: Human experimentation in dental research. Aust. Dent. J. *26:*92, 1981.

655. Wittrock, J.W.: Ethics and health care in capitalism. J. Law Eth. Dent. *3:*3, 1990.

656. Wittrock, J.W.: Prevention and ethics: Going upstream. Va. Dent. J. *59:*34, 1982.

657. Woodall, I.: Don't deny AIDS victims dental care [editorial]. R.D.H. *8:*8, 1988.

658. Woodall, I.: Legal, Ethical, and management aspects of the dental care system. 3rd Ed. St. Louis, Mosby, 1987.

659. Woodall, I.: Values and victories [editorial]. R.D.H. *5:*7, 1985.

660. Wotman, S.: The changing compact between the health professions and society. J. Dent. Educ. *51:*91, 1987.

661. Young, L.J., and Newell, J.: A model for the development of educational materials for facilitating ethical development. Educ. Dir. Dent. Aux. *9:*22, 1984.

662. Young, R.S.: Professional misconduct of individuals. J. Am. Coll. Dent. *41:*45, 1974.

663. Zinman, E.J.: Informed consent to periodontal surgery—advise before you incise. J. West. Soc. Period. *24:*101, 1976.

Index

Page numbers in *italics* indicate figures.